No More Hysterectomies

VICKI HUFNAGEL, M.D., is an obstetrician/gynaecologist and gynaecological surgeon in private practice in Los Angeles. She received her medical degree at the School of Medicine of the University of California, San Francisco, and completed resident training at the Albert Einstein School of Medicine in New York. As the Medical Director of the Institute of Reproductive Health in Los Angeles, she co-authored and worked to pass a California Senate bill that requires women's informed consent prior to hysterectomy. This bill is now law.

SUSAN K. GOLANT is a writer specializing in medical issues. She lives in Los Angeles.

No More Hysterectomies

A woman surgeon explains how unnecessary
hysterectomies can—and should—be avoided . . . and gives
straightforward advice on the latest alternatives—both
preventive and reconstructive

Dr Vicki Hufnagel
with Susan K. Golant

Thorsons Publishing Group

First published in the USA in 1988 by NAL Books, a division of Penguin Books USA Inc., 1633 Broadway, New York, NY 10019.
This edition published 1990

British Library Cataloguing in Publication Data

Hufnagel, Vicki
No more hysterectomies.
1. Women. Uterus. Hysterectomy
I. Title   II. Colant, Susan K.
618.1453

ISBN 0-7225-1958-3

Published by Thorsons Publishers Limited,
Wellingborough, Northamptonshire NN8 2RQ, England

Typeset by Harper Phototypesetters Limited, Northampton
Printed in Great Britain by Woolnough Bookbinding Limited,
Irthlingborough, Northamptonshire

1 3 5 7 9 10 8 6 4 2

Contents

To Robert and Tara

Acknowledgements

Update: Lost Heroes

Prior to publication, I lost two mentors: Dr Robert Mendleson and Dr Robert Greenblatt.

Dr Mendleson supported my work and encouraged me to 'go for it!' He had lived through years of controversy in medicine and had developed a sense of humour that allowed him to face adversaries with equanimity. He wanted to be part of the Women's Health Care Rights crusade and told me I could call him anytime. When I did, he would tell me wonderful historical anecdotes, followed by appropriate adages. Somehow, his humour always put things in perspective. Last April, he passed away. His brilliance and genius will always remain; for those who knew him, his enthusiastic activism remains an enduring force.

Dr Robert Greenblatt was a pioneer in female endocrinology. He did years of research which proved women had sexual desires and secreted a variety of hormones. His views were met with resistance from the medical community; he was labelled a medical heretic. He continued to write and lecture despite his early textbooks being banned from his university. With the slow passage of time, his visions became accepted reality. Many times in my career, when events seemed overwhelming and impossible, Dr Greenblatt would smile and reach out to comfort me. He would hold my hand and say, 'You can do it; don't let them get you down.'

Both Dr Mendleson and Dr Greenblatt were true healers, kind and loving men whose egos were not dependent on a medical degree. Their encouragement helped me continue with this work. Both Roberts taught me to see the vision of 'the child'—an idea that needs protection and nurturing, an idea that will grow despite all adversities because of its parent's unconditional commitment to its being. The child's being is truth.

Men like Drs Mendleson and Greenblatt honour the beauty of life itself. My heroes are gone, but I will continue on the path they have shared with me.

—Vicki Hufnagel, M.D.

I feel grateful for having had this opportunity to work with Dr Vicki Hufnagel. I would like to thank my fellow writer Raquel Skolnik for having had the foresight to bring Vicki and me together; my attorney Linda Lichter for watching over my interests; our publisher at New American Library, Elaine Koster, for her enthusiasm; our editor, LuAnn Walther, for her tireless attention to detail; and Trish Aude for her technical assistance.

My husband, friend, and soul mate, Dr Mitch Golant, and my daughters, Cherie and Aimee, have provided the wellsprings of support without which this work could not have been accomplished.

Finally, I would like to single out my mother and father, Mary and Arthur Kleinhandler. Survivors of Dachau and Buchenwald, they taught me about pain and strength, injustice and hope. Facing the depths of despair with the utmost courage, they inspired in me a deep respect for the resiliency of the human spirit and the value of life. It is through their experiences that I have learned to understand the necessity of *Tikkun Olam*, the quest to make a 'correction', to 'heal the world'. This book is but one small offering in that quest. My contribution to the book is dedicated to them—and to all others who have suffered needlessly—with love.

—Susan K. Golant

Introduction

When I started my research into options for hysterectomy, I began collecting all the textbooks I could find. My shelves are lined with ageing leather-bound texts, some of them so old that pages fall out or crumble as I read them. Having such a collection gave me a historical view through the various opinions expressed by surgeons of times past.

One surgeon, Dr Victor Bonnie from England, stood out above all the others. He had surgically taken on the task to conserve the uterus. Unlike other doctors of his time, his books and journal articles spoke to the spirit of women. He wrote with love and respect of the beauty of women and their ability to have children. When he was ready to retire, he was given a large 'BIRTHday' party. Among the many people present were all of the babies he had helped to create by saying 'NO' to hysterectomy. Imagine the joy felt and shared with this man who dared to stand alone against all others. I had not come across anyone else in all my readings who seemed as dedicated to this subject as Dr Bonnie. Reading his work inspired me.

I knew that writing No More Hysterectomies would produce a change in women. I was not only going to publish a text that would reveal established surgical abuse of hysterectomy but I was also looking into why these abuses began and flourished, and how this could be reformed to benefit everyone —doctors and women alike.

I began to speak aloud about the abuses I had witnessed pertaining to unnecessary hysterectomies and against established authority in the medical community. I had never felt so clear-visioned and purposeful as I felt then, and still feel now, and I focused my energies with a passion for doing what I believed was right . . . no matter what the odds were.

I felt that legislation would help to protect women. I entered into a political arena to work toward actualizing these beliefs. I was warned that I was taking a step from which there would be no return and that my life would no longer be the same. I felt I would be able to withstand any personal assault against me because I was doing what was right. The confidence and passion I felt helped in making SB835, the Informed Consent for Hysterectomy Statute, a new law in the state of California. This took several years, during which time I finished this book.

When No More Hysterectomies was published and released I was booked on a national TV network morning show to discuss the issues. The producers of the show flew me to New York and put me up in a hotel. After a hectic afternoon of radio interviews, I returned to my hotel room to find an urgent message from my publisher. There would be no show. It was cancelled. I found out later that the show had been set up to interview me and another doctor, sent as a representative of the medical establishment. He had stated that he was going to attack me personally on the air, refusing to address the issues the show had prepared. He convinced them that I was 'too controversial'.

I am not a radical feminist attacking the medical establishment, I am a conservative surgeon. I am 'too controversial' because I can debate against arrogance and ignorance. I am a threat to those who don't know of my work because they think I am attacking men and medicine. Their immediate response is hostile and offensive. The fear that a woman surgeon had written a book with the title *No More Hysterectomies* was all that was needed to inflame this small, but powerful, minority of physicians.

My pain and suffering through this entire event are universal to all women. The work in which I am involved is the healing of women: educating them to have choices, giving options where there were none, and helping them have babies that could so easily never have been.

Despite efforts to keep *No More Hysterectomies* from getting national coverage, women found the book, read it, and shared it with others. The first printing was sold out in a few weeks. The changes it created have spread across the nation. Soon it will reach across the ocean as special editions for the United Kingdom, Canada, France and Australia are published. Women will not let the issues die. The message lives on through *No More Hysterectomies* ... and through you.

PART 1

Hysterectomy:
Separating Myth from Fact

This book is for you

- If you have been told you need a hysterectomy
- If you have problems that may lead to hysterectomy in the future
- If you want to be fully informed about a health decision that could affect the rest of your life

Why? Because all women are at risk of losing their reproductive organs! This book is for you and me—for all women and their daughters. It will empower you by educating you about female health care and the risk of hysterectomy. It will help you in your discussion of options with your doctors. It will show you why hysterectomy should no longer be blindly condoned as the norm for all women.

I'm frustrated and angry at what I see is the accepted standard of medical care for women. I'm angry at the needless suffering, illness, and emotional trauma that are caused by my own colleagues—professionals who often mean well but whose practices, in actuality, cause irreparable harm for millions of women and their families. I'm angry because often I feel alone in my struggle to effect change within the 'good old boy' medical system.

I'm telling you this because, perhaps ironically, *No More Hysterectomies* is not an angry book, although from time to time, I'll get up on my soapbox to vent my frustration. Indeed, this book has been written out of concern—the concern that I feel for women and their plight at the hands of an often uncaring profession. It is written out of the concern that women have shown me over the years as I've helped them to maintain the integrity of their bodies.

CHAPTER 1

The Revolution in Women's Health Care

'In my experience it is the woman who is most terrified and has the most lurid fantasies that is the one least able to question whether she needs a hysterectomy or not and if she does need one to ask about the effect the operation is going to have on her—physically, emotionally or sexually. Her anxieties may relate to her mother or grandmother's experience or her own sex life with her husband or partner. Such a woman should realize it's her body and her life, take a friend along for support, remember that indirectly it is she who is paying for the doctor's services. Even though it may be difficult to ask questions such as "how will it affect my sex life, doctor?" she should still ask and if she doesn't get an answer (and not all doctors *know*) she should ask to be referred to someone who can give her one.'
Dr Prudence Tunnadine, gynaecologist and Scientific Director of the Institute of Psychosexual Medicine, London.

The following letter is typical of the hundreds I've received from patients whose organs I've saved:

Dear Vicki:
What I thought was going to be a nightmare turned out to be one of the most positive experiences of my life. As you know, being 46 years old and healthy all my life, I was appalled to be told during a recent routine exam by my doctor that my 'useless' uterus would have to be removed because of a benign tumour mass (fibroid) and 'at your age you really don't need it anymore'. I saw a succession of doctors but everywhere I turned, nobody seemed to offer any alternative except hysterectomy. I was continually admonished for wanting to retain my organs as being 'silly and ridiculous' since I was 'way past childbearing age and the risk of cancer was growing daily' as I got older.

Then I happened to be watching TV and there you were, telling the world exactly my sentiments: that gynaecological procedures as practised in this country today are archaic and too many women are suffering needless butchery.

You said that because of advances in technology, you had developed a procedure called Female Reconstructive Surgery which, with the exception of cancer, can correct and restore many female problems—fibroids being a speciality. Using the latest equipment, laser and microsurgery, there is minimal blood loss and very minimal shock to the body. You said hospital stays were usually three to four days with full resumption of daily activities in ten to fourteen days. This was for me!

I saw you as soon as I could. After using ultrasound, you reconfirmed the presence of the fibroids and asked me what I wanted you to do. I was impressed that you weren't dictating orders to me but wanted my input.

'Can't you fix it?' I asked, and then you

explained in great detail how you were going to do just that. You indicated that you would videotape my operation so I could review it later.

During what turned out to be a four and a half hour operation, you skilfully removed eight large but benign tumours from inside my uterus, one of which was the size of a watermelon and was twisted around my other organs. Not only did you fix them, but you removed a cyst on one of my ovaries, and some endometriosis, and then resuspended all of my organs.

Four days later, I was up and at 'em. After ten days I was just about back to normal, including driving my non automatic car. None of my friends who had had hysterectomies could believe it! Now, six months later, it's as if I never had surgery. My periods have returned to normal and I am completely energized and feeling terrific.

I am very, very grateful to you. [. . .] How wonderful to be instrumental in enhancing the quality of lives. Continue the 'good fight'. You have all of my support.

Love, Fran

With letters like that it's hard for me to remain angry for long! But then I'm reminded of the facts behind hysterectomies —facts that few women are privy to—and I begin to feel that same sense of injustice.

Hysterectomy—why all women should question it

'All unnecessary surgery is bad: some gynae-cologists, for example, routinely remove the ovaries during a hysterectomy if the woman is over 45; some never would. Male gynae-cologists would certainly not be happy if along with a hernia operation the testicles were removed to prevent possible testicular carcinoma. The ovaries, even in a post-menopausal woman, contribute to her hormonal health. Oestrogens prevent osteo-porosis and heart disease and your own hormones come in a more measured, natural and continuous dose than those in a pill or in a patch. As for cancer, we can now screen women using ultrasound scanning.' Professor Stuart Campbell, Head of Department of Obstetrics and Gynaecology, King's College Hospital.

NEARLY THREE QUARTERS OF A MILLION WOMEN CASTRATED IN THE U.S. LAST YEAR

Imagine reading that headline in your local newspaper. You would be aghast that such barbarity were occurring in your civilized country, wouldn't you? Well, look again. This headline is true.

Hysterectomy is the surgical removal of the uterus, often accompanied by oöphorec-tomy, or the removal of the ovaries. Fre-quently, the ovaries are removed by the surgeon simply because we 'might as well take them since I'm "in there" anyway'. These organs are portrayed as having no function beyond your desire to bear chil-dren, but this is plainly not true. Your ovaries continue to secrete hormones for a dozen or more years after menopause. Oestrogen helps ward off oesteoporosis and heart disease, whereas testosterone augments sexual desire.

The words *hysterectomy* and *oöphorectomy* can be a euphemism for *castration*. Of course we could not call a procedure performed on nearly three quarters of a million American women a year castration, because that label would probably force a reexamination of the practice. Incredible as it may seem, in 1983, 13,000 women lost their reproductive organs because they complained of premenstrual tension (PMS), a condition that could have been treated with hormone therapy, nutritional supplements, and exercise. Other reasons listed by surgeons are cancer (which often *does* require hysterectomy), as well as endometriosis, fibroids, and prolapse (which may not).

One wonders whether castration of the *male* would be as prevalent if men grew fibroid tumours of the testicles or if men suffered from monthly depressions. I think not. If as great a proportion of the male population were faced with castration as the female population is, I venture to say there would be a branch of medicine dedicated solely to the saving of male organs.

The uterus is the only part of the human anatomy that lacks a constituency determined to preserve it. Although the 'solution' to the problems of female disorders was found ninety years ago to be hysterectomy, generations of doctors have staunchly continued to remove those organs as if hysterectomy were the perfect, immediate, and only solution. In fact, to my knowledge, they rarely inform the potential hysterectomy patient of the serious negative consequences, both physical and emotional, that may affect many post-hysterectomy patients.

The shocking facts about hysterectomy

According to one British study[1] hysterectomy is now one of the most commonly performed surgical operations, offered mainly for the control of heavy bleeding, to 50 per cent of US women, 20-25 per cent of British women and 40 per cent of women in Australia.

Because of this prevalance, especially in the United States, statistics now project that within a few years every woman will have a 50-50 chance of losing her female reproductive organs by the time she reaches the age of 65.[2] If you have been told that you

might need a hysterectomy, or if hysterectomy looms in your immediate future, you may feel confused and vulnerable. Knowledge about your body is essential to making any choices. Before you rush into surgery, here are some facts that you ought to know:

● You may experience a loss of physical sexual sensation, desire, or arousal as a result of hysterectomy.
● Your uterus holds many of your internal organs in place. After hysterectomy, they may cave inward or prolapse, causing pelvic pain, sexual difficulties, pressure on your bowels and bladder.
● Hysterectomy's long-term consequences, in addition to operative dangers and complications, include:
     osteoporosis
     increased risk of heart disease
     bone and joint pain, immobility
     chronic fatigue
     urinary tract infection, frequency, incontinence
     emotional changes, depression

This short but potent list explains, in part, why I'm angry. It is clear that hysterectomy is a surgery that should be avoided if possible because of its serious, long-term consequences. And yet *hysterectomy is the most performed major gynaecological surgery*. In my opinion, and I'll get into the statistics in Chapter 5, a vast number of hysterectomies are done unnecessarily. They can and should be avoided. Studies have shown that surgeons remove perfectly healthy organs.[3] Only cancer, emergencies, and incurable, recurrent diseases should necessitate the removal of your uterus and/or ovaries.

In fact, with the exception of these life-threatening situations, hysterectomy should be regarded as the last possible option—not the first line of treatment. Wouldn't you elect a conservative surgery using a local anaesthetic before choosing something more radical? Of course. The risks are lower, the side effects less severe. Similarly, you should do everything possible to save your organs. If more conservative measures fail, then—and only then—should you consider a hysterectomy. But first consider the options.

HOWEVER—and this is a big HOW-EVER—if you choose to seek alternatives to hysterectomy, you must be responsible. That means regular cervical smear tests and, as you grow older, uterine biopsies and ultra-sound exams of your ovaries. When you empower yourself and participate in your own health care, you and your doctor must create a preventive programme and screening system to detect any problems early. This approach can save your life.

Should you consent to a 'possible hysterectomy'?

Gladys had fibroids. Her gynaecologist, Dr M., promised exploratory surgery and implied that with his surgical skill, he could 'preserve everything'. Gladys checked into the local hospital, feeling prepared for what lay ahead. Just prior to surgery, however, the nurse brought in the consent form (Appendix 3). On it was written, 'possible hysterectomy'. Gladys had not been told that her exploratory surgery might result in the loss of her female organs.

The nurse was adamant; if Gladys didn't sign the consent, they would not proceed. Imagine her confusion and dismay at being confronted with the possibility of hysterectomy on such short notice.

Did Gladys have the opportunity to discuss the procedure with her gynaecologist? Did they review together the possible operative and postoperative complications? Did they explore the long-term hormonal, emotional, and sexual effects? Did she have

a day, a mere 24 hours, to consider fully what such an operation would mean to her in the long run?

Of course not. Gladys signed under duress without adequate education. She awoke from the operation with 'everything out'.

The function of denial

When the truth becomes too frightening to bear, it is our natural inclination, at first, to deny the facts. We can't and then won't believe them. Psychologists tell us that this happens frequently when a loved one dies. How can we accept the idea that the person is gone?

The same can be said for the shocking facts about hysterectomy. No one wants to believe that such an enormous segment of the population has been made to suffer for so many years. 'How could this be occurring today, on such a large scale?' you might ask, and your scepticism is justified. 'After all, we have laws. Women are educated and liberated. There are even women doctors. Certainly we should have heard of this before now. Why are you the only gynaecologist against hysterectomy? You must be some kind of feminist kook'.

Mass hysterectomy is just too horrible to be true, so it isn't true. Or, if it's happening, it has to be valid. After all, if everyone approves of it, it must be OK.

Imagine the rage we would feel once we realized how we have been victimized; how our mothers and friends and even how we ourselves have been made to suffer needlessly; how our rights have been abrogated. Better to believe that all the hundreds of thousands of hysterectomies performed are absolutely necessary. Better to buy the line than to question. Yet I have seen the pain of thousands of women. It is essential, I feel, to put an end to the denial.

How I started questioning my own medical training

During my training as a resident physician, making the rounds with the technically swift surgeons, the gynaecologists known for the fastest hysterectomies, I learned the bedside sales pitch for hysterectomy. It was repeated so often to vulnerable women in such a rote and essentially insincere manner that it rendered me suspicious.

'You won't have those messy, unpleasant periods anymore'.

'You'll finally be rid of those cramps'.

'No more worry about unwanted pregnancy, especially at your age!'

'By taking everything out, you'll never get cancer'.

'If you want, I can do your hysterectomy through your vagina so you won't have an ugly abdominal scar. No one will ever know'.

I had absorbed the party line for merchandizing a hysterectomy, but I couldn't espouse it, perhaps because being female, I identify with women. Besides, it could happen to me.

At that time, I only had contact with hospitalized patients, immediately before and during surgery. When I began my private practice as a gynaecological surgeon, however, I became aware of the full picture and I learned the truth about hysterectomy. I was startled to find a multitude of hysterectomized women with various complaints filling my office. In fact, 80 per cent of my patients who had been hysterectomized by other surgeons consulted with me for post-hysterectomy problems.

I began to question my medical training. Hysterectomy had always been the first and easiest answer. Yet something had to be wrong with the way I had been educated. A few 'crazy' women made sense. But this onslaught of distraught, hysterectomized women bearing the same woeful tale was completely out of proportion with what I had been led to expect.

Had my medical training dehumanized and defeminized me to such an extent that I, like so many of my colleagues, had been deaf to the truth? Finally one day things became very clear: There the truth sat, in the person of a patient named Joyce, opening up her heart to me. Would I finally be the one to hear her? Would I believe her? And, could I help her?

Is it all in your head?

When Joyce noticed sexual problems and pain after her hysterectomy, she returned to her surgeon, seeking advice. What she received was denial.

'Everyone knows that the removal of the uterus cannot cause any of these problems,' he said. 'The uterus and ovaries are needed for reproductive purposes only.'

Admonished for acting out of line, Joyce was told to 'Shape up!' That was all the comfort she could expect.

Joyce became desperate and changed physicians, abandoning years of trust and loyalty. But soon she heard a more insidious line from her new gynaecologist. Because the hysterectomy wasn't at fault, the crisis of the surgery must have uncovered a latent emotional illness in Joyce, suddenly triggering all her deep-seated neuroses to make themselves evident. The woman was advised to seek psychiatric counselling.

Frantic, without answers, without alternatives, Joyce, like so many others in her predicament, traipsed from one doctor to another, praying that someone would listen, someone would care. What did she gain from this? Nothing. In the end she lost her credibility, her self-respect, even, ultimately, her marriage. She was labelled 'hysterical'. Since she couldn't even stay with one doctor for any substantial amount of time, *she must be crazy.* With 'unstable' medical records, Joyce became a classic example of a 'difficult patient'.

I shuddered at the thought that I, too, had contributed to the senseless hysterectomies and unfounded accusations of mental illness. If I were to be a part of the 'good old boy' system, I, too, should have turned a deaf ear to Joyce. Doing what everyone else did would make me acceptable, one of the 'guys'. All I had to do was prescribe tranquillizers, sleeping pills, and refer her and women like her back to her original doctors and to a therapist to help her with her frigidity and assorted other neuroses.

The trouble was, I couldn't. As I listened to Joyce's and my other patients' stories, as I paid attention to what they were *really* saying, I found the whole situation intolerable. In case after case, the pathology reports showed that the removed uteruses were normal or had had minimal pathology. The truth had been kept from these patients who had never read or been taught to understand their own medical records.

The majority of these women had had other options, including *no* surgery. The majority of the complaints were justified. These women had real physical problems and now they suffered emotionally from feeling so powerless in their own lives and from being labelled 'neurotic'.

No, the wholesale castration of these women was wrong—and painfully, in too many cases, there was no strong medical indication for the surgery. I could no longer be part of this conspiracy. There had to be another way.

My own breakthrough

In my years as a physician, I have realized that when you look at problems with openness, creativity, and a willingness to learn, alternatives do make themselves available and answers can be found. In breaking the rules and actually listening to my 'hysterical' patients, I found that I could create solutions —or at least try. Much of my inspiration came from my patients themselves.

One woman, Nora, a well-educated, active, trim blonde in her late forties, had been told by at least five gynaecologists that she required a hysterectomy for a prolapsed uterus. Prolapse is a condition in which the uterus is no longer adequately suspended by its ligaments.

Women with prolapse have legitimate complaints. Most often, the descended uterus causes them to lose bladder control. These women can't leave the house without wearing incontinence pads. Given the choice between a life of fear and embarrassment and surgery, hysterectomy seems a welcome relief.

I was taught that prolapse was cured only by hysterectomy. Every attending physician, every professor, every modern textbook confirmed that. But Nora didn't want the operation. Although she had no intention of having more children, she wished to preserve her uterus. And her case was severe. Her uterus had fallen so drastically that it took up all of the space in the vagina. Sex was out of the question. In fact, if she pushed or strained at all, her cervix would emerge through the vaginal opening. Yet she simply looked me in the eye and asked me to find a way to fix it.

I had performed a D & C, and found that the lining of Nora's uterus was completely normal. Physical examination and ultrasound also showed everything to be the correct size and shape. It appeared that her organs were perfect, but the ligaments that held the female organs had stretched out. What was I to do?

Let's look at a simplistic analogy. Imagine that you've bought an exquisite designer silk skirt—the kind you save for and purchase once in a lifetime. Now, suppose you send this skirt to the dry cleaner and, to your distress, the dry-cleaning agents cause the elastic in the waistband to deteriorate. Suddenly, the garment is large enough for two. Do you toss out your prized skirt or simply fix the elastic?

Several of the surgeons whom I consulted told me that it was impossible to tighten the ligaments. In reviewing the medical literature, however, I found that during the late nineteenth century, operations had been performed to correct prolapse. Yet nowhere could I find recent information on ways to repair the loss of elasticity in the ligaments that held the female organs in place. Nora's request had forced me to wonder why gynaecologists had abandoned fixing the organs rather than just removing them.

It made perfect sense to me that if prolapse was a result of weakening ligaments, all one would have to do was strengthen or shorten those 'elastic bands' to resolve the problem. What if I merely resuspended Nora's female organs, restructuring the whole support system?

I discussed my idea with my patient and she decided that she could always have a hysterectomy later—she wanted me to see if I could strengthen her ligaments. I performed a laparotomy (I opened her abdominal cavity) and found the stretched ligaments. Using permanent sutures—stitches that would not dissolve but would stay in her body—I restructured the ligaments, resuspended the uterus in the proper position, and brought the uterus (which had prolapsed) upward to its original position.

Then we discovered that part of Nora's bowel had also prolapsed and had fallen into the vaginal cavity. My dexterous assistant, a general surgeon, helped to reposition the bowel. After two hours of surgery, Nora's 'insides' were back to the way they had been some twenty years earlier. Before I closed her up, I looked at it all and was amazed. We had re-established Nora's anatomy.

Would it hold?

The true test was gravity. Everything looked wonderful on the operating table and in the hospital bed. But would the correction hold once Nora got up and resumed her active life? I am delighted to say that indeed it did! Basic anatomy and surgical procedures have eliminated the need for hysterectomy in many cases like Nora's.

In fact, not only had I corrected the problem but I had improved Nora's condition markedly. With her vaginal walls pulled up higher and into their normal position than would have resulted from a hysterectomy, Nora could resume her life without the dire consequences of organ loss. She is now a functioning, sexual, active woman whose intact ovaries continue to produce the hormones her body needs. And should she require a hysterectomy in the future, that option is still open to her.

Since Nora's surgery, I have performed many prolapse repairs. Most have withstood the stress of the earth's gravitational pull. And, more significantly, all of these women have retained their precious organs.

The psychology of victimization

Some women have been so socialized or so terrorized that they cannot take action or control in their lives. They seem to make choices that eventually will be hurtful. They become accomplices in their own victimization.

I have encountered women with abnormal cervical smears or bleeding who refuse to return to their doctors for diagnosis and treatment. These women risk the development of cervical and endometrial cancer in the future—diseases that would necessitate hysterectomies. Yet they are too uneducated or frightened to take the action necessary to alter the course of disease.

Others opt for the hysterectomy and the other surgeries to remove their reproductive organs. It's hard for me to believe that women could want to be victimized, but they defer to 'authority' figures without doing their own evaluation. As women, we have been well trained in self-sacrifice. The needs of others must come before our own.

How we sacrifice ourselves

Dana came to see me after learning about my work from a friend who had done beautifully after Female Reconstructive Surgery (FRS), a form of surgery where the emphasis is on repair and reconstruction rather than ablation (surgical removal) of tissue. Dana had already been scheduled for a hysterectomy with her gynaecologist and was seeing me for a second opinion about her multiple fibroids.

In my office, she expressed fear about her impending surgery. She didn't want it. She knew that she could encounter problems as a result of the hysterectomy. I assured her that FRS could probably resolve her medical condition without the loss of her organs.

Dana went home in confusion. She informed her husband that now she had options—either hysterectomy or FRS. She wasn't sure what to do, so he made the decision for her, insisting that she have the hysterectomy because it had already been scheduled. If the surgery was rescheduled, his business plans would be disturbed. They had planned their holiday around the surgery.

Dana had the hysterectomy. She couldn't bear to confront her doctor of seven years. And, worse still, she couldn't disappoint her husband who had fitted the hysterectomy into his schedule. His business plans were more important than her health and well-being. According to him, postponement of surgery would put more stress on the family. But what about Dana and her needs? What about the stress that hysterectomy would put on her body?

Why in the world do some women allow and even encourage this kind of treatment? Perhaps it's a pattern of abuse, stemming from childhood. If you have been victimized as a child, it is easy to fall back into an old mode of behaviour. You are used to the situation. As painful and destructive as it may be, victimization is still a known quality, and reassuringly familiar. Unfortunately, women who are continually victimized cannot understand that perhaps there is another way to deal with the world.

The coming revolution

A majority of the women who enter my practice do so as if they are prisoners on death row, hoping for a reprieve. These women have received two, four, even twenty-four opinions prior to seeing me. Each opinion rendered by a gynaecologist is similar—you need a hysterectomy, but not to worry because:

- Your uterus and 'ageing' ovaries are useless after childbearing years and may become cancerous in the future.
- Replacement hormones will correct all of the after-effects of your hysterectomy.
- PMS and dirty, nasty, interfering menstrual periods are inconvenient and better off eliminated surgically.

- This 'consequence-free' form of birth control enhances your sexuality.
- Most women benefit from undergoing a 'spring cleaning'.

My patients are lucky, for their persistence has led them to my office and the education and reprieve they sought. Sadly, most women succumb to the pressure, eager to please their trusted doctor, uneducated about the true nature of their female problems, and frightened by the ugly spectre of cancer. I am shocked that so many are not informed of the severe and irreversible consequences of this serious surgery. Once the organs are amputated, there is no way to put them back!

So I have gone public with my message. After being interviewed on the 'Phil Donahue Show', and other television programmes, radio, and newspapers, I've received thousands of letters from women, describing their private ordeals, asking for help and education, and wanting to help others avoid their own fate.

Why not give women a choice?

I openly advocate giving women a choice. I claim that the uterus has many functions other than childbearing, and that whenever possible it should be repaired and not removed. Because this stance is contrary to preconceived notions, I have been challenged to 'prove' that the uterus should be repaired whenever possible.

Therefore, among other things, I have researched the relevant medical journals, I have interviewed hundreds of women; I have worked for two years on a study of the National Hospital Discharge Survey for the years 1965-1984. I have consulted leading professionals who are working in women's health.

I believe the research substantiates my claim that the uterus is a vital organ and should be removed only if there is no alternative. This book is an expression of the conclusions I've reached both in my practice and my research. It is not presented as a final report, but rather as a basic introduction, and is written for the average woman, not for my peers in the profession—though I hope they will read it too.

I believe there needs to be a revolution in women's health care. The battle cry? *No More Hysterectomies!* What must be changed is very simple: how we in the medical profession and how women themselves perceive the female body and psyche. Having done this, we can use new medical and scientific technology to improve women's lives, and perhaps most important, women themselves can be empowered to make responsible decisions about their own bodies in concert with their physicians.

In a way, I hope you become angry too. This is a call to action. The aim of this book is to inform you of the many options open to you, including new surgical techniques and medications that would help avoid the unnecessary loss of your organs. Armed with the facts and knowledge of the risk factors involved, you, too, will be clamouring for a change in the way things are done.

Hysterectomy and birth control

In the US and elsewhere hysterectomy is still used by many as a method of birth control (see Chapter 7). A woman who has completed her family looks at having a hysterectomy from an entirely different point of view from that of a woman who has not yet had children. This fact means that the removal of the uterus to prevent pregnancy is still a 'selling point' for hysterectomy for many women. For women who belong to religious denominations which do not permit the use of birth control: Orthodox Jews and Catholics, for example, the removal of the uterus is viewed as an acceptable standard procedure. For Orthodox Jewish women hysterectomy also makes their lives easier in that they no longer have 'unclean' days when sex is not permitted. In figures presented to the American College of Obstetrics and Gynecology in 1988 it was disclosed that in one predominantly Catholic area of Germany the rate of vaginal hysterectomy (suggesting that the uteri removed were normal) had soared to 80 per cent.

'Indications for carrying out hysterectomy in the US are certainly broader than they are in the UK: in fact it's one of a class of operations known locally as a "remunerectomy". In the US hysterectomies are often carried out for pelvic pain of unknown origin. This does not in general reflect the UK experience: in this country hysterectomy is carried out because there is a need for it, given that there may be various interpretations of the word "need".'
UK Medical-legal expert

'There are many reasons for suggesting hysterectomy: a woman, especially a Catholic woman, may be desperately anxious to avoid another pregnancy, for example: she produces pelvic pain symptoms, obtains a hysterectomy and thus she's sterilised—she doesn't have any more children. Her anxiety having been resolved, her pain disappears. Her uterus may be perfectly normal.'
Ex-gynaecologist

What is my background?

You may be asking what my credentials are

for making these strong statements. I have been operating on women since 1980, and to date I have performed nearly 400 Female Reconstructive Surgeries. Many of my patients come from around the country for Female Reconstructive Surgery and then return to their local gynaecologist for continuing care.

Most of my formal medical training took place at the University of California, San Francisco's School of Medicine. Later, I continued as Chief Resident in Obstetrics and Gynaecology at the Albert Einstein School of Medicine in the Bronx, New York. During my schooling and early training, I learned how to perform the surgery that was a required part of my medical schooling and, in my early years as a doctor, I admit that I did perform hysterectomies where now other options exist.

Combining my experience with my patients' needs, however, I was able to improve upon traditional surgical techniques and originate new ones. As one of the pioneers in the use of ultrasound,[4] for example, my work led to the practice of using ultrasonography during surgery. This procedure gives the surgeon 'eyes' and direct moment-to-moment visualization of the uterus, its contents, and the adjacent pelvic organs. It limits and reduces potential complications such as the perforation of the uterine wall.

Today, of course, I do perform hysterectomies on women suffering from cancer. In such cases, hysterectomy is a necessity. Better to lose the uterus than allow the disease to spread to other vital organs. Indeed, when it comes to cancer, hysterectomy saves and improves the quality of women's lives. I have developed new techniques to be used during hysterectomy, including pelvic suspension. And I perform surgical corrections for post-hysterectomy patients.

Over the years, I have coupled my training

and experience with the latest technological advances to create alternatives to elective hysterectomy—Female Reconstructive Surgery (FRS)—which I will explain in detail throughout this book. I have simply *rein-stated the concept of saving women's organs,* using various existing and new techniques to reach this goal.

It's time to break free of the myths. It's time to empower yourself with knowledge.

CHAPTER 2

What is a hysterectomy?

'Since the risk of having hysterectomy is greater than the risk of not having it why have it at all unless you're among the 5 or 6 per cent who really "must" have it? As a purely prophylactic [preventive] measure it's a big operation for little benefit—perhaps 3-6 weeks of life. This is hardly a strong argument to set against the discomforts of major abdominal surgery.'
Dr K. McPherson, Department of Community Medicine, University of Oxford

Hysterectomy is a relatively quick procedure, usually requiring an average of 60 to 90 minutes or even less of an experienced surgeon's time. In most cases, it's easy because it involves the simple cutting out of tissue.

It's a matter of routine . . .

Hysterectomy is an *elective* procedure for benign diseases—diseases that are non-malignant and are not immediately life-threatening. Yet it is almost always recommended for the following benign conditions:

- Fibroid tumours
- Prolapse

In addition, hysterectomy is frequently performed to 'cure':

endometriosis

pelvic pain
ovarian cysts
adhesions
menstrual pain
adenomyosis
benign ovarian tumours
infection (salpingitis)
endometrial hyperplasia
menstrual disorders
premenstrual syndrome

We will see, in subsequent chapters, the results of hysterectomy on these various conditions.

There are many kinds of hysterectomies

The term *hysterectomy* comes from the Greek *hystera*, meaning uterus and *ektome*, meaning to cut out. There are several kinds of hysterectomies and, as is true of most women's medical issues, a great deal of confusion exists as to what the medical terminology means (Figs. 1, 2, 3, 4).

- *Hysterectomy* refers to the removal of the uterus and, most commonly, the attached Fallopian tubes.
- *Total hysterectomy*, contrary to popular belief, does not mean that the ovaries are removed with the uterus. Rather, the medical term indicates the removal of the uterus and the cervix.

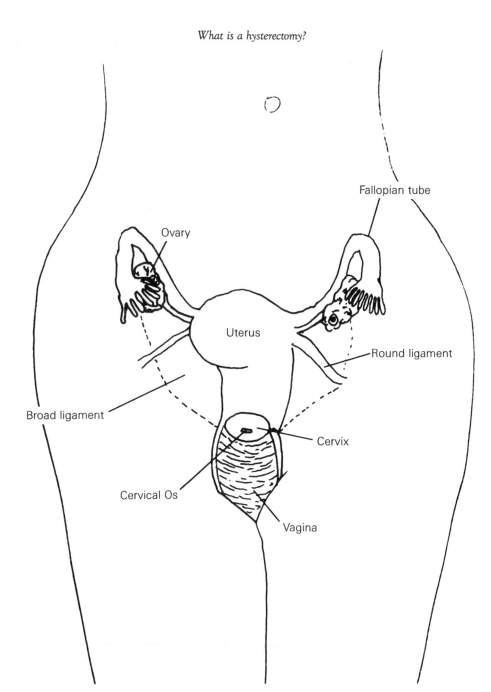

Fig. 1. The normal female reproductive organs.

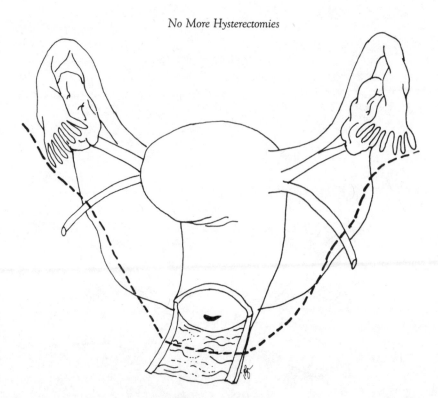

Fig 2. *Hysterectomy with bilateral salpingo-oöphorectomy: the uterus with cervix, ovaries, and fallopian tubes are removed.*

- *Subtotal or partial hysterectomy* is the amputation of the uterus above the cervix—the cervix is left in place. Again, the ovaries are not in question.
- *Oöphorectomy* denotes removal of one ovary.
- *Bilateral oöphorectomy* means both ovaries are taken.
- *Salpingo-oöphorectomy* indicates the loss of a fallopian tube and the ovary on one side.
- *Bilateral salpingo-oöphorectomy* refers to the loss of both ovaries and both fallopian tubes.

Most frequently, the surgery is achieved through a 6- to 8-inch midline incision running down from the navel, or across the lower abdomen near or below the hairline (known as a 'bikini cut'). This is called an *abdominal approach.*

Vaginal hysterectomy is the removal of the uterus through the vaginal canal, rather than a surgical opening of the abdomen. This procedure is most often performed to resolve prolapse (because the uterus has already descended into the vaginal canal) or when the uterus is not enlarged, so that it can be pulled down and out through the vagina.

If the hysterectomy is being performed because of fibroids (benign tumours), the abdominal approach is usually advised. Fibroids which are so large that they call for the sacrifice of the uterus are generally too large to pass safely through the vagina.

When hysterectomy can't be avoided

No matter how dedicated I am to saving women's reproductive organs, when invasive cancer of the female organs strikes (including cancer of the ovaries, uterine lining, and cervix), there is no alternative but to perform a hysterectomy. Lifesaving measures necessitate different priorities. I perform hysterectomies when patients are suffering from malignancy. Often women with cancer come

to see me because they know that if organs can be saved *safely*, I will do that. For example, in cases of cervical cancer, there are times when I can preserve healthy ovaries.

The terror of cancer

Cancer is dangerous—we all know this. The very mention of the word brings forth terrifying images for all of us. Who among us has not lost a dear friend or loved one to this horrible and wasting disease? As a surgeon, I have seen first-hand how cancer can ravage a woman's body. It is a destructive disease, no question about it.

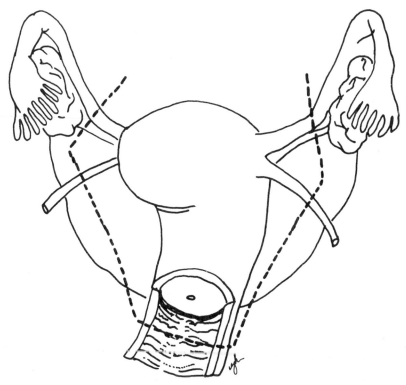

Fig 3. Total hysterectomy: the uterus and cervix are removed together with supporting ligaments. The ovaries and fallopian tubes remain.

When you're told you 'may' get cancer

I do want to make it clear, however, that having cancer is vastly different from being told that you *may* have or *may* get cancer in the future. Your doctor's comments might imply or even insinuate that your female organs hold the potential seeds for cancer and death. Because the very mention of the word brings on terror, often you are unable to make a reasoned decision in the doctor's office.

Normally, when presented with a difficult problem, you would ask basic questions such as:

● Why or how did I get this?

● What are my options?
● Could there be a mistake?
● Where can I learn more about this?

When it's a question of the *possibility of cancer*, on the other hand, you may, out of fear, agree to anything.

The purpose of this book is to aid you in making responsible decisions when you discuss your options with your doctor—decisions based on the latest technology and research. You may choose to conserve your reproductive organs or you may choose to have them removed, being fully informed of the risks, consequences, and alternatives. So, if you've been told:

● 'At your age, female organs are likely to

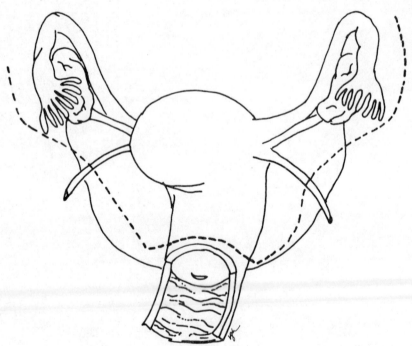

Fig 4. Subtotal or partial hysterectomy with bilateral salpingo-oöphorectomy: the uterus is amputated at the cervix; ovaries and fallopian tubes are also removed. The cervix remains.

become cancerous. You don't need them anyway . . .'

- 'You may be the one in ten women who get cancer. Why take chances?'
- 'This is a precancerous state. We caught it just in time. All we have to do is a hysterectomy.'
- 'While we remove the uterus, we can simply remove your ovaries. You don't need them and one day they'll probably become cancerous and kill you.'
- 'Your fibroid tumour grew rapidly. It might be cancerous . . .'

Take heed. And talk to your doctor about the options I will be discussing throughout the pages of this book. Hysterectomy for women with cancer—YES. But hysterectomy for benign female problems? Wait! You may have options.

Helping your body ward off cancer in the first place

Of course, one of the best ways to avoid a hysterectomy is to short-circuit the creation of cancer by your body. Although no one holds all of the answers to this dread disease, of course, certain life-style changes and nutritional alternatives can work on your behalf.

- *Hormone imbalances*, especially excess oestrogen, have been shown, over time, to cause endometrial cancer. The imbalance can be treated with the addition of progesterone.
- *Obesity* is a factor in both endometrial and ovarian cancers. Maintaining an ideal weight is essential to your health.
- *Cigarette smoking* may increase the incidence of cervical cancer by as much as 50 per cent.
- *Sexually transmitted diseases* like venereal

warts, herpes, and chlamydia, which come from having unprotected sex, have been linked to cervical cancer.

Isn't it time to stop some bad habits now?
Many vitamins, minerals, and food supplements may also boost your general nutritional status to assist your body in fighting carcinoma. Indeed, our knowledge of nutrition and the use of supplements is still very limited.

I have been fortunate to have as colleagues several biochemists who specialize in nutrition. They have kept me abreast of what is new in this field. They suggest that the addition of selenium, vitamin C, folic acid, amino acids, vitamin A, beta-carotene, vitamins E and D to the diet does have some positive effect in the body's fight against cancer.

Life-style and nutritional changes cannot be a substitute for surgery, if cancer does occur. However, with a carefully designed programme combining innovative approaches to traditional medicine and a new awareness of nutrition, you and your doctor can create individual healing programmes based on your body chemistry and known pathology.

Hysterectomy is no guarantee against future cancer

Many doctors use hysterectomy and oöphorectomy as a 'guarantee' to their patients that they won't get cancer in the future. This is plainly misleading. No one is omniscient enough to make such a prediction. It is possible to get other female cancers after a hysterectomy.

Vaginal and vulvar cancers, for example, have been known to occur in women who have had hysterectomies for benign diseases.

In one study advocating the continued use of cervical smears even after hysterectomy, an investigation of 87 women with vaginal cancer revealed that 31 of the cancer patients had had a previous hysterectomy for non-cancerous diseases.[1]

The false security created by doctors pitching hysterectomy to their unsuspecting patients can prove to be dangerous. Another investigation found that carcinoma of the vagina following hysterectomy for benign disease tends to be more advanced at the time of diagnosis than similar cancers in women whose hysterectomies were performed because of prior cervical or uterine cancer.

I imagine that the cancer is diagnosed late because the post-hysterectomy patient erroneously assumes she no longer needs gynaecological care, because she is without a uterus. And so she falls outside the system, eluding our most helpful cancer-screening device—the cervical smear—until it's too late. As with all cancers, the later the diagnosis, the less optimistic the prognosis for full recovery.

There have even been cases in which a woman's uterus and ovaries were removed if she got breast cancer, based on the belief that oestrogen caused the cancer. Although oöphorectomy may have been a viable treatment for advanced breast cancer in the past, today's chemotherapy is safer and more effective. Breast cancer itself is not prevented by hysterectomy-oöphorectomy. Studies have shown that women hysterectomized for benign disease can contract this female cancer, too.[2] Don't be misled. Hysterectomy does not necessarily protect you.

Hysterectomy during childbirth

Uncommon problems during childbirth can necessitate a hysterectomy. During labour,

the uterus may rupture and at birth it can *invert*. When it is a matter of saving a woman's life over saving her uterus, the choice is obvious.

Placenta accreta is an abnormal bonding of the placenta (the network of blood vessels and tissue that connects the foetus to the womb) to the underlying uterine wall. Diagnosis of this condition is made on the delivery table, only after the baby is born. If the obstetrician is unable to remove part or all of the placenta, and severe haemorrhage occurs, a split-second decision must be made. As late as the 1950s, hysterectomy was the only course of action. This was a lifesaving measure.

Today, with advances in technology, blood banking, and antibiotics, the uteri of many women have been saved with conservative approaches. In cases of massive bleeding, however, hysterectomy may be the only answer.

Tuberculosis

Tuberculosis of the reproductive system, although rare in the United States, does occur in many countries around the world. When TB ravages the female organs, it can destroy the tissue beyond repair. Antibiotic drugs such as *streptomycin*, and rest and good nutrition can be used to control the disease in its early stages, especially if the woman's tubes are still open and she wishes to conceive. If the destruction is severe or if the symptoms recur, however, hysterectomy is the only alternative. In order to reduce the complication rate, treatment with antibiotics is usually necessary before surgery.

Vaginal hysterectomy: a questionable cosmetic promotion

At 33, Cheryl had a vaginal hysterectomy for

falling of the bladder. After her operation, she had constant pain and her bladder fell even further. During her FRS, I found that her ovaries had been pulled down and had adhered to the top of her vagina.

Now Cheryl is doing much better with her bladder problem corrected and her ovaries back in place. But she suffered for four years, because her gynaecologist told her there was nothing wrong with her except that she didn't like sex.

Vaginal hysterectomies have been hyped as the ideal surgery. The uterus is removed through the vaginal canal so there is no incision on the abdomen and no scar. Twenty-five to 40 per cent of all hysterectomies are accomplished vaginally, depending on one's age at the time of surgery. Some physicians promise their patients a less-complicated, faster-healing, cosmetically pleasing surgery.

I do not agree. A 1981 landmark study published by the US Congress, weighing the costs, risks, and benefits of hysterectomy states that women undergoing vaginal hysterectomy are more likely to have postoperative fever and to receive antibiotic treatment. Other studies have shown a significantly greater risk of postoperative wound infection, bleeding, and infection of the ovary following the vaginal approach. What's more, vaginal hysterectomy patients may undergo further surgery at a rate as high as 5 to 10 per cent.[3]

Why is this so? The vaginal hysterectomy is performed by grabbing the cervix and literally pulling the uterus out through the vagina. As the physician pulls, (s)he cuts the ligaments and supporting structures alongside the uterus, until all the supporting structures are free. These ligaments are drawn down and eventually sewn into the vaginal closure. The original pelvic configuration and angle is never reapproximated.

The surgeon is, in effect, operating with a blindfold on. (S)he cuts but can't see into the body beyond the instruments and the tissue at hand. Operating in a confined area, the surgeon risks catching a ureter, missing the ligature (closure) of an artery, cutting the bladder or bowel, or accidentally removing an ovary.

In addition, when the support tissue is pulled down into the vagina, the ligaments often are not properly restructured. At worst, if your ovaries are pulled down on top of your vagina like Cheryl's, you may experience pain during intercourse. (At least, in the abdominal approach, the surgeon can pull upward on the ligaments and attempt to resuspend them and the ovaries in a more normal fashion.)

When the internal support structures are gone, other pelvic organs—including the vagina itself—can collapse inward, creating a secondary prolapse. In fact, vaginal vault prolapse is frequently considered to be a complication of a vaginal hysterectomy.

Although I don't condemn all vaginal hysterectomies, because they do often shorten your hospital stay, I believe these negative aspects must be addressed to help you in your decision making.

The myth of the 'intact' ovaries

Suppose you're about to have a hysterectomy and your gynaecologist offers to spare you the loss of your ovaries even though (s)he feels your uterus must come out. Should you feel relieved, protected? Most women do. And, I'm sad to say, that for many, this may be only a false protection and a false hope. Why? Because in more than a third of the cases, the ovaries simply die following a hysterectomy and menopausal symptoms ensue.[4]

In a recent sophisticated investigation in

West Germany, gynaecologists mailed questionnaires to nearly 250 premenopausal women who had been hysterectomized during the preceding ten years. About 40 per cent of the respondents reported typical signs of ovarian failure:

hot flushes	weight gain
nervousness	irritability
vertigo	sleeplessness
anxiety	palpitations
headaches	aching joints
depression	

Only a small number had reported the complaints before their surgery. In cases where only one ovary was left intact, the incidence of menopausal symptoms was more than 50 per cent. Many other American and international studies corroborate these findings.[5]

Perhaps even more interesting were the hormone studies that the West German doctors undertook on a selected number of patients. Although they found the women were still cycling, their oestrogen and progesterone levels were 'markedly lower' than in healthy women in the same age group. This corresponds with findings by the late Dr Robert Greenblatt, one of the foremost endocrinologists in the United States, who stated, 'We do see patients undergoing earlier menopause when hysterectomy is performed.'[6]

What happens to the ovaries after hysterectomy?

Why should the ovaries cease functioning after a hysterectomy? We are not sure of all the reasons, but probably a combination of effects creates the problem.

To begin with, organs that lie next to each other in the body often share the same blood supply, which is essential to their functioning and health. In the case of the ovaries, they and the fallopian tubes are fed by two arteries—the uterine and ovarian. However, these two blood vessels do not share the load equally in every woman. For some, up to two-thirds of the ovaries' blood comes from the uterine artery—that is, directly from the uterus. It stands to reason, then, that the massive dissection occurring during a hysterectomy interrupts a great deal of the blood supply to the ovaries of many women.

Other problems may combine with the loss of blood supply. The ovary may require stimulation by the cyclic changes in the uterus to keep it functioning. The loss of *prostaglandins* (a chemical produced by the uterus, which contributes to ovulation and uterine contractions) after hysterectomy may be a factor in the disruption of ovarian cycles. Ovulation may cease, based on the messages the ovaries get from the pituitary gland alone.

The ovaries left behind can become encased in thick adhesions or scar tissue following the hysterectomy. This tissue traps the ovaries and prevents them from developing and releasing eggs and ovarian hormones into the pelvic cavity. Painful pelvic masses known as *post-operative residual ovary syndrome* can develop. One or both ovaries may degenerate. This can happen even with excellent operative technique.

When I'm called upon to perform FRS on women who have had major complications following hysterectomy, I frequently discover those organs encased in such bands of scar tissue—so thick, in fact, that the ovaries are hidden. They are wrapped up and stuck onto the back wall or side of the pelvis or on top of the vagina. In some cases, the ovarian tissue is hardened and sclerotic. Sometimes, when I remove the adhesions, my patient improves. For many, however, ovulation and hormone production have diminished.

Intercourse is impossible, because the ovaries are hit with each thrust of the penis.

Ovarian failure is confirmed by blood tests which indicate that no follicles are being developed in the ovaries. Yet the tests show detectable amounts of oestrogen present, which leads me to believe that these women were manufacturing oestrogen in their body fat as well as their adrenal glands—but not, to a great extent, in their ovaries.

What does this mean to you? The potential of post-hysterectomy death of the ovaries is most distressing, especially because many gynaecologists do not recognize this as a possible consequence of the hysterectomy and do not inform their patients. You may have been led to believe that your body will hardly be disturbed by the removal of the uterus and fallopian tubes alone. I agonize over the number of post-hysterectomy women that are suffering from physical symptoms which they do not attribute to their surgery, and who continue to believe they are personally somehow at fault.

As the West German research team so aptly put it in their seminal study, 'Even after hysterectomy with both ovaries left intact, ovarian failure phenomena may follow, and these patients *should not undergo psychotherapy but rather hormone therapy*'.[7] I might add that psychotherapy may be necessary to help combat the dramatic changes that accompany organ loss, leaving a woman to feel both chemically and emotionally disturbed (see Chapter 3).

For your own good . . .

Vaginal hysterectomy and ovarian failure are not the only problems. Abdominal hysterectomies can cause multiple complications, both during and after surgery. Women undergoing abdominal hysterectomies are more likely to receive blood transfusions and anticoagulants during their hospital stay. And their recuperation time is longer. The use of conservative surgical techniques like FRS (Chapter 6) is one way of minimizing these problems.

Nevertheless, how many times have hysterectomies been portrayed as beneficial in the long run for a woman with benign disease? Your own doctor might have told you, 'We'll do this for your own good.' You may believe that you are travelling the right course.

Yet these potential complications are physiological as well as emotional. They can last a lifetime and can be life-threatening in themselves. Rarely are they mentioned to the woman about to undergo the procedure. Is this also done 'for her own good'? The less she knows, the better?

What you don't know can hurt you. The vital information about post-hysterectomy complications should no longer be kept from you 'for your own good'. Rather, it is in that spirit, and with your own very best interests at heart, that we take a closer look, in the next chapter, at what can go wrong during and after hysterectomy.

'Women are being sold hysterectomy as being the end of their problems—they go into it thinking just that—but it's major surgery; there's a 3 to 6 month recovery period afterwards, and in many cases—for instance where there is pelvic infection or ovarian scarring—it doesn't solve the problem.'
Enquiry worker, Women's Health and Reproductive Rights Information Centre

Complications: why I believe you should know about the alternatives to hysterectomy

'Many women don't realize they're going to end up with a hysterectomy—a doctor will refer them to a specialist for heavy bleeding and a specialist will assume the doctor has mentioned it. After such a shock announcement, even when a choice is given and a consultant says "go away and think about it", a woman will often assume that it really is "vital"—why else would a doctor suggest it?' Ann Webb, Health Visitor and founder member of the Hysterectomy Support Group.

Alice's gynaecologist had diagnosed fibroid tumours. Premenopausal and experiencing some pelvic pain, Alice consulted with me on the phone. Based on this diagnosis, I offered FRS, an alternative to hysterectomy.

Alice did not choose FRS. She was persuaded to have a hysterectomy by her doctor and her daughter, Linda, who had just finished residency in family practice. Linda had never heard of my work to save the female organs. Her med-school professors confirmed, predictably, that hysterectomy was the answer for women with fibroids.

The day following the surgery, a family member phoned me with regrets and bad news: *complications*. The surgeons began by performing a vaginal hysterectomy. They removed the uterus, but couldn't find the ovaries. In the confusion, they thought they cut a ureter, one of the tubes that takes the urine from the kidneys to the bladder.

Now, this would have been troublesome enough, but in order to repair the ureter and complete the surgery, the gynaecologist opened Alice abdominally, endangering her further by making two incisions. Ultimately he removed normal tubes, normal ovaries, and according to the pathologist's report, a normal uterus. Alice didn't have fibroids at all—only a retroverted uterus (her uterus was angled in a posterior direction). She needed no surgery—or at most a suspension—30-minute repair with a low risk of complications and only two days in the hospital.

Weighing the risks

Your doctors may be doing you an injustice in promising that hysterectomy will resolve all of your problems without adequately informing you of the possible consequences of the surgery. And, you may have become so imbued with the 'naturalness' of hysterectomy, that you may not even question whether it is absolutely necessary or even whether the correct diagnosis has been made.

Outdated concepts should be evaluated. A 1985 study of over 8,000 Massachusetts women between the ages of 45 and 55 documents how these women perceive menopause. Thirty per cent of the group had been hysterectomized and these women reported significantly more chronic illness

36

than those experiencing menopause naturally. In addition, they used twice as many prescription medicines, including sleeping pills, tranquillizers, and hormones. They were more likely to describe their health as 'worse than that of others'.

This same researcher, Dr Sonja McKinlay, following a sample of 2,500 women, found that menopause itself doesn't cause poorer health or the increased use of health care but rather the '*occurrence of a surgically induced menopause is the primary menopause-related change associated with subsequent perceived health status and [health care] utilization behaviour*'.[1] That is, it was the hysterectomy that brought on the problems. In fact, in a personal phone call, she expressed her belief, from the data she had gathered, that hysterectomy had very far-reaching and dangerous effects.

Just how bad are the aftereffects of hysterectomy? Estimates of the relative rate of diseases and complications following hysterectomy vary. A 1983 study of hysterectomy in the United States by the American College of Obstetrics and Gynecology and the US Department of Health and Human Services, states that 'one fourth to one half of all women who undergo hysterectomy develop some morbidity [disease], with fever and haemorrhage the most common type'. The Congressional report quoted earlier cites complication estimates as high as 81 per cent.[2]

One woman in a thousand dies as a result of her hysterectomy. This seems rather low, but the figures can be misleading. The actual number of hysterectomies performed is so large that approximately 600 women die of its complications each year.

Hysterectomy carries an additional risk of re-operation. A 1984 Canadian investigation found that there is a significant risk (40 per 1,000 cases) of complications requiring hospital re-admission during the two years after hysterectomy and associated repair procedures. Although women visit their doctor less frequently with gynaecological problems after surgery, they visit more frequently for psychological problems, urinary tract infections, and menopausal symptoms.[3]

It's clear that hysterectomy for benign disease can create more problems than it solves. The hysterectomy as 'cure-all' harkens back to the late nineteenth century, when castrations were performed wantonly for all possible female disorders from headaches to sore throats to indigestion to orgasm.[4]

Your risks may be compounded by pre-existing factors such as advanced age, obesity, diabetes, and various pulmonary and cardiac diseases. Even for women who are healthy before the hysterectomy—women like Alice—hysterectomy can have tragic, life-threatening results.

Operative complications

The operative and post-operative complications of hysterectomy are easily found in any gynaecology text. The following discussion is based on several standard training guides, on various medical research papers, and on my own clinical experience. It is crucial that you understand the potential risks *before* surgery. Also, bear in mind that these surgical complications *can* occur with Female Reconstructive Surgery; however, they have been less evident.

Blood complications: transfusions haemorrhages, and clots

Blood Transfusions. Transfusion is common during hysterectomy. Some gynaecologists routinely transfuse before surgery simply because a woman is anaemic, rather than changing the way in which they operate so that less blood is lost. Others require transfusions during surgery. Surgical technique may not be careful enough to prevent blood loss.

The rate of blood transfusions varies from 8 to 19 per 100 hysterectomies. Actually these figures may be quite low. Some less-skilled surgeons may require blood transfusions in 50 to 100 per cent of their hysterectomies.

Haemorrhage. The average blood loss during a hysterectomy is estimated at between 400 an 500 ml (about a pint). Massive bleeding, however, can occur and may cause varying degrees of shock. This would require transfusion and even re-operation. Abdominal bleeding may occur as late as 10 to 14 days following hysterectomy. If such is the case, the surgeon must perform emergency abdominal surgery, to find and tie off the bleeding vessels. If the surgeon cannot see the bleeding vessel clearly while (s)he clamps it, (s)he can run the risk of damaging a ureter.

Haemorrhage is not confined to a hospital setting. Once home, the repair of a woman's vaginal vault can be disturbed during intercourse. Such cases require emergency surgery to reclose ruptured blood vessels.

Blood clots. These may form at least one week after the hysterectomy. The symptoms can be vague. A low-grade fever, discomfort in the thigh, swelling, and other medical signs are used to diagnose this complication. The clots may take the following forms:

Haematoma. Haematoma is an area where blood has collected and organized. It is a common, if not somewhat delayed post-operative complication of hysterectomy, more frequent among younger women who have an abundant blood supply. Although symptoms are elusive, a rise in body temperature and a drop in the red blood cell count can be indicators.

The haematoma may be absorbed naturally by the body. It can be removed with further surgery, but the doctor must be careful not to create new problems by injuring the bowel or bladder in the corrective procedure.

Thrombo-embolism. Thrombo-embolism is a serious, disturbing complication of hysterectomy. Any trauma to the pelvic veins may lead to *thrombosis*, or blood clot in the leg. The clot can remain in place or it may break away from the formation site and travel within the circulatory system, settling in a vital organ. Because of the vagueness of symptoms, often the thrombosis is not caught until this has occurred. Such an eventuality is dangerous because the clot may lodge in the lungs, causing a *pulmonary embolism*. The latter can obstruct vital blood vessels in the lungs and may cause death. Thromo-embolism can be treated with blood thinners (*anticoagulants*), but this treatment must be balanced by the risk of haemorrhaging.

As you can see, blood complications can cause serious health problems and are a risk factor that must be considered before agreeing to an elective hysterectomy.

Bladder, kidney, and urinary tract complications

Urinary tract complications are most frequently caused by gynaecologic surgery. The rate varies from 1 to 10 per cent of all cases. Injury to the ureter (the tube taking urine from the kidneys to the bladder) is a common cause of malpractice suits against gynaecologists.

Urinary Retention and Infection. At the time of Pam's hysterectomy, a catheter or small tube was introduced into her urethra in order to help her empty her bladder automatically. This is standard procedure. After five days, the catheter was removed, but Pam still found herself unable to urinate. Each time her bladder needed draining, the catheter was reintroduced. Finally, an indwelling catheter was left for six weeks, until Pam's bladder function returned. She suffered from several infections during that time.

Urinary retention is a common complication of hysterectomy, particularly after a vaginal approach with anterior repair. Because the urine isn't adequately expelled, bacteria can multiply within the bladder, causing *cystitis*, or bladder infection. If the infection works its way up to the kidneys, high fever and chills result. In severe cases, a kidney can be lost.

Ureteral Fistula. A ureteral fistula is an opening or cut in the ureter. It often occurs when the ureter is not properly identified during surgery. Seventy to 75 per cent of ureteral fistulas are related to abdominal hysterectomy. Many of these injuries don't create immediate symptoms, and therefore go undetected.

If the fistula has not been discovered during the surgery, the leakage of urine into the pelvis may cause otherwise unexplained fever, pain, abdominal distension, bowel obstruction, and urine dripping from the vaginal vault with eventual loss of a kidney. This prolongs the period of disability and dims the expectation of a complete recovery. Further corrective surgery is often required.

Infections

Febrile morbidity. Febrile morbidity, or fever following surgery, is one of the most frequent complications of hysterectomy, occurring in about one-third of abdominal hysterectomy cases. The infection rate after vaginal hysterectomy is even higher because of contamination by the bacterial flora of the upper vagina and the proximity of the bowel and lower urinary tract to the uterus.

Indeed, contamination by bacteria within a woman's body, most commonly from the vagina and rectum, may occur at the time of any gynaecological surgery, despite vigorous washing and preparation. Prolonged hospitalization with therapeutic antibiotics and often a second operation may be necessary before a woman recovers.

Peritonitis. Following her hysterectomy, Harriet became very ill from peritonitis, an infection of the membrane that lines the abdominal cavity. She experienced pain, muscle spasms, and fever. Fortunately, she responded to antibiotic therapy. Other women require re-operation to drain pelvic abscesses. Some have gone into irreversible endotoxic shock, resulting in death.

Ovarian Infections. Ovarian abscesses and infection are associated with vaginal hysterectomy. They occur when bacteria from a post-operative pelvic or vaginal cuff infection invade an ovary during ovulation. The infection may not become evident until months after the surgery in women who have been previously healthy. In many cases, once an ovarian infection occurs, the surgeon often must re-operate to remove the affected organ(s).

These ovarian problems can be avoided using aggressive treatment with antibiotics and adequate drainage after the hysterectomy. Many doctors perform hysterectomies without irrigation solutions, antibiotics, or drainage.

Lung complications

If you suffer from respiratory diseases such as chronic bronchitis, asthma, and emphysema, you are at risk for developing breathing difficulties after any surgery. In addition, postoperative coughing spells may endanger the integrity of the stitches and wound repair.

Even if you have a healthy respiratory system, you may suffer a collapse of the lungs following surgery. And despite preventive measures, like the administration of antibiotics, bronchitis and pneumonia occur in some cases.

Bowel complications

Abdominal surgery may lead to disruption of normal digestive function. Michelle suffered from *paralytic ileus*, a condition that is caused by the failure of *peristalsis*, the normal, successive waves within the digestive tract that carry the digested material forward. As a result, her hospital recovery was marred by painful abdominal distension due to gas, frequent vomiting, and dehydration. She was treated with bowel stimulants and enemas, in order to get things going again.

Janna's problem was more serious. She too suffered from postsurgical nausea, profuse vomiting, and a distended abdomen. At the time of her hysterectomy, a loop of her small intestine was inadvertently fastened to the closure of the vaginal vault. This *mechanical obstruction* prevented her bowels from functioning normally and required corrective surgery.

Other post-surgical complications

Electrolyte Imbalance. This complication arises from the use of intravenous fluids during and after surgery. The natural balance of blood chemicals such as sodium, potassium, and chlorides may be upset. Overenthusiastic use of intravenous fluids may put a cardiac patient into heart failure.

Evisceration. Although evisceration is relatively rare, it is a severe complication with a 20 per cent mortality rate. It is the complete or partial tearing of the abdominal incision, which can occur with straining following surgery. In addition, if severe infection sets in, preventing the incision from healing, the wound may open up and the body contents may come spilling forth. Evisceration requires additional exploratory surgery to repair the tear.

Nerve Injury. Nerve damage is a common side effect of hysterectomy, occurring at the rate of 11 per cent. In particular, the *femoral nerve* in the leg can be affected, especially when a particular surgical tool, *self-retaining retractors*, are used during surgery. (These instruments are standard for hysterectomy but are not used routinely during FRS.)

Nerve injury can cause numbness in the thigh and leg, instability of the knee during walking, and pain in the hip joint area following surgery. Some women are unable to raise the affected leg off the bed, have decreased sensation of touch and pain, and a decreased or absent reflex response when the kneecap is tapped. Symptoms can last from six months to six years.

Prolapse of the Fallopian Tube. This is a rare complication of hysterectomy, but it can occur when the tube falls through the top of the vaginal vault. This problem creates varying degrees of discharge and discomfort.

Long-term post-operative losses

Not only can hysterectomy pose an immediate threat during and shortly after surgery, but its long-term consequences can be just as pernicious. In a questionnaire given three years after surgery, one researcher asked 56 hysterectomized women and 56 women who had undergone gallbladder operations, appendectomies, or partial mastectomies how long it took them to recover. Hysterectomy patients reported an average of 11.9 months, compared to 3 months for the others.[5]

In my own practice, I find that 70 to 80 per cent of the post-hysterectomy patients who come to me for help have problems. The long-term consequences of hysterectomy can take various forms and are quite serious. The effects of the loss of oestrogen can be life-threatening when you look at them realistically.

Severe Adhesions. Adhesions are thick bands of scar tissue that can form after any surgery. They often result from the use of catgut and clamps and the rough handling of tissue. Post-hysterectomy adhesions can change one's internal anatomy and can result in long-term pain and small bowel obstruction.

Irrigations to flush out blood and debris after surgery help prevent the formation of this scar tissue. Many patients come to me for FRS after hysterectomy to remove the adhesions that create chronic pelvic and abdominal pain.

General Prolapse. In Chapters 6 and 11, I will discuss how the removal of the uterus can cause the other pelvic organs—including the intestines, bowels, bladder, and vagina—to collapse downward. This can occur as soon as several days or as long as ten years after the hysterectomy.

Loss of ovarian function

With the loss of your ovaries following a hysterectomy-oöphorectomy, the female hormones that stimulate your menstrual cycle, including oestrogen and progesterone, stop circulating abruptly. Your body is forced into a state of 'surgical menopause'—menopause caused by surgery. In truth, you have been castrated.

However, even ovaries left behind may fail in 30 to 50 per cent of hysterectomy cases (see Chapter 2). The disruption of your ovarian function can be catastrophic to your health and well-being. Many of the long-term complications arising from hysterectomy result from this loss, including:

osteoporosis
arthritis
cardiovascular disease
hot flushes
insomnia
depression
loss of sexual desire
masculinization
chronic migraines
bowel dysfunction
generalized fatigue
neurological complaints
increased allergies
loss of normal body fat pads
loss of orgasm
severe PMS
rapid ageing of skin
bloating
cyclic oedema
obesity
thyroid dysfunction
memory loss
loss of sex drive

Osteoporosis. Osteoporosis is one of the most common bone diseases, affecting 10 million American women and *26 per cent of all women over the age of 60*. Bone is living tissue that is constantly being broken down and rebuilt. Osteoporosis is the gradual thinning and weakening of the skeletal system. Bones become brittle and break easily.

Women suffer from osteoporosis more frequently than men because, in women, the absorption of calcium into the bones is dependent on oestrogen. Without oestrogen, the calcium supplements you take will not ward off this bone disease. Bone calcium content declines at menopause because of the gradual loss of this hormone. Immediately following oöphorectomy, however, there is a sudden drop in oestrogen levels and an equally rapid demineralization of the bone. If your retained ovaries have failed, a similar situation will result.

The consequences of osteoporosis can be serious. The collapse of the vertebra, the bones of the spine, causes pain, immobility, and loss of stature. About 25 per cent of all white women over the age of 60 develop these spinal compression fractures because of osteoporosis. A simple fall, resulting in hip fracture, may, in some cases, bring on pulmonary emboli, pneumonia, and death. Some women with the disease are afraid of leaving their homes, especially in colder climates where the risk of slipping and falling on icy pavements is great.

Women must have oestrogen, yet many of the post-hysterectomy patients whom I see have never taken hormone replacements. Typically, they do not know about the positive effect oestrogen has in fighting osteoporosis or they fear oestrogen replacement will cause cancer. Women who receive oestrogen coupled with progesterone, however, have been shown to suffer from cancer less frequently than women who take no hormone replacement at all.[6]

Arthritis. Scientists in the Erasmus University, Rotterdam, the Netherlands, have found that middle-aged women who take replacement oestrogen have a four-fifths reduced risk for rheumatoid arthritis than women who do not. They believe that the oestrogen has a 'protective effect' that prevents the onset of the disease. Other recent studies with laboratory animals have shown that oestrogen suppresses the development of collagen-induced arthritis.[7]

The loss of your ovaries would halt oestrogen production and thus may trigger or exacerbate arthritis.

Cardiovascular Disease. Many recent studies have confirmed a link between a premenopausal hysterectomy and cardiovascular disease (including heart attacks and high cholesterol). In 1981, for example, The Nurses' Health Study, an ongoing investigation into the health of 121,964 women, found that premenopausal hysterectomy with the ovaries left intact was associated with significantly increased risk of heart attack later in life.

We are not entirely certain why this is so. The loss or failure of the ovaries seems to be a factor, however, because oestrogen may protect the circulatory system. A recent investigation reported in the *New England Journal of Medicine* concluded that the removal of both ovaries increased the risk of coronary heart disease, probably because of the loss of oestrogen. In addition, the chemical *prostacyclin* (PGL), may be created in the uterus and may provide some protection against coronary heart disease.[8] The US Framingham study found that women with premenopausal hysterectomy had relative odds of new-onset cardiovascular disease that were 2.7 times greater than other premenopausal women of the same age.[9]

In the United States, the death rate from heart disease caused by fat-clogged arteries is four times greater than the combined death rates of breast and uterine cancer.

Hot Flushes and Insomnia. Hot flushes

have become a symbol of menopause, and are the most common reason that post-menopausal women seek medical attention. Changes in skin temperature, skin resistance, core temperature, and pulse rate have been measured during flush episodes. At night, hot flushes contribute to insomnia, which can create great emotional distress.

It is believed that the hot flushes are triggered by oestrogen deficiency and decreasing *luteinizing hormone* (LH). During natural menopause, oestrogen levels decline slowly over a dozen or more years. Women who undergo hysterectomy, however, may experience abrupt loss of oestrogen. They do not have the benefit of the natural hormonal slowdown that normally occurs.

Most clinicians have observed that hot flushes and heavy sweating in hyster-ectomized-oöphorectomized women are more severe and more sudden in onset than those seen in natural menopause. The symptoms begin within 24 hours of surgery while the women are still hospitalized. For some women, hot flushes and night sweats increase significantly after hysterectomy, *even when the ovaries are preserved*.[10]

The real, but never discussed, emotional complications

Depression. There have been dozens of articles associating hysterectomy with psychiatric problems. The likelihood of hysterectomy causing you severe psychological problems, including depression, depends on:

- Why your surgery was performed (women who undergo hysterectomy because of cancer are less likely to be depressed).
- Your psychological state before the operation.
- Your marital adjustment and happiness.

- Your desire to bear children.

In addition, the absence of your uterus and menstruation may represent a loss of strength, vitality, and self-esteem. There is grief over this loss.

Here are the sad statistics from just one study:

- Women undergoing hysterectomy in the absence of pelvic disease were referred for psychiatric care twice as often as those who had had pelvic disease.
- Women who had psychiatric care prior to their hysterectomy were ten times as susceptible to further mental illness after the operation.
- Women who had a history of marital disruption were six times as likely to be referred for psychiatric care after a hysterectomy.[11]

Linda was less than 30 years old at the time of surgery, and she suffered from intense depression and insomnia because of the sudden hormone loss. When hysterectomy is performed at such an early age, the abrupt chemical change is a shock to the system.

Karen's hysterectomy was performed because of prolapse. Her organs had been healthy. Now, she was depressed because her physical discomfort had not let up. She felt confused and betrayed by her doctor.

Colleen had dreamed of mothering a large family—five children, at least. Imagine her emotional and spiritual anguish when her doctor informed her that she would have to limit her family to one child: in his opinion, she needed a hysterectomy because of fibroids. Suddenly she had lost her dream.

Did you know that a hysterectomy is followed by a two- to threefold greater incidence of post-operative depression than other elective pelvic operations? In one study, the psychiatric referral rate four years after hysterectomy was more than twice as great as that of women who had had their gallbladders removed and three times greater than women in the general population.[12]

Why is depression so prevalent? Is it *all in your head*, as your gynaecologist may suggest? No. The mood doesn't just result from the fact that you have undergone surgery. Rather, it is caused, in part, by the loss of hormones due to oöphorectomy or ovarian failure. In addition, recent studies suggest that an imbalance in certain neurohormones is associated with mood changes such as crying spells, irritability, nervousness, and changes in sexual desire (libido). The metabolism of these hormones within the brain is now believed to depend on oestrogen levels.

In fact, when scientists study the effect of oestrogen on post-menopausal women's mental states, they have found that depression, anxiety, and headaches are alleviated for some women by hormone replacement therapy.[13] Why? The answer lies within the complexities of brain chemistry.

Researchers have demonstrated that plasma levels of the amino acid *tryptophan* are low in depressed menopausal women (and by association, oöphorectomized women). Tryptophan breaks down into other agents in the brain, including the neurotransmitter *serotonin*, whose decrease has been associated with depressive illnesses. The levels of tryptophan are set aright by the administration of oestrogen, which I prescribe in conjunction with tryptophan and other amino acids. Even the uterus may contribute its own (as yet unnamed) hormones to the delicate balance.

In addition to these neurochemical factors, depression can also result from the physical loss. When the uterus is removed, many women experience diminished or absent orgasm because the uterus, itself, can be an orgasmic organ.[14] Add to that the

pain, complications, loss of childbearing ability, sense of helplessness, and loss of femininity that women experience and you can understand why hysterectomy is in a class by itself.

Normal 'manageable' stress after a hysterectomy usually lasts six to eight weeks and includes weakness, fatigue, excessive drowsiness, changes in appetite, labile (unstable) mood, and bowel irregularities. If symptoms such as

- Agitation
- Crying spells
- Insomnia
- Mood swings
- Inadequate re-establishment of significant relationships

persist after six months, you may need hormones.

It's difficult to separate what is physical from what is emotional, so you may wish to see a psychologist to help you adjust to:

- Profound physical and neurochemical changes
- Sense of loss (especially of childbearing)
- Problems of cancer
- The deep shock to the mind and body brought on by surgery

These certainly are not deep-seated neuroses that suddenly come out of hiding following your hysterectomy. They are real emotional losses that need to be dealt with. You may want to find support to help you cope.

Loss of Libido (sexual desire). As early as the Renaissance, doctors recognized the loss of sexual satisfaction that can be brought on by a hysterectomy. Dr Jacopo Berengario da Carpi (1460–1530), a professor at Bologna, Italy, and doctor to Benvenuto Cellini, described a surgery he observed his father perform: a prolapsed, gangrenous uterus was removed. The patient lived for many years and was able to resume relations with her husband, but the doctor noted *there was an absence of coital gratification.*[15]

Modern researchers reiterate this fact. Many studies show deterioration in sexual activities after the operation. Frequent complaints include:

- A decrease in sexual desire
- A decrease in coital activity
- Loss of orgasm
- Loss of lubrication
- Painful intercourse

The complaints worsen with time. In fact, one investigator simply comes right out and says, 'The operation of hysterectomy, with or without conservation of ovaries, was found to affect libido deleteriously.'[16]

Why is this so? Part of the answer is hormonal. The depletion of oestrogen and progesterone at menopause (and surgical menopause) has been associated with a decline in female sexual interest, capacity for orgasm, and coital frequency. Conversely, studies in oestrogen-replacement therapy for menopausal women have shown that 'oestrogen stimulates sexual desire, enjoyment,

Fig. 5. Normal anatomy.

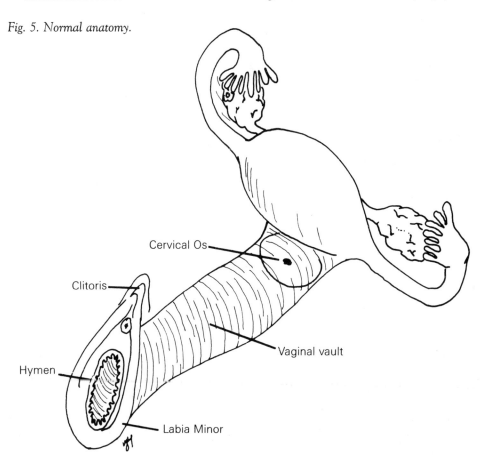

Cervical Os

Clitoris

Vaginal vault

Hymen

Labia Minor

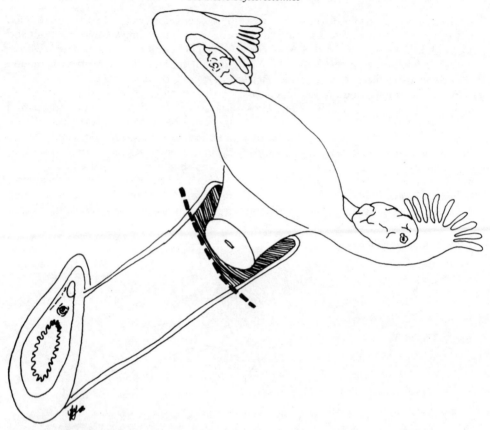

Fig. 6a. The dotted line shows where the vagina is cut during hysterectomy; shaded area indicates lost vaginal length.

vaginal lubrication, and orgasm . . .'[17]

In addition, the loss of oestrogen can cause progressively worsening vaginal atrophy. If you experience atrophy and are sexually active, you may complain of vaginal dryness and painful intercourse.

Testosterone depletion can also be devastating. Testosterone, a hormone (*androgenic*) produced by the ovaries, is essential for positive sex drive in both men and women. In a British study of 100 women, it was found that the testosterone levels in the blood were significantly lower after oöphorectomy than after normal menopause, 'presumably due to the loss of ovarian androgens'.[18] Furthermore, there was a greater incidence of depression, painful intercourse, and loss of libido with oöphorectomy as compared to natural menopause.

The sudden loss of oestrogen and testosterone because of oöphorectomy can cause sexual diminishment; however, that may not be the whole story. Female sexual response is not dependent on hormones alone.

Sex therapists have found that at least some women are at risk for decreased sexual

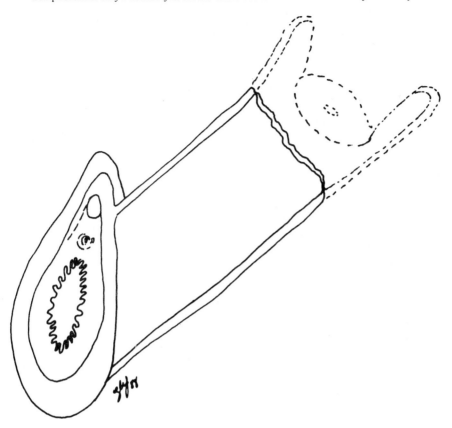

Fig. 6b. Actual vaginal length lost after final healing from hysterectomy.

pleasure following their hysterectomy because of the loss of the uterus and cervix. Women who feel uterine contractions at orgasm will feel both a quantitative and qualitative decrease in their sexual pleasure following hysterectomy. Although it has been assumed that the cervix has no important function during coitus, some women feel less pleasure after the cervix is removed.[19]

Pain during intercourse may also be caused by the surgeon's failure to reapproximate the vaginal canal's former contours. Surgeons frequently neglect to maintain the correct length and comfortable shape of the vagina after hysterectomy (see figs. 5, 6). The doctor may not leave enough structural tissue to preserve the normal anatomy. A Scandinavian study showing a highly significant reduction in the frequency of orgasm, speculated that nerve damage, the alteration of the shape of the vagina, and perhaps scar tissue in the vagina in addition to psychological reactions caused this loss.[20] I have also found that women who have given up their children for adoption as well as women who are victims of incest have a particularly high rate of hysterectomy with problems beginning at a very young age. Gynaecologists must become sensitive to this issue and work towards the conservation of these women's reproductive organs; they should recognize that these women often see their sex organs as evil or dirty and wish them to be removed in order to remove their painful experiences of the past.

I will discuss sexual misconceptions about hysterectomy and the uterus as an orgasmic organ in Chapter 7. We can only imagine how many marriages have been disrupted by this surgery.

Divorce. After her hysterectomy, Nancy felt as if she were going berserk. She hated everything and everyone around her. She withdrew. She was bitter. She became non-sexual. Who would want to live with such a person? Certainly not her husband.

Hysterectomy can place tremendous stress on a marriage. Women are told that sex will be better after hysterectomy—and may wake up with no sexual desire or response at all. Rapid ageing, depression, insomnia, physical complaints, incapacitation add to the brew. Divorce is a common 'side effect' of this surgery.

'Hysterectomy spells the end of fertility; the ending of an era for a woman. For women who have had any psychological or physical problems with their fertility: childless career women, lesbians or women who have lost babies through termination or miscarriage, it is even more important that they are counselled and given the opportunity to grieve for what have might have been as the woman who has borne children.'
Dr Prudence Tunnadine, gynaecologist and author of *The Making of Love*

'Many women undergoing hysterectomy may already have had relatively low lying wombs for some time—as a result of fibroids, pregnancies or prolapse. Lovemaking for them (and for their partners) afterwards will be different—and it is an important part of their recovery and their future enjoyment of sex that they relearn some part of their technique.'
Dr Prudence Tunnadine

Why do hysterectomies continue to be performed?

If hysterectomies can have such negative, life-threatening consequences, you may ask, why do they continue to be performed on such a large scale? Why, indeed? That's a question I've been asking over and over again to no avail, for the past ten years. Even my standard gynaecological text, which advocates hysterectomy for benign problems, states, 'the only way to avoid these [complications] is to avoid the practice of surgery'.[21] Well then, why not avoid surgery if we can?

After giving this problem careful thought over many years, I believe the answer is largely sociocultural and economic. That is, historically, we as a society have been culturally conditioned to accept the unacceptable. It may be that we have been urged on by economic necessity on the part of the medical profession but, more likely, hysterectomy has become acceptable because it's simply what's *done*. The next two chapters will explore these issues. Maybe that will help you understand why we have come to consent to hysterectomy so readily.

CHAPTER 4

The conspiracy against the uterus: making a change

A Glasgow study[1] showed that almost twice as many younger women (35-40) underwent hysterectomy in 1980 than in 1970. The researchers put this increase down not to an increase in gynaecological pathology—ie more disease—but to a change in gynaecological practice: in 1980 there was no increase in the incidence of pelvic tumours nor in the majority of cases of demonstrable organic disease and the number of repair operations actually fell. The increase was due 'solely or primarily' for pelvic pain: patients were requesting relief of symptoms and were offered hysterectomy.

A life rescued

It seems I was a medical student a lifetime ago. Yet I still vividly recall an incident that occurred while I was rotating through gynaecology. The patient, Marie, was in her early twenties and had been suffering from pelvic pain every month with her periods. She was a novice nun and celibate.

During the operation, moderate endometriosis was found. I remember the attending doctor, an excellent surgeon, thinking out loud. 'Well,' he mused, 'she is young—but she has pain. She's a nun so childbearing isn't a concern here. Perhaps we should just take everything out. She won't have to worry about messy, painful periods anymore . . .'

I was only a medical student and relegated to the role of retractor holder. The attending doctor looked up at the resident assisting him with a quizzical expression. 'What do you think we should do?'

Yes, the resident agreed that everything should come out. They started to place a clamp on the ligament that holds the uterus.

Medical students are to be seen and not heard. My job during this surgery was to hold the retractor, observe, and remain silent. Yet I realized, as we all stared into this young woman's pelvis, that these men were planning to remove all of Marie's reproductive organs based on the fact that she was a nun.

How could I hold my tongue? I asked softly if anyone had discussed with the patient her desire to have children. Both men looked at me with surprise. No, neither had ever broached this young woman's future childbearing plans with her. They had simply assumed that she was a nun and wouldn't care if her organs were removed.

The attending doctor began to laugh. The resident, not knowing how to respond, stood stock still, at attention. I was fearful about the meaning of the laughter. But then the senior surgeon removed the clamp. He cleaned out the endometriosis rather than the organs. He was laughing at himself.

After the surgery, Marie told us that she had made a mistake in her choice of a vocation. She was leaving the church and had planned to marry a young priest, who

49

was similarly disillusioned. Her recovery went well. Her pain was alleviated by the surgery. She married her young man and had several children, never knowing how close she had actually come to losing it all. A 'happily ever after', wouldn't you agree?

But what a harsh lesson for me. *One person's beliefs in the operating room could lead to unnecessary organ loss.* And as time went on in my training, the lessons became more and more difficult, the stories more and more tragic.

As a resident, I loved the operating room. I enjoyed the opportunity of being able to change someone's body and then watch the healing process take place. Yet I was struck by the sheer number of uteri that were surgically removed without any pathological findings. I learned the hard way that I should not question my superiors about the wisdom of hysterectomy for benign problems. This was accepted practice.

Had I missed something? Perhaps I was naive in thinking that I had become a doctor to heal women. It was too late when I found out that much of my profession of healing had little to do with the ideal, but, rather, with belief systems, economics, and institutionalized conformity.

For the last century there has been an unspoken conspiracy against the uterus. I don't believe it is a premeditated conspiracy to hysterectomize all women, but, instead, a psychosocial attitude concerning the female reproductive system. The uterus, *the only organ for which no analogous male structure exists*, remains a source of fascination. It is the focus of many of our beliefs.

Beliefs and social attitudes we 'buy' about hysterectomy

You may have been socialized to accept that:

- It's a fact of life: most little girls will grow up to *need* a hysterectomy. (After all, so many of our mothers, aunts, grandmothers, sisters, and cousins have had the surgery . . .)
- The post-childbirth uterus is a useless organ of no value, producing bloody and painful discharge, rendering us undesirable once a month.
- Hysterectomy causes no adverse side effects and enhances sexuality by removing the fear of pregnancy.
- The uterus is strictly a procreative organ and has nothing to do with a woman's sexuality.
- Women over 30 (or 40) should no longer bear children.
- Our female organs are all potential cancer sites that should be removed to avoid future danger.
- Any woman who wants to keep her organs is hysterical or superstitious or worse.

These beliefs make themselves evident in the way your doctor treats you and in the way that you perceive your own body. After all, with such powerfully negative beliefs and stereotypes, what self-respecting, modern woman would want to hang on to her uterus, anyway?

Misery loves company

Women themselves sometimes perpetuate the 'need' for hysterectomy in a sort of 'misery loves company' conspiracy. Their reasoning goes something like this: *'If I've had to lose my organs, and go through Hell to boot, what makes you think you should get off scot-free?'* Not a very generous attitude, I admit, but one that appears all too frequently.

I spent an hour one afternoon consoling

Wendy, whose fibroids were removed and uterus put back into its normal condition during Female Reconstructive Surgery (see Chapter 6). Physically Wendy looked great. She had had a perfect surgical outcome. Her scar had healed. Her uterus was back to its normal size and was no longer tender. Her examination showed nothing abnormal. Emotionally, however, she was a wreck.

Her complaint? When Wendy returned to her job, her female colleagues could not believe that she had healed so quickly and was looking so healthy. All the women who had had hysterectomies, bad experiences, residual problems with their bodies, began harping on her. It wasn't possible for her to be doing so well, they said. Here she was back at work full time in just a few weeks. They insisted that Wendy would destroy all of the surgical work and get massive adhesions if she didn't stay in bed for six to eight weeks. They had had hysterectomies and they had had problems, so certainly she should too.

The upset created by Wendy's friends was greater than the stress and pain of FRS. We had to deal with her emotions for the next several months. Her colleagues didn't let up on their scare tactics.

Wendy had taken a new approach—one that defied the commonly held myths and beliefs which our society holds so dear—and in doing so, she alienated her 'sisters' who had accepted their own suffering as part of a woman's lot in life. How sad for everyone concerned.

Doctors are not immune

Your doctor perceives you and the other women in his or her practice according to a personal set of social beliefs. Those beliefs are reflected in the medical care you receive. We are all products of our society and culture. And our cultural conditioning regarding the womb began with the Greeks, whose complacent attitude held that the uterus was *not required for life*. According to Dr Don Sloan, Director of the Sex Therapy Center at New York Medical College, 'The "UUS" or "useless uterus syndrome" has been given as proper indication for surgery by many surgeons . . .'[2]

But who can determine when a uterus is 'useless'? The decision regarding the age at which a woman should undergo a hysterectomy is often arbitrary. I have had one disturbing altercation after another with gynaecologists who ascribe to the beliefs about hysterectomy, proclaiming them to me and their patients, as if citing from the Ten Commandments.

In one such incident, I was treating Betty, a member of an ethnic minority in her early forties, for abnormal bleeding. I performed a D & C (a scraping and analysis of the uterine lining) and ruled out uterine cancer. I diagnosed a fibroid uterus. Betty asked if I would please just remove the tumours and leave her uterus, fallopian tubes, and ovaries intact, which I was perfectly willing to do, provided everything else checked out free of cancer.

Betty was lying on a trolley in the hallway of the operating suite, ready for her surgery. She had consented to a laparotomy (an incision into the body), fibroid removal, and the reconstruction of her uterus. She also agreed to having her ovaries biopsied, for evaluation purposes.

The assisting surgeon approached the trolley and was horrified when he read Betty's chart. 'Why didn't you consent her for a hysterectomy?' he yelled over her head, as if she were a piece of furniture. 'She's 43.' I didn't respond. What was I to say? She didn't have cancer. She wanted to keep her uterus. Why should I have her sign a consent form for a hysterectomy? She didn't want or need one.

He pulled me aside into an adjoining room

where he proceeded to excoriate me in front of nurses and the anaesthetist. 'She's too old. She doesn't need her uterus anymore, anyway. These women are all alike . . . they think it's some kind of magical organ. They're all ignorant and superstitious.'

It wasn't the first time that I had heard such words. This doctor wasn't practicing medicine—he was practicing myths, stories, beliefs. Was it ludicrous to think of removing Betty's fibroids? Had I used poor judgement? Was Betty a woman with no sensibility, no intelligence, no innate consciousness to make her own decision about what she wanted?

And, I remain dumbfounded at how this one organ, so vital to women's health and essential to the species, can be labelled worthless and useless after childbearing age is past. As you will see in Chapter 7, it continues to serve many functions.

Playing God?

What if a woman has postponed having a family until she's over 35? Again, we have another set of beliefs. Medically speaking, the biological reproductive age for women can range from one year after menstruation begins to three years following menopause. This is not to say that women at either end of the spectrum would want to or benefit from bearing children—only that they are capable of doing so.

Beliefs about the appropriate age for motherhood vary from region to region and from doctor to doctor. For example, in America the incidence of hysterectomies among younger women is twice that in the South as it is in the Northeast.[3] Does the Southern environment engender more gynaecological problems? I doubt it. It's more a sociocultural issue. Perhaps a single, childless young woman with no immediate pros-

pects for marriage is thought of as a spinster in a Southern state, with little further use for her reproductive organs.

This concept comes from the nineteenth century, when women over 30 were thought to be sterile or capable of bearing only defective children. *What is childbearing age today?* Thirty? Forty? Forty-five? Studies have shown that although there may be more complications for women who bear children at 40 years of age and more, infant outcomes for women of normal weight and few pregnancies are comparable to those of infants born to women in their twenties.[4]

Today millions of women are giving birth to children at 35 and older. I had my first child at the ripe old age of 37. The latest technology and genetic screening have changed what our society accepts as the norm for reproductive capabilities.

If a woman seeks medical attention because of a gynaecological problem, the deciding factor about whether or not to perform a hysterectomy may depend—not on the health of her uterus, not even on her reproductive capabilities—but on the doctor's personal belief about the appropriate age for childbearing—given his or her propensity for viewing the uterus as an organ exclusively needed for reproduction.

In one case, I was treating Sheila, a vivacious woman of 42 who had complained of chronic pelvic pain, but who also wanted me to reverse a tubal ligaton. She had remarried and desired a child with her her new husband.

Again, an assisting physician responded to his own beliefs during surgery. After glancing at Sheila's chart, Dr J. exclaimed, 'This woman is 42! Why are you doing this? Women who are 42 should not be having children.' He stated this with such conviction that I held my tongue. I just asked why he felt that way.

Dr J. went on to explain that he was 41 and

his wife was 38. They already had two children and he would not want to start again. Besides, he and his wife would be too old to care for a teenager when they were in their sixties. 'You can't be an adequate parent when you're that old,' he explained matter-of-factly.

Frankly, I couldn't help wondering whether anyone who is so dogmatic would be a great parent at any age! I imagined that he had had a fight with his wife that morning over the kids. After all, doctors are only human. They have family problems and insecurities. Had I not been in the operating room, some hapless patient may have paid the price for Dr J.'s family squabble.

Whether or not my fantasy was true, it was quite clear to me that Dr J. had given this 'problem' much thought. However, just because he had chosen not to have any more children, did that mean that no one else could either? Nowhere have I seen it carved in stone that over 40, thou shalt not bear children. But, I learned from this man's persistence and intensity that for him, and the women in his practice, this was a rule.

The evolution of belief systems

Belief systems are personal and societal ways of understanding and explaining the universe. When a particular belief system is in vogue, people will organize their thoughts and actions to conform with it. Until a belief is substantiated by medical fact, however, it remains just a belief—and not the truth.

As medical knowledge evolves, beliefs change. At one time, for example, babies were thought to emerge from tiny *homunculi*—little people contained in the sperm or egg. We can all remember beliefs about the use of bloodletting to cure infections. And, less than 100 years ago, many doctors in the

United States advocated castration for women who enjoyed sex. [5]

We consider these beliefs archaic and laughable. Yet many still exist regarding the uterus and hysterectomy. Where do the rules, beliefs, and myths come from? A brief look at the history of gynaecology will answer that question and help you understand why hysterectomy has flourished during the past century.

The uterus as an 'animal'

Historically, the womb has been regarded as a mystical entity with fascination and awe—the source of both life and death. How can it be that life takes shape and emerges whole from within another being? And yet, since the beginning of time, women have died horrible deaths from the complications of childbirth and problems within the female reproductive system.

In prehistoric times, the uterus was imbued with mystical and magical powers. Later, the Egyptians, who were well acquainted with female disorders, regarded it as an independent animal, capable of movements within a woman's body and having a mind and preference all its own.

The Greeks had equally interesting ideas. Hippocrates stated that the uterus often went wild when not fed with male sperm. Indeed, *hyster-*, the root of the modern word *hysteria* (meaning excitability, unmanageable fear, and emotional excess) can be traced back to the ancient Greek name for the uterus. From that time almost till the present day, all gynaecological and emotional disturbances were thought to originate in that organ.

Over the ages, fascinating theories were evolved to explain the workings of the reproductive system. These, too, were based on beliefs. During the Middle Ages, for example, the uterus was thought to contain seven separate compartments: male embryos were imagined to develop in the chambers on the right, whereas females developed on the left. The middle cell was reserved for hermaphrodites. The organ was also thought to have horns and testicles. One proponent of this theory, Mudinus, (AD 1270-1326), said of the uterus:

It is made chiefly for conception, and consequently to cleanse or purge the whole body from superfluous undigested blood. This is the case in human beings only. Other animals do not menstruate, and in them such superfluidities are consumed by the production of hide, fur, claws, beaks, and feathers and the like, of which man is deprived.[6]

Hysteria: the tyranny of the insatiable womb

During the early fourteenth century, a French surgeon compared female anatomy to 'a penis turned inside out'.[7] But there was at least one difference between these two anatomies. For although the penis was regarded as the seat of such positive attributes as masculinity and strength, the womb was the cause of *hysteria*. Hysteria, in fact, was frequently diagnosed as a 'disease' and the principal cause of all female complaints including: epilepsy, asthma, breathlessness, flatulence, tiredness, convulsions, and painful menstruation, among others.[8]

According to Germaine Greer in her ground-breaking feminist work of the early 1970s, *The Female Eunuch*, 'Women were assumed to be by nature subject to the tyranny of the insatiate womb, and to suffer symptoms from which men only suffered if they indulged in excessive self-abuse'.[9]

Why wasn't this tyrannical organ re-

moved, then, as a matter of course? It was simply a question of medical technology. Hysterectomy was considered incompatible with survival until 1768, when Joseph Cavallini successfully removed the uteri of pregnant dogs and sheep. At the moment of his triumph, he predicted, very correctly, and to my great dismay, that one day the womb 'may be plucked out with impunity from the human body'.[10]

The age of the womb

Toward the middle of the nineteenth century, vast numbers of middle- and upper-class women suffered from a sort of invalidism—symptoms included headache, muscular aches, weakness, depression, menstrual difficulties, indigestion—which required complete rest. Social historians believe this was brought on by a 'lady's' new social role to be a reproductively active ornament to her husband. She was required to do nothing, and so, 'sickness became a part of life, a way of filling time'.[11]

Female ills of all sorts continued to be interpreted as *uterine sympathies*. Doctors still believed that the uterus was the *controlling* organ in the female body. As one prominent doctor stated:

Thus, women are treated for diseases of the stomach, liver, kidneys, heart, lungs, etc.; yet in most instances, these diseases will be found on due investigation, to be, in reality, no disease at all, but merely the sympathetic reactions or the symptoms of one disease, namely, a disease of the womb.[12]

Society was so obsessed with female disorders that in 1868 French historian Jules Michelet characterized the nineteenth century as 'the age of the womb'.

In her informative book about women's health care during that era—*Female Complaints*—social historian Sarah Stage explains that despite the demonstration of the ovaries' function two centuries earlier, doctors continued to equate menstruation with the elimination of superfluous blood. 'This lead some physicians to label the uterus as "the sewer of all the excrements in the body"'.[13]

Although minor operations on the female genitalia date back to ancient times, in general the practice of gynaecology did not include much surgery until the late nineteenth century.

Assault against the ovaries

Although the uterus was responsible for a woman's physical ills, the beliefs of the nineteeth century held that a woman's personality was directed by her ovaries, and any abnormalities, from irritability to insanity, could be traced to some ovarian disease. Castration was performed most often to modify female personality disorders. Among the reasons given for ovariotomy (later called oöphorectomy) were 'troublesomeness, eating like a ploughman, masturbation, attempted suicide, erotic tendencies, persecution mania, simple "cussedness", and painful menstruation'.[14]

Abuse was rampant. One doctor, Dr Robert Battey, took it upon himself to rid women of 'mania' by removing healthy ovaries. His hope was to 'uproot and remove serious sexual disorders and re-establish the general health'.[15]

Sexual desire in women was regarded as an abnormality and thus a perfectly good reason for castration. One of the early practitioners of ovariotomy called women's orgasm a *disease*. Indeed, he felt it was irrelevant to a woman's feelings whether she had sex organs or not. He advocated castration for women who masturbated or showed uncontrollable sexual desire.[16]

Ovariotomy became very popular, despite dubious results, in part because it was an easy operation that a young surgeon could master. Doctors boasted of the thousands of operations they had performed at professional meetings and displayed ovaries on platters to admiring audiences. By 1906, a leading gynaecological surgeon estimated 150,000 women in the United States had lost their ovaries to the scalpel.[17]

The struggle to popularize hysterectomy

If the ovaries were an easy target, could the uterus be far behind? One doctor at the end of the nineteenth century stated it clearly: 'After you have laid violent hands on the ovaries, it matters not what becomes of the uterus.'[18] Abdominal hysterectomy was successfully accomplished for the first time in June 1853 by Walter Burnham of Lowell, Massachusetts. When surgery became a viable option in the late 1800s and early 1900s, more conservative procedures were abandoned.

Indeed, by the end of the century, hysterectomy had become a frequently and commonly performed surgery. Admittedly hysterectomy saved many lives. Microbiology was a newborn science. Antibiotic treatment for 'the pox'—gonorrhoea and syphilis—had yet to be developed. There were no screening programmes for early detection of cancer. Microsurgery and sophisticated endocrinology as we know them today were unheard of. Hysterectomy was the only means of dealing with female disorders at a time when the uterus and the ovaries were considered unrepairable.

Understandably, however, women were

fearful of the new medical speciality called *gynaecology*. Misdiagnosis was rampant. In the prudishness of the era, false modesty got in the way of safe medical practice. Doctors were permitted to touch the female genitalia but not to expose them to view. Besides, women dreaded losing their organs. The uterus, seat of all life, *has* some mystical qualities. Women equated hysterectomy with death itself.

The male medical establishment considered women's fears to be unfounded and 'hysterical'. When hysterectomy became an option, male doctors ridiculed women severely for wanting to keep their uteri. Besides, surgeons specifically view human organ systems without personal attachment. They are most critical of the natural affection we feel for parts of our own bodies, especially if they are the potential source of disease and, in fact, historically had been equated with disease.

Physicians had seen too many women die from the scourge of cancer and suffer from severe pelvic infection. Yet women resisted, even if their lives depended on the removal of their diseased organ. And so, surgeons developed a near hatred for the 'mystical uterus'. It became the object of a massive re-education programme, coming under direct attack. The uterus alone was seen as the evil instrument for women's self-destruction.

Thus is the medical model, the uterus involved only one function. It was to serve as the vessel for procreation. When childbearing ended, so did the need for the uterus—a troublesome organ which, when left intact, would only create problems. The uterus lost its powerful, mystical position. It became useless.

Hysterectomy today

I believe that we have not kept up with the times, but rather, apply medical standards and habits adopted ninety years ago to modern women. The procedure of hysterectomy, as first performed before the turn of the century, remains virtually unchanged today.

In fact, within the last twenty years, new 'justifications' have evolved to substantiate increasing the number of hysterectomies performed. Legal and social changes in the late 1960s, for example, led to an acceptance of hysterectomy for the purpose of sterilization. As recently as 1969, a gynaecologist, Dr R.C. Wright, explaining why tissue committees were presented with such large numbers of uteri completely free of pathology, wrote:

> To sterilize a patient and allow her to keep a useless and potentially lethal organ is incompatible with modern gynaecologic concepts. Hysterectomy is the only logical approach to surgical sterilization . . . The uterus becomes a useless, bleeding, symptom-producing, potentially cancer-bearing organ, and therefore should be removed.[19]

Truly, this attitude does not differ appreciably from our nineteenth-century predecessors.

Making changes in medicine

As we make strides in medicine, our practice must reflect these breakthroughs. Changes, however, are never easily tolerated, whether in the healing disciplines, or in life in general. And medicine is an institution, just like any other. Its forms and conventions are based on what has worked in the past. No one welcomes change. My own struggle to alter the course of medicine seems overwhelming, at times. Yet I persist, because I know that I am making a needed correction.

I am most grateful to all of the doctors and nurses who have supported me, allowing Female Reconstructive Surgery to grow, and develop. At least they did not let the beliefs and economics of the hysterectomy industry get in the way of each woman's right to have a choice.

The rule to have no rules

The evolution of medical beliefs has taught me to make no rules! I try to be flexible because what is unusual today may be commonplace tomorrow. Every day medical science advances. Every day we learn more and more about how your hormones function, about what makes your fibroids grow, about the mysteries of your uterus, about how genetics come into play, about how technology can help you. In many fields, we are just beginning to find the keys that unlock the doors to knowledge and not myth.

The old rules stem from thoughts, individual preferences, fear, and socialized myths, which exert a powerful influence on your thinking. Breaking these conventions is difficult. When you understand how your beliefs have limited your vision, however, you can begin to take greater responsibility for your own health. You can see the medical facts with clearer eyes. Then, not only is there a great outcome, physically, but mentally, too.

My patients participate in their own care and take charge of their lives. They no longer accept the belief that hysterectomy is inevitable but understand that there are other options available. And if hysterectomy is chosen, it is done so with all the options considered and all the cards on the table.

Update: the times they are a-changin'

Everyone thinks the local university medical centre is a great place to get your medical care because it has the image of having the 'best'—the 'best' staff and the 'best' facilities. This image was called into question for me in January, 1989, during regular weekly grand rounds, when a typical case was presented.

P.C., a black twenty-seven-year-old childless female, woke up from her supposed myomectomy to find her uterus removed. The female resident on this case had been eager to remove the enlarged uterus she found. She never thought of cutting into the uterus to look for a fibroid that may have been deep within the walls; it was easier to remove the whole organ. The pathologist opened the uterus after it had been removed and found a large submucosal fibroid central inside the uterine cavity.

When a sensitive male member of the staff confronted the resident with the fact that she could have removed the fibroid and conserved the uterus, she shrugged it off. Her attitude was, 'So what?' This was simply part of her medical training. The patient was later told by the team of university doctors, 'Nothing else could have been done. You needed a hysterectomy . . .' A room full of residents, students, and attending staff let this one go—as they had always done. 'So what? It was just a uterus'.

The pain this young woman was to experience because of her desire to have a child someday had not been felt by her resident surgeon. Even in this modern day, residents are not being educated on the extended roles of the uterus and the general importance of the reproductive organs in the daily functioning of a woman's body. Hysterectomy was the quick, simple answer in this patient's case because the medical school system had not yet offered young residents a concept of reproductive health rights, nor the full understanding of the role of the uterus.

The surgeon that spoke up did feel the pain of the patient. He didn't win any popularity contests with his questioning, but he *did* question, and he showed his concern for this woman. Perhaps there were other doctors who heard him and also understood. They may have even asked themselves the same question. Someday there will be no questions to ask . . . just options to offer women.

CHAPTER 5

The hysterectomy industry

'According to researchers at the University of Sheffield[1] the growth of private fee-for-service surgery in the UK has resulted in an increase in the number of hysterectomies carried out in the private sector: from less than 15 per cent in 1981 to approaching 24 per cent in 1986. This fact is accounted for not so much by an absolute increase in the number of operations carried out but by women electing to go privately rather than to wait for surgery.'

Private health sector business analyst

It's simple economics

Interesting how loosely and frequently we use the term obstetrics and gynaecology without thinking about it. The two specialities, obstetrics and gynaecology, deal with the same territory, the female reproductive system, yet they are different disciplines.

When young obstetricians and gynaecologists first qualify, they usually begin by delivering babies. The obstetric part of the training helps to make contacts and gain referrals of young women. This builds the practice.

Then, perhaps when it's time to take life a little easier and earn more money, some abandon the childbirth aspect of the practice (often to younger associates) in favour of the gynaecological side. In their book entitled *Gynaecology, Sex, and Psyche*, Dr Lorraine Dennerstein and a team of gynaecologists and psychiatrists at the University of Melbourne, Australia, examine the possible reasons for the high hysterectomy rate. They suggest that 'hysterectomy is one of the few major operations done by the gynaecologist and pride, technical practice, and financial incentive may generate a bias towards this'.[2] There is also the fact that many western women, especially, according to the statistics, those from social classes A and B, go out and seek a hysterectomy as a kind of status symbol. A woman can separate herself from others in her community by boasting that she had a hysterectomy by a private surgeon—many women wear this kind of surgery like a medal. Psychosocially we are 'educated' to use possessions like jewellery and designer clothes to replace a more healthy self-esteem. In much the same way, especially I believe in the UK where two healthcare systems operate side by side, women can show off their economic and social status through the performance of a hysterectomy.

Why the situation is worsening

Today, many doctors do not want to do obstetrics. It's a high-risk procedure with little financial return. Each time a doctor takes on an obstetrics patient, given today's malpractice climate, (s)he places a career on the line. Some communities in this country have lost the services of their obstetricians altogether, because of skyrocketing malpractice insurance costs. And in the end, 30 to 40 per cent of the huge sums awarded by the courts find their way into the pockets of the lawyers and not the victims. It's a self-perpetuating system.

The risks are great because anything that happens during the delivery can be construed as the obstetrician's fault. Even an excellent obstetrician who has established a practice that brings love into the delivery room can be destroyed by one poor outcome. The obstetrician may have nothing to do with it, but our society wants to blame someone.

What does this mean to you? Simply that many obstetricians and gynaecologists are now opting to limit their practices to gynaecology. Obstetrics is growing at less than 1 per cent a year. The costs of running a quality gynaecology office, which include, machinery, staff, and malpractice insurance, mean that in order to exist, obstetricians and gynaecologists *must* do surgery. The standard operation is hysterectomy. So, they must do hysterectomies. And, being an 'old boys' group, everyone—men and women—must stick together and support the hysterectomy industry.

Deeper motivations

Aside from economic necessity, I believe several other issues motivate doctors to perform these surgeries. First is the belief that they are doing no harm. After all, hysterectomy is simply the way things have been done and continue to be done. It must be OK.

Second, there is an ego gratification. Some male doctors need to control women and feel

power over their organs. In the nineteenth century, the castration frenzy revealed a 'profound anxiety about female sexual appetite'.[3] The doctor knew best. A woman's participation in the decision about castration constituted a symptom in itself and her empowerment, a form of dementia.

Even today, if the rate of hysterectomy were purely dependent on pathology and physical problems, then the sex of the doctor should have no effect on the number of hysterectomies performed. This may not be the case. In a Swiss study, female gynaecologists performed half as many hysterectomies as their male counterparts.[4] This has psychosexual implications, which can result in victimization of women.

A statistical look at hysterectomy

Hysterectomy rates, viewed internationally, vary considerably, but they have risen in Canada, Australia, various European countries and in England, Wales and Scotland as well as in the US.[5] The operation is performed three times more commonly in the USA than in Britain and twice as often in Australia than in Britain.[6] In Australia the lifetime risk of hysterectomy is now as much as 40 per cent (in the US it's 50 per cent), that's 400,000 hysterectomies per year. Why? In a prominent Australian study[7] this number was found to be related to the number of gynaecologists in practice (Australia has four times as many obstetricians and gynaecologists per head of the population as the UK).

In Canada rates in 1971 were 600 per 100,000, just under those of the US. A review committee from the College of Physicians and Surgeons of Saskatchewan investigated the reasons for the increase and re-classified the operations into what they considered 'justified' and 'unjustified'; they then publicized the results and the rates dropped by almost 33 per cent in a 4-year period.[8]

According to Swiss researchers[9] variations in the frequency of hysterectomy seem to be best explained by 'factors such as medical and surgical bed density, insurance and payment systems, professional uncertainty, surgeon's sex, control and review of surgical indications, medical auditing and second opinion programmes, rather than differences in morbidity, mortality and other socio-demographic characteristics of the population studied. They suggested that a drop in the 35 to 49 age group (when most operations are done) was caused by gynaecologists themselves using a "change in indications"'. Once again, at the start of their study rates showed an increase (of 57 per cent). Once they publicized these results the annual rate dropped by 25.8 per cent overall and by 33.2 per cent in the 35 to 49 age group.

In 1985, only 62.8 per cent of all American women over the age of 65 had intact uteri.[10] According to one report, 'the incidence of hysterectomy is increasing so rapidly in the US that within a few years 50 per cent of women younger than 65 will no longer have their uterus'.[11] Other researchers have found that one of every four American women reaches menopause through surgery.[12]

According to epidemiologist Elaine Meilahn of the University of Pittsburgh, the incidence of hysterectomies in the US population is related to racial and socioeconomic factors. In a random survey of 2,137 Pittsburgh-area women, she found that black women undergo twice as many hysterectomies as whites. Although she was careful to point out that black women may choose this surgery as a form of sterilization, she did 'wonder when the differences are so great by race and education and you don't see any differences in disease which can explain these differences'.

Meilahn found that the hysterectomy rate for all white women in her survey decreased as educational levels increased.

● . . . 38 per cent of high school graduates (with no further education) had been hysterectomized.
● 20 per cent of all college graduates were hysterectomized.
● Only 13 per cent of the women who had done postgraduate work were hysterectomized.[13]

It seems the more informed *you* are and the more you participate with your doctor in medical decisions, the less likely you will be subject to unnecessary surgery.

The survey

Because of these startling statistics and my belief that the medical profession should re-evaluate elective hysterectomy for benign disease, I decided to learn as much as I possibly could about hysterectomies in the United States. I wanted to know:

● How many hysterectomies are performed each year for cancer, and how many for benign diseases?
● At what age are hysterectomies most common?
● In which geographic area are they most frequent?
● What is the cost of these surgeries?
● How many normal uteri are removed?

With Robert Pokras, a medical statistician at the National Center of Health Statistics, I studied the hysterectomy statistics on the Federal Hospital Discharge Survey supplied by the Department of Health and Human Services. In the United States, there are approximately 6,000 civilian inpatient hospitals where patients stay less than 30 days. Our survey is based on a random sampling of 500 of these hospitals, selected by region of the country and number of beds. The data I'll be sharing with you in the following sections exclude military and federal hospitals, so the true numbers are about 2 per cent higher than the ones I cite.

All of the following statistics, except as noted, were published in 1987, in a government document, by the Department of Health and Human Services. Our report is entitled 'Hysterectomy in the United States: 1965–1984'.[14]

How many hysterectomies a year?

According to our survey, hysterectomy is one of the most frequently performed major surgical procedures in the United States. This is all the more disturbing when you realize that only half of the population is eligible for the procedure. From 1965–1984, a total of 12.6 million hysterectomies were performed. We have estimated that over 670,000 hysterectomies occurred in 1985, the lastest year for which statistics are available. By way of comparison, look at other common surgeries done that year:

- 506,000 lens extractions for cataracts
- 485,000 cholecystectomies (gallbladder removals)
- 469,000 repairs of lower abdominal hernias
- 361,000 prostatectomies
- 202,000 coronary bypass procedures

Hysterectomy was surpassed only by caesarean section (813,000)—not a completely compariable procedure because it's a non-elective obstetric operation. If your baby is in distress, you must have the C section, but if you have fibroids, you can opt to have treatments other than hysterectomy.

The number of hysterectomies nearly doubled between 1965 and 1975 to a high point of 724,000. Recently, the rate has been declining. This is due, most likely, to women's growing awareness of the excessive abuse of this surgery. Other researchers have found, however, that the more surgeons and the more hospital beds available in a region, the greater the number of hysterectomies. When hospitals are audited, hysterectomy rates decline sharply.[15]

Who gets hysterectomized?

According to our study, and contrary to popular belief, this operation is not reserved for 'older' women. Here are the facts:

- The majority of women who lose their uteri are between 19 and 44 years of age—when women are reproductively active. (In 1984, 15.4 per cent of all hysterectomies were performed on women under 30, and 60.2 per cent were accomplished on women between the ages of 30 and 49.)
- The frequency of hysterectomy rises dramatically as women approach the age of 30, peaks for women in their thirties and forties, and drops markedly from 50 years of age on.
- From 1965 to 1984, only 23 per cent of all hysterectomies were performed on women over the age of 50.

As mentioned earlier, the Southern States have the highest overall rate of hysterectomy, and women in that region are more likely to undergo the operation at a younger age.

Regional variations must also be taken into account outside the US. In 1985 in a survey of 14 English regional health authorities numbers varied from a low of 12.2 per 10,000 of the population in the North to a high of 17.5 per 10,000 in East Anglia. This was put down in part to variation in whether hysterectomy was offered or not but was 'more likely' to be the result of variations in clinical judgement since consultant gynaecologists vary in their opinions as to when surgery is indicated . . . and GPs referral behaviour also varies.[16]

Why are women hysterectomized?

All of the information in our survey concerning why the hysterectomies were performed was taken from patients' records where the surgeon records his or her reasons for the surgery. Here is what we found in our study:

Medically Indicated Hysterectomies. From 1970–1984, 10.5 per cent of all hysterectomies were performed because of cancer.

Elective Hysterectomies. Between 1970 and 1984, 89.5 per cent of all hysterectomies were performed for benign deiseases:

20.9 per cent	prolapse of female organs
26.9 per cent	fibroid uterine tumours
14.8 per cent	endometriosis
6.2 per cent	endometrial hyperplasia
20.0 per cent	other indications

'Other indications' includes disorders of menstruation; infectious or other diseases of the pelvis, cervix, ovaries, or fallopian tubes; benign tumours other than fibroids; obstetrical catastrophes. Abnormal bleeding is a symptom, not a disease.

Oöphorectomies were performed during more than a third of the hysterectomies studied. Although our data did not show whether cancer or other ovarian pathology prompted the oöphorectomy, we can assume that the majority of these removed ovaries were normal because no pathology was listed.

In my estimation, 10.5 per cent of all hysterectomies were necessary and medically indicated. In other words, up to 90 per cent of all the hysterectomies performed in the United States between 1970 and 1984 might have been avoided, had other options been explored.

In the UK, as in the US, the vast majority of the hysterectomies are carried out for non-life-threatening conditions.[17] In the UK, the main indications for hysterectomy are excessive menstrual bleeding and/or fibroids. The rising hysterectomy rate in Australia has in part been put down to increasing pressure from women themselves.[18] One British study[19] showing a breakdown of the reasons for hysterectomy (where the majority of women were under 45 years) gave the following figures: cancer or suspected cancer 5 per cent; excessive menstrual bleeding 38 per cent; excessive menstrual bleeding associated with fibroids 37 per cent; prolapse 6 per cent; endometriosis 6 per cent, other 8 per cent. According to this breakdown 2-3 out of every 4 operations are for menorrhagia (heavy bleeding), a common finding.

To some extent the performance of hysterectomies is seen by many cultures as a reflection of their nation's advancement to be more like the USA as a leader in medical technology. This socialization of medical practice fails to even question the standard practices of what can only be called female vivisection. It is claimed that in Japan surgeons have turned hysterectomy into an assembly line operation. Much of the pressure comes from women themselves, especially if hysterectomy is seen as a high status operation, but some comes from women's lack of education about the workings of their own bodies and their fear of cancer in the future, a fear that doctors do little to dispel. Women have been led to believe that a hysterectomy has no negative effects and will only benefit them.

Questionable diagnoses

From my clinical experience, I have found that the diagnosis written on the surgical record sheet can indicate a major problem, whereas the pathology report found within the chart discloses a normal uterus. Furthermore, I suspect that many of the charts labelled 'uterine cancer' may have been simply benign hyperplasia, a non-cancerous, medically reversible thickening of the cells lining the uterus (see Chapter 10).

Recently, I received a letter from a colleague, Dr Phillip S. Alberts, in Portland, Oregon, which documents an abusive diagnosis. It read, in part, as follows:

[. . .] She was seen by another physician about itching and burning after coitus and was immediately evaluated with a diagnostic laparoscopy with the findings of a cystic ovary that was aspirated. Upon conclusion of these studies, the patient was told that she had a severe uterine prolapse [with complications] and was advised to have a vaginal hysterectomy.

The only thing that I could find upon examination was a reddening of the vulva, including the clitoris, along with reddening of the vagina . . . There was no evidence of any pelvic floor relaxation. I was quite surprised to hear that a hysterectomy had been recommended to this patient, particularly because she had no symptoms to even cause one to consider something like this.

Fortunately this woman was spared the hysterectomy. But what about the thousands of others?

These are not isolated instances. The 1981 Congressional report mentioned in Chapter 2 confirms my findings:

For many reasons, the true indications for hysterectomy are often not included in a patient's hospital charts. The reasons include peer review; nonreimbursement; and patient, physician, or hospital religious affiliations which make it expedient at some hospitals to write in only approved indications such as 'abnormal bleeding' and 'prolapsed uterus'.[20]

One study documents how indications for hysterectomies reported on hospital charts have changed over the years. In 1945, for example, only 4.4 per cent of the hysterectomies performed at a community hospital were for prolapse (the falling of the uterus due to stretched ligaments), whereas in 1972–1973, that number had increased to 37.9 per cent.

Was this dramatic rise in the diagnosis of prolapse due to a sudden loss of muscle and support ligament strength in the women of that community? Of course not! The researcher attributed the increase to a change in hospital policy, which accommodated elective hysterectomy for sterilization at a time when insurance payments for hysterectomies for sterilization were unpredictable.[21] In other words, the doctors misrepresented the diagnosis on the operative reports in order to collect from the insurer.

An investigation, published in 1983 by doctors at the Centers for Disease Control in the US Department of Health and Human Services, again reconfirms my experience.[22] Hysterectomies of 1,851 women were studied. The researchers found that, overall, only 52 per cent of the hysterectomies were performed for reasons that could be validated later by a pathologist. Forty-eight per cent of the pre-operative diagnoses could not be confirmed by a pathologist. These included menstrual bleeding disorders, pelvic relaxation (prolapse), and pelvic pain.

This means that abuses can run rampant. The researchers found that 22 per cent of hysterectomy specimens had *no substantial abnormalities on post-operative pathological examination.* Most of the fallopian tubes were normal, whereas functional ovarian cysts were the most common ovarian problem. A hearty proportion of normal uteri and ovaries are amputed each year because of misdiagnosis or abuse.

Hysterectomy . . . at what cost?

Women who undergo hysterectomy pay an average of $4,710[23] (the cost of having the operation privately in the UK is around £2,500) for the operation. In Los Angeles, where I work, the cost to a patient is $3-4,000 for the surgeon's fee and around $15,000 for the hospital stay. Each hysterectomy requires an average stay of about seven days (nine days in the UK).

The costs under the British National Health Service are also literally incalculable. Estimates of the cost of hysterectomy vary from a flat £1,000 per operation to £10,000 per operation. Health economists have worked out that if the operation is a straightforward one and can be done when an operating theatre session is free (ie when all the necessary personnel are already there) it can be done at minimal cost. If, however, an operation is so urgent that it has to be fitted in when theatres are already full, or it necessitates additional staff being brought on duty, costs rise. Then there are post-operative complications, longer than average stays in hospital, as well as the number of visits to a consultant, pre-op hospitalization for tests, general health checks, etc. Then there are the costs of follow-up visits after the operation and any home nursing required while the patient is recovering: all of these send costs soaring to the higher end of the scale.

'It has been calculated that if the British rate of hysterectomy was to rise to US levels, at an estimated cost of £1,000 per hysterectomy, it could cost an additional £60 million a year'.[24]

In the American situation, when we multiply the number of hysterectomies by the number of days spent in federal and nonfederal hospitals and the costs, the totals are staggering. In 1984:

- Women with hysterectomies were hospitalized for an estimated 4,781,000 days of hospital care. This amounts to almost 2 per cent of all hospital inpatient days, nationwide.
- Inpatient care of women with hysterectomies cost $3.16 billion.

I should point out that these estimates cover just the hospital expenditures. They exclude doctors' fees, pre- and post-operative tests and care, costs associated with complications, and other expenses related to hysterectomy including the long-term human and financial costs of hysterectomy's hidden side effects.

The bottom line: is hysterectomy cost-effective?

It is impossible to translate the quality of human life into dollars and cents. Yet some investigators have drawn correlations between the prevention of cancer by hysterectomy and the number of lifetime years saved with the economic costs of surgery and possible complications incurred. The costs would include medical expenses, potential adverse metabolic and psychiatric problems, osteoporosis, and increased risk of cardio-vascular disease.

On the whole, it is not an even exchange. The chances for cancer are small when weighed against the chances of post-hysterectomy complications and problems. According to a 1983 study, any savings of life from the prevention of uterine cancer (an uncommon disease) may be outweighted by loss of life from cardiovascular disease (a common condition), which increases follow-ing hysterectomy. In addition, the removal of normal ovaries at the time of hysterectomy prevents future ovarian cancer in the 1 per cent of women that might otherwise have died of this disease. Because diagnosising ovarian cancer can be difficult, this may seem advantageous. However, some or all of this advantage may again be offset by the side effects of hormone loss.[25]

I would have to agree with the American College of Obstetricians and Gynecologists that 'neither the prevention of cancer nor contraceptive sterilization appears to justify elective hysterectomy in asymptomatic women'.[26] To me, the evidence is over-whelming that benign problems should be treated with alternative methods.

The next chapter brings you good news about a surgical breakthrough—finally, an alternative to hysterectomy! And, those that follow examine diseases for which hyster-ectomy has become the treatment of choice. In each case, I will provide you with options to help avoid hysterectomy.

Update: censorship

When Bob Pokras and I finished our paper reviewing the national statistics on hyster-ectomy rates ('Hysterectomies in the United States, 1965–84', *American Journal of Public Health*, 7/88) we knew that doctors needed to know about the numbers of hyster-ectomies being performed and why. The American College of Obstetics and Gyne-cology (ACOG) was a primary target for the data. While writing papers to help create a consent for female surgeries in California, I continued to submit more data, write papers, and give talks to open the dialogue with other doctors to persuade them to re-evaluate their beliefs.

These efforts met with continual rejection. On one occasion, I was invited to speak on informed consent at a discussion held through the ACOG. After writing and preparing this paper, I received a letter withdrawing the initial invitation. I was blacklisted because I had spoken out against the existing standard. Persistence in sub-mitting data I had collected over a four-year period seemed to spark some interest from the ACOG, who finally responded by putting together a Hysterectomy Task Force. Again, I was denied any participation in it. A few powerful doctor colleagues felt I was attacking them by taking the position of a patient advocate; actually, what I was doing helps doctors.

Interestingly, psychologists, psychiatrists, and experts in sexuality openly sought out this data and invited me to present the statistics and other clinical material. These humanistic branches of medicine both needed and welcomed the data because they were the caretakers of hysterectomy's failures. The work confirmed what they saw in everyday practice: depression, physical dysfunction, loss of libido and orgasm.

I will continue to furnish academic medi-cal information to husbands concerned about their wives, mothers concerned about their daughters, and university professors wishing to share this research with their students to pave a new future.

CHAPTER 6

What is female reconstructive surgery (FRS)?

'Major surgery such as hysterectomy for benign conditions is highly controversial: for conditions such as cancer of the endometrium and uterus, serious prolapse or unacceptably prolonged heavy bleeding, most people are agreed; for other more borderline indications: slightly heavy periods, sterilization, pelvic inflammatory disease (PID) and endometriosis, there is still considerable debate, especially now that we have newer, more reconstructive techniques using microsurgery, and techniques such as TCRE (trans cervical resection of the endometrium) and HEAL (hysteroscopic endometrial ablation by laser)—although not in themselves reconstructive— to offer women.' Head of department of obstetrics and gynaecology, London

Your right to choose

If I have been successful in conveying to you that hysterectomy need no longer be perceived as inevitable, then half the battle is won. The second half? You need to know that there are alternatives—both medical and surgical—that can alleviate your female problems in a less-invasive way. You do have options.

The miracle of female reconstructive surgery

Years ago, if a finger or limb were severed, the only solution was to sew closed the stump. Major advances in microsurgery have been made, so that now delicate tissue, nerves, and muscle can be reattached in order to avoid amputation. In the past, a face or other part of the body crushed in an accident would have resulted in a lifetime of disfigurement. Now, utilizing microsurgical techniques, many body parts can be rebuilt to approximate normality. Hearts, lungs, and kidneys can be transplanted. Surgical breakthroughs over the past twenty-five years are dazzling.

Your uterus, ovaries, and associated tissue and organs can also be repaired rather than amputated in cases of benign disease. Using modern surgical techniques to remove uterine tumours and ovarian cysts, resupport pelvic structures that have fallen, open fallopian tubes, and rebuild other internal and external organs, Female Reconstructive Surgery or FRS can provide an alternative to hysterectomy for you.

FRS is conservative, avoiding many of the usual complications that follow a hysterectomy. And it respects your desire to remain whole. FRS restores and conserves your body, so that following the procedure, it returns as nearly as possible to its original condition. Flora, one of my satisfied patients, referred to her operation as 'internal plastic surgery'. Indeed it is. The uterus is a very strong organ with amazing regenerative powers and it is repairable.

Fig. 7. *Your female organs don't exist alone, disconnected from other systems.*

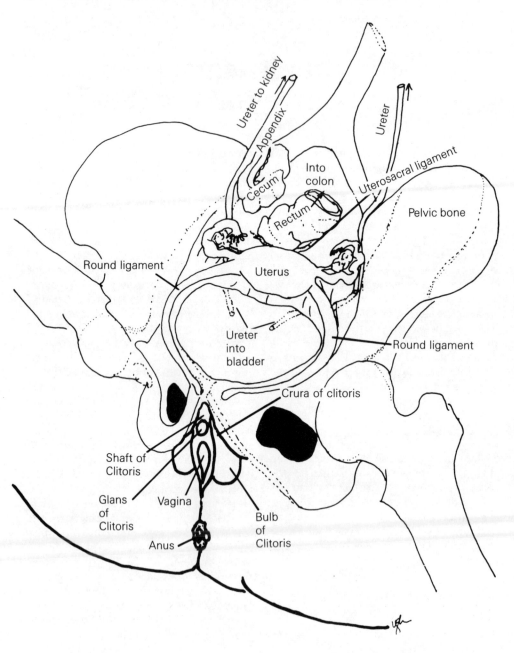

What's involved?

FRS is much more than just a surgical technique. It is a new way of conceptualizing and honouring your body. Traditionally, many gynaecologists have considered the 'female' part of a woman as distinct from the rest of her. But your female organs do not exist alone and disconnected from other systems. The dynamics of a working system include both anatomy and physiology. To restore and repair your female organs often requires that other areas of your body be examined and repaired, as well.

FRS evaluates your entire female pelvic system and its relationship to other systems. This may involve abnormalities in both internal and external organs. Therefore, surgery may be performed inside and outside the pelvic cavity to correct the problems (see fig. 7).

Internal Pelvic Organs	External Pelvic Organs
Uterus	Clitoris
Ovaries	Labia majora
Fallopian tubes	Labia minora
Broad ligaments	Anus-rectum
Uterosacral ligaments	Vaginal oriface
Cardinal ligaments	Cervix
Round ligaments	Urethra
All supporting structures	Vulva
Appendix	Hymen
Small bowel	Perineum
Large bowel	
Rectum	
Bladder	

How FRS seeks to restore function internally

In Britain, alternative techniques such as trans cervical resection of the endometrium (TCRE) are now gaining acceptance. Here an instrument like a wire loop is used to shave away cells from the womb lining (endometrial cells). The whole procedure is controlled via an endoscope, an instrument that allows the surgeons to see what (s)he is doing so that cells can be removed selectively. The result is no or lighter and shorter periods and a return to normal activity within 2-3 weeks. TCRE has been called the elegy of the hysterectomy for menorrhagia (heavy bleeding).[1]

Anne came to see me at the age of 31. She was bedeviled by a variety of benign problems. Her pelvic area was covered with adhesions from a prior pelvic infection. Endometriosis was evident on her ovaries, and she had three large fibroids growing within the wall of her uterus. Because of these problems, she had a good deal of pain during menstruation and she simply stopped having sex, even though she yeared for a child. She wanted to know whether I could help her.

The traditional approach to this multiplicity of problems would have been to remove Anne's uterus and ovaries. The outcome, however, could have been less satisfactory, especially since Anne was quite young and would have suffered from the loss of her childbearing ability and her hormones.

In performing FRS, the following occurred:

- Anne's ovaries were inspected for disease —they were cancer-free (and could be saved), so I obliterated the endometriosis that was growing on them, using laser surgery.
- I removed the fibroid tumours, using the techniques that I have perfected.
- I removed the pelvic adhesions, again with the laser.

After surgery, I prescribed medication to help reduce the chances of the return of endometriosis. The result? Anne's pain is gone. She is once again sexually active and has even noted improved uterine orgasm after the fibroids were removed. She has also become pregnant.

FRS's new techniques, which I'll explain later, allow for a return to normality. Throughout this book, I will be discussing cases where I've applied the principles of internal and external FRS successfully to treat fibroids, ovarian cysts and benign tumours, prolapse, endometriosis, pelvic pain, external deformities, and other non-malignant female problems.

Reconstructive surgery of the vaginal vulva area

Jane came for help after consulting more than fifteen gynaecologists in the last eight years. After the birth of her son, sex was always accompanied by pain so intense that Jane feared intercourse. Each gynaecologist she saw told her that she needed psychiatric help because there was nothing wrong physically.

During Jane's examination, I noticed that she had a large defect in her vulva with a buildup of scar tissue. When I touched this area, Jane winced in pain. There was no guarantee that FRS could cure her, but after eight years of difficulty this woman felt it was worth a try. At surgery, I found many cysts under the scar tissue. They had caused the problem. I removed this area and reconstructed the entire opening. And now Jane enjoys sexual relations again.

Perhaps because of its sexual import, no area may be as sensitive and difficult to discuss with your doctor as congenital abnormalities and damage (due to childbirth or biopsy) of the vulva. Yet such problems can be devastating physiologically, emotionally, and sexually.

Many women suffer from congenital defects, such as elongated labia, which prevent them from functioning normally. These can cover the entrance to the vagina, making routine intercourse painful and difficult. The labia can even be torn during sexual activity.

Often biopsies on the vulva are performed simply by using an instrument resembling a biscuit cutter. It leaves a circular hole in the delicate tissue. If several samples are necessary, numerous holes can result, and this can disfigure the vulva. Indeed, the vulva is often treated as if its appearance is inconsequential.

During childbirth, whether natural or with the aid of forceps and episiotomy, tears of the tissue are allowed to occur. Repairs may be done haphazardly or not at all. Scar tissue, cyst formation, a failure of the tissue to close or reapproximate in a normal manner can result. Torn muscles retract, and lose strength, structure, and tightness. If the muscle layer is destroyed, the whole area becomes lax.

If you have any of these problems, you may be too embarrassed to seek medical care. Or, you may find that your doctor does not respond in a warm or sympathetic manner to your special needs. In fact, you may have been told that there is nothing wrong or that you will have to live with your condition because nothing can be done. This may leave you feeling like a freak of nature.

During Female Reconstructive Surgery, I rebuild all damaged areas, restoring the function of your external organs. The same treatment accorded your face as a result of a car accident, or to your breast after mastectomy, can now be given to your perineal, vaginal, and vulva areas.

The surgical team

I operate with several surgeons. Dr Peter Taleghany is trained as a gynaecological oncology (cancer) surgeon; Dr Edward Austin is a paediatric and general surgeon; and Dr Brian Novak is a plastic surgeon. They are enthusiastic about my work and support the fact that I am offering women options. Each comes from a different technical world, being experts in different areas. Their extensive experience in other fields has allowed me to incorporate new surgical techniques into the practice of gynaecology.

Dr Taleghany is an expert's expert. He has operated with America's finest surgeons. In addition to being a superb surgeon, he is a cultured and compassionate person.

Dr Austin is a wealth of information and expertise on microsurgery. An infant's organs are tiny, and his handling of tissue and organs is very delicate. He has taught me to use instruments and handle tissues in ways not normally practised in routine gynaecology. Also, his experience in general surgery and paediatrics always brings a fresh perspective and exciting ideas.

Dr Novak has helped me to transform women's lives. One example is Dorothy, who came to see me after her hysterectomy. She had gained weight, was depressed, and had pain during intercourse because her vagina had been improperly repaired and was falling. In her obese state, her abdominal fat was pushing down on her bladder. Together, Dr Novak and I resuspended Dorothy's internal organs and reconstructed her abdomen.

Recently, I saw Dorothy at one of my teaching conferences in Oregon, and I hardly recognized her. We had removed a good deal of fat and I had fixed her organs. After surgery, I balanced her hormones. As a result, Dorothy lost 75 pounds. She looked beautiful and had a new lease on life. There was no mistaking her happiness.

Preparation

Before any patient undergoes Female Reconstructive Surgery, or even considers it seriously, I require that she learn everything about the surgery she can. I have developed a large videotape library showing the various procedures and explaining the entire process surgically and anatomically. I also advise patients on nutrition, vitamins, exercise, creating an emotional support system, and making the hospital stay as personal and individualized as possible.

Length of surgery

FRS is more complex than many procedures routinely performed by gynaecologists. It stands to reason, therefore, that the length of time needed for FRS will be entirely dependent on the amount of repair needed. No two surgeries are alike. In most cases, FRS takes from 2 to 4 hours, depending on the complexity of presentation. The operations can be quite involved, requiring many procedures in order to restructure the anatomy and highly integrated, multiple techniques to attain the best outcome (see figs. 8, 9).

How it's possible to reduce adhesions

During one long Thursday spent in surgery, I operated on Dana, whose pelvic cavity was scarred by old infection. Adhesions had obliterated the tubes and ovaries so that I could not visualize them during laparoscopy (the insertion of a small, lighted 'periscope' through the abdomen, which allows the physician to view the pelvic organs). During FRS we removed adhesions, using the laser, and then reconstructed these organs. This

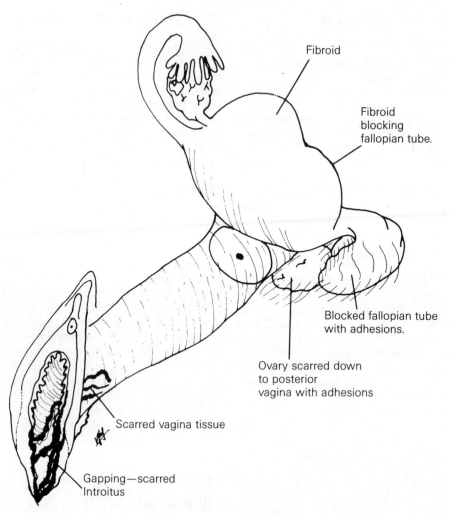

Fibroid

Fibroid
blocking
fallopian tube.

Blocked fallopian tube
with adhesions.

Ovary scarred down
to posterior
vagina with adhesions

Scarred vagina tissue

Gapping—scarred
Introitus

Fig. 8. Female reconstructive surgery may require many procedures, both internally and externally.

was a 4-hour operation.

On that same day, I removed multiple tumours—over 20 of them—from within Bernice's uterus. Her fibroids had begun to degenerate—they were dying. Her surgery lasted 4 hours, as well. Both women rested Friday and Saturday in the hospital. By Sunday, both were released, and went home

to recuperate.

Time and time again, I have been questioned about how I can do such extensive internal work without the creation of serious post-surgical problems—adhesions and scar tissue.

Many factors, working together, help to minimize adhesions. To begin with, I initiate the care by placing patients on vitamin and amino acid programmes associated with their deficiencies, specific for each individual, prior to surgery. Once in surgery, technique is of the utmost importance. Gentle, meticulous handling of the tissue is a must, as is precision cutting using laser beam. And, during the operation, I infuse solutions that aid in healing and in preventing adhesions.

Laser surgery

In Britain as well as in some parts of Europe—although not in the United States —laser ablation is becoming an accepted technique in gynaecological surgery, particularly the technique known as HEAL (hysteroscopic endometrial ablation by laser). Here the laser, monitored by an endoscope, is used to coagulate the cells of

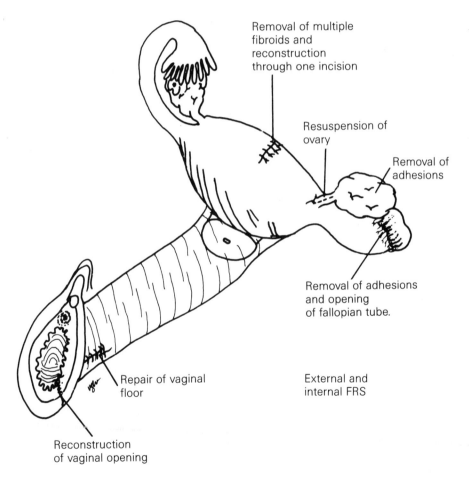

Removal of multiple fibroids and reconstruction through one incision

Resuspension of ovary

Removal of adhesions

Removal of adhesions and opening of fallopian tube.

Repair of vaginal floor

External and internal FRS

Reconstruction of vaginal opening

Fig. 9. The female reproductive system shortly after FRS.

the endometrium. Laser equiment is expensive but it can be used in many branches of surgery so the costs can be shared. Although this is still a new and relatively unpractised technique outside the United States, studies have shown that after such laser treatment up to 87 per cent of women no longer require a hysterectomy and only 9 per cent require further treatment.

Personally, I see the use of a laser for conditions such as heavy bleeding as nothing less than a hoax (see Chapter 10). Dr Milton Goldrath, in his review of the pathology specimens for hysterectomies performed for heavy uterine bleeding, found that the uteri removed frequently showed no pathological abnormality. In simple terms those uteri were normal. He saw the problem and sought an answer ... looking for another way to treat uterine bleeding. Dr Goldrath pioneered laser ablation.

In laser ablation, Goldrath states, '. . . the uterus shrivels to nothing ... we are producing an Asherman's syndrome (where scar tissue forms inside the uterine cavity) . . .' Goldrath felt that the technique for laser ablation could replace up to 30 per cent of the hysterectomies performed in the US. Interestingly, Dr Goldrath was taken aback when other doctors did not jump on this bandwagon. Laser ablation certainly has its place when a major operation could have high morbidity, in women with cardiac disease, obesity, and bleeding disorders.

Dr Baggish, a laser specialist, has pointed out another problem with ablation. Residual tissue of the endometrium could become trapped in the uterus, and since no pathological specimens are taken during the procedure, what actually may be occurring to the uterus over time is unknown. It will be years before one can fully evaluate the long-term consequences of ablation. Dr Goldrath had the right general concept to begin with. To many normal uteri were being removed

for bleeding problems. This is the area that we need to focus on. What causes bleeding problems; how can we prevent and treat them?

The laser beam has many benefits. It has become a precise and indispensable tool for the surgeon. Depending on how it's used, it can cut tissue, 'weld' it, and even vaporize unwanted growths. It prevents bleeding by sealing the edges of a wound closed, as it cuts. During Female Reconstruction Surgery I use the laser to excise fibroids and adhesions, obliterate endometriosis, and even seal open the fringe-like ends (or *fimbria*) of the fallopian tubes, in cases where they have been closed. Other advantages of laser surgery include:

- Bloodless surgery
- Precision destruction and cutting
- The ability to reach otherwise inaccessible areas
- Preservation of more normal tissue than traditional surgery
- A decrease in tissue injury[2]

Solutions are part of the solution

During surgery, exposed tissue can become dehydrated; the cells will die if they are not kept moist. Thus, I bathe them in solutions used most often during infertility surgery while operating to prevent drying. In fact, I use different solutions at various stages of the operation. One actually contracts the blood vessels so that there will be no bleeding during the surgery. When blood loss is kept to a minimum, there is less adhesion and scar formation later.The medications that I use, however, are potent and must be handled very carefully.

Other solutions combine fluids consistent with the body's own chemistry. In these solutions, I float antibiotics and anti-inflammatory agents. These chemicals prevent swelling and adhesion formation. When I find that the internal organs have become diseased, especially in cases of old infection, I see the tissue change from a yellow, pale discoloured look to a pink, healthy look with the use of these solutions. By bathing, the tissues come into immediate contact with the fluids to promote healing. I routinely give antibiotics intravenously in all cases.

Sometimes I use materials that stop blood from clotting. These keep any blood that stays in the cavity from sticking together, thus further preventing adhesions.

With each patient, I may modify not only what is in the solution, but the amount of the solution. But what is routinely consistent is that I use solutions liberally. In fact, I use up to 5 to 6 litres on an average case.

When I close the incision site, I may use another 2 to 3 extra litres to irrigate the body, making sure that all debris has been washed out. Debris includes old blood clots, adhesions, mucus, inflammation tissue that may have remained in the body. Of course, I don't merely put the fluids in—I also remove them. I'm actually cleaning the pelvic area.

Post-operative care

Again, post-operatively, I administer vitamins and amino acids that promote healing. In addition, I prescribe medication to stop inflammation and help tissue elasticity so when the tissue heals, it does so in a soft, stretchy manner. The typical hospital stay for an FRS patient rarely exceeds five days, as opposed to a week to ten days in the case of hysterectomy.

A post-operative protocol, which often includes medications to assist the healing process, must be followed. Just as each surgery is different, so is each post-operative protocol. In the majority of cases, the patient can return to her normal routine within two to three weeks.

Future care

Removing tumours and reconstructing the uterus do not change a woman's risk for developing other problems in the future. New fibroids can grow in five, ten, fifteen years. No one can predict. Endometriosis can recur.

Therefore, if you have undergone FRS, you will need to have a routine biannual examination with cervical smear and, if you are on hormone replacement, an endometrial biopsy. Surveillance and careful screening are the keys to detecting uterine, cervical, or ovarian cancer. And, should the need so arise for any reason, a hysterectomy can always be performed in the future.

You may be reassured to know, however, that in a survey I conducted of 200 patients who received FRS in my practice (100 women responded to my lengthy questionnaire), less than 10 per cent noted new gynaecological problems. None required further surgery related to their Female Reproductive Surgery procedure. The new problems included: the aspiration of an ovarian cyst, a caesarean section, a Bartholin gland cyst removal, and two D & C's for bleeding. Of the 96 women who answered the question, 'Do you consider your Female Reproductive Surgery a success?' 95 answered affirmatively and 93 said that if they had to, they would do it over again. I do know, however, of a few patients who had a hysterectomy following FRS, but who did not answer my questionnaire.

PART II
The Uterus

CHAPTER 7

Why is the uterus important?

According to Finnish research[1] the uterus may have some hormonal or other secretory function which helps prevent coronary heart disease in premenopausal women.

The 'dumb organ'

You may have heard the expression, 'Hysterectomy is when you take out the baby carriage but leave the playpen behind', a statement that glamorizes hysterectomy—and trivializes your uterus and ovaries, which are important parts of your body. It also ignores the miracle of conception and childbirth. Yet, routinely, doctors and women consider the uterus a simple organ whose sole purpose is to carry a pregnancy to term. We are led to understand that its function is not complex relative to other organs. Once childbearing is completed, the carriage becomes obsolete and the uterus transforms into a bothersome, dangerous, expendable nuisance.

Not only is your uterus portrayed as useless, but it is still seen as the source of those messy and painful periods. Comments published in a 1980 medical journal, instructing doctors about patient care, reveal these attitudes:

The uterus can be a tremendous nuisance after it has finished its childbearing function. If a woman is willing to withstand the nuisance, well and good; let her keep her uterus. But if she wants freedom from its problems, her wish should be honoured.[2]

When we undergo a hysterectomy, we are freed from all of this unpleasantness and the concomitant fear of unwanted pregnancy. Indeed, institutionalized medicine has taught some women to greet an upcoming hysterectomy with relief or as a future goal. Finally to be rid of 'the curse'! Although it's true that the abatement of heavy bleeding and pain *may* be a relief for some, this cure needs to be weighed against the short- and long-term consequences of hysterectomy. Besides, other, less-invasive cures can be sought before resorting to this surgery.

Viewing hysterectomy as a form of 'liberation' is a negative attitude to take toward one of your organs. And doctors are guilty of it as much as anyone—maybe more. Even in the field of gynaecology, the uterus is often maligned. There is nothing intriguing about it and, consequently, little research has been done concerning such problems as adenomyosis and fibroids because of the prevailing attitude that hysterectomy will suffice. Other fields such as reproductive endocrinology have attracted much more attention.

I have already alluded to the fact that this simplistic and negative view of the uterus is very limited and ultimately dangerous. Indeed, this organ has many far-reaching functions that have been ignored. Many are still yet to be discovered. How sad that we have not truly appreciated the importance of our female organs for our overall health and well-being. It's time to reject archaic and irrational beliefs and fears and look at the facts.

Your uterus—from conception

At conception, the egg and sperm join, forming a single cell that divides billions of times to create a baby. Interestingly, we are all potentially female in our earliest embryonic stages. The sex organs in males and females come from the same rudimentary cells, which develop and cluster to form organs. The distinction between male and female gonads becomes evident at about the seventh week of gestation. In male foetuses,

specialized inhibitory masculine hormones begin working to prevent the development of female organs.

Because of their common origins, the sex organs are analogous: the female clitoris corresponds to the male penis; the ovaries to the testes; the labia (the outer opening to the vagina) to the scrotum (which holds the testicles). However, *there is no male organ analogous to the uterus*. Can this be why it is under attack?

The anatomy of the uterus

The uterus is a thick-walled, upside-down, pear-shaped organ, about 3 inches long, where a fertilized egg grows into a baby. The *fundus* is the main body of the uterus, whereas the *cervix* is the mouth that opens into the vagina during labour to allow the baby to be delivered (fig. 10).

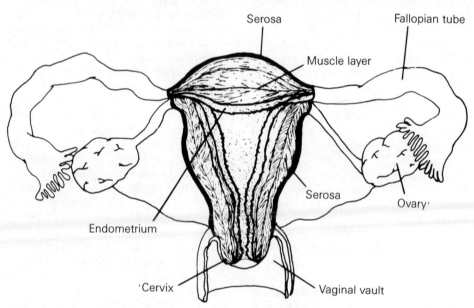

Serosa   Fallopian tube

Muscle layer

Serosa

Ovary

Endometrium

'Cervix   Vaginal vault

Fig. 10. The three layers of the uterus.

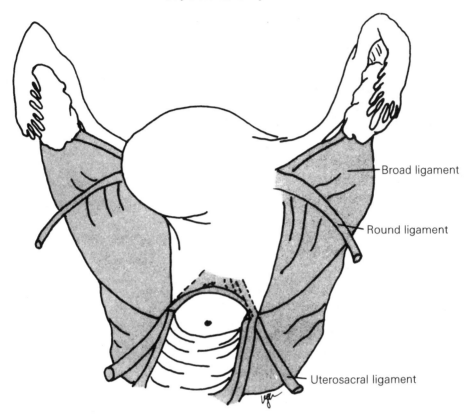

Fig. 11. The shaded areas show the support ligaments of the pelvis and their attachment to the uterus.

The uterus is composed of three layers:

- *Serosa*: the smooth outer surface
- *Myometrium*: middle layer, composed of three sheets of muscle, wrapped one on top of the other, in different directions
- *Endometrium*: the inner lining that receives the fertilized egg and sheds during menstruation

Your uterus and its surrounding ligaments—the cardinal, broad ligaments, uterosacrals, and round ligaments—serve as a vital support structure, helping to keep your female organs separate from your intestines, much like the diaphragm in the chest isolates your lungs from the abdomen. This allows your bladder, rectum, and vagina to maintain the correct position within your body, ensuring their proper functioning (see fig. 11).

The uterus as a mystery reproductive organ

Moment to moment, day to day, year to year,

81

I change, I revise, I learn more about medicine. Rather than viewing gynaecology as an advanced science for which we have found all the answers, I am continually struck by how little we actually know about the true function of the incredibly complex uterus. So few answers exist.

For example, we cannot as yet answer the fascinating, perhaps Nobel prize-winning question of why the uterus allows the implantation of the early, developing embryo in the first place. After all, isn't it foreign tissue, like a heart or liver from another donor? And, on the other hand, why, in some cases, does that rejection occur?

What mechanism in the uterus permits the foetus to create a placenta, a blood supply, and grow? And, in contrast, if the implanted embryo is chromosomally abnormal, and not developing correctly, how does the uterus recognize this and create a miscarriage? Many miscarriages have been shown to be caused by an abnormal number or arrangement of chromosomes.

This question is no trifling matter, for not only would its answer gives us the key to reproduction but would also provide insight into still unsolved problems in immunology, biochemistry, protein synthesis, and hormone interaction with the whole system.

We must view this organ as an integrated unit which, in its reproductive capabilities, has many specific activities, including the production of proteins and protein-like hormones. And these substances may have an effect on other parts of the body.

The uterus as part of the hormone 'team'

Until recently, little attention was given to the uterus and the endometrium as a source of hormone secretion. You may have been told that your ovaries are the only important organs for hormone function. The newest medical data indicate otherwise.

Increasingly, the evidence suggests that endometrial tissue may play a major role in the complex functioning of endocrine signals governing female fertility[3] and in the endocrine system itself. Your uterus serves as a receptor site for oestrogen and progesterone and works as a feedback mechanism with the pituitary gland. The loss of your uterus disrupts the production and circulation of these hormones. In fact, one recent study shows that the uterus manufactures and releases oestrogen, just as the ovaries do.[4]

We should keep in mind, however, that uterine biochemistry affects more than just the reproductive process. Procreation is just one aspect of these chemicals' importance. The uterus produces other agents that are active throughout your bodies and that help to maintain your overall health.

Several proteins, *blastokinins* and *uteroglobins*, have been identified in the human uterus. These play an important role in suppressing the immunological response of the uterus in order to allow the fertilized egg to implant without being rejected as foreign tissue. Is it possible that these relatively newly discovered agents have an effect on other body functions? At least one team of researchers speculates that since these agents have important endocrine and immune functions, they may enjoy some larger, as yet unrecognized importance.[5]

Prostaglandins are produced by the uterus and act on the muscles of that organ, creating contraction and relaxation. They also act on the joints of the body, both increasing and decreasing inflammation. One form of orally administered prostaglandin has been used successfully to reduce the chronic and acute inflammation of arthritis. Would the absence of this form of prostaglandin exacerbate arthritis?

There has been heated debate and speculation about early menopause and the correlation to heart attack. I, for one, believe that premenopausal hysterectomy *does* increase the incidence of heart disease. Studies have suggested that the uterus, without benefit of the ovaries, may have some protective role in the prevention of coronary heart disease. One researcher speculates that this is due to the hormonal function of the uterus which, operating independently of or in conjunction with the ovaries, prevents *atherosclerosis* (the laying down of fatty deposits in the arteries) in premenopausal women.[6]

The uterus as a support structure

As I mentioned earlier, your uterus and its surrounding ligaments play a vital role in maintaining proper pelvic anatomy. When your ligaments slacken or are cut, as in the case of a hysterectomy, your surrounding organs can fall or 'prolapse'. This occurs especially in cases where the ligaments have not been sewn in such a way as to reapproximate the natural pelvic structure. Prolapse can intensify with time, depending on your own tissue elasticity (see Chapter 11). Loss of the uterus often results in secondary complications such as:

- Constipation
- Inability to have sexual intercourse
- Bloating of the abdomen with intestines falling
- Discomfort during bowel movements
- Urinary incontinence with 'prolapse' of the bladder

The uterus as a 'sex' organ

How often I have heard touching and truly sorrowful accounts of patients whose sex lives and marriages have been disrupted by their hysterectomies. Naomi Stokes, in her book *The Castrated Woman*,[7] documents the tragic stories of hundreds of women whose gynaecologists had promised them that the surgery would have no effect on their sexual enjoyment. Rather, the physicians claimed, pleasure would be enhanced by eliminating the fear of pregnancy. For many women, this is just not the case.

The underlying misconception is that the reproductive organs are separate in function from the sexual organs, in which case they can be removed without any change in your sexual satisfaction. The prevailing theory, first formulated in a study published in 1947 and often repeated by physicians to their preoperative patients, stated that neither the uterus nor the ovaries were necessary for climax. Thus, any changes in sex drive after hysterectomy were attributed to psychological factors.[8]

The psychological causes were thought to be based on a woman's experiencing her loss of her sexual organs as emotional castration or loss of femininity. This would, of course, cause psychological stress that could inhibit sexual response. It was also believed that if the diminishment of sexuality was a result of hysterectomy, then all women undergoing the surgery would suffer the same loss, which in fact, they do not.[9]

Because not every woman loses her sex drive after hysterectomy, and the findings of many studies conflict, physicians blithely told their patients that the uterus and ovaries had nothing to do with sex. Now, women not only suffered the loss of their organs, but many were made to take the blame for their loss of sexual pleasure, as well. All the psychotherapy in the world will not compensate for missing hormones and absent organs.

Indeed, the loss of sexuality can be very

real. Studies in the United Kingdom show that 33 to 46 per cent of women report decreased sexual response after hysterectomy-oöphorectomy.[10] Let's examine why this is so.

Hormones. As early as 1943 it was established that androgens, in the form of testosterone, enhance women's *libido* (sexual desire) by increasing susceptibility to psychosexual stimulation, heightening sensitivity of the external genitals, and creating greater intensity in sexual gratification. For years it was assumed that testosterone was produced only by the adrenal glands. But now we know that your pre- and post-menopausal ovaries are instrumental in creating up to 50 per cent of that hormone.[11]

Doctors had been relying on oestrogen replacement therapy after hysterectomy to enhance sexuality, but you can see how this would fall short of providing sufficient testosterone. In fact, in cases where pellets of testosterone were implanted after oöphorectomy, women reported a restoration of their lost libido.[12]

Another myth held that the ovaries became old and nonfunctional after menopause and so could be removed with little or no effect. Again, this has been disproven. Your ovaries continue to produce hormones for at least a dozen or more years after the onset of menopause.[13]

The famous offer, 'We might as well take the ovaries while we're in there', ought to be carefully scrutinized if you are facing a hysterectomy-oöphorectomy for benign disease. You may be losing more than you bargained for!

The Orgasmic Uterus. Many hysterectomized women in my practice have similar complaints. They no longer experience orgasm or at times only feeble response—the ghost of their former pleasure—following their hysterectomies.

This correlates with the famous Kinsey Report, made in the 1950s, which found that 'the cervix has been identified by some of our subjects . . . as an area which must be stimulated by the penetrating male organ before they can achieve full and complete satisfaction in orgasm'.[14]

Other medical researchers and sex therapists have pointed out that 'an internally induced orgasm occurs when the penis presses hard and repetitively against the cervix, causing movements of the uterus and its broad supporting ligaments, and stimulating the surrounding peritoneal membrane, which has great and pleasurable sensitivity'.[15]

Masters and Johnson's pioneering work in the 1960s and 1970s on sexual responsiveness of the uterus to stimulation elaborates on Kinsey's earlier findings. They and other researchers on human sexuality state that the uterus is a contractory organ—that is, it elevates during the excitement phase of intercourse and then *contracts during orgasm.*[16]

I believe the media and the public's focus on Shere Hite's research regarding clitoral stimulation has unwittingly done women a great disservice. *The Hite Report* drew the public's awareness to the clitoris. But, in the process, we forgot that the vagina, the upper area of the vagina, and the uterus are also stimulated during intercourse, and that for many women the uterus often contracts during orgasm. As a result, many physicians tell their patients, 'Well, you still have your clitoris, so if we remove the uterus, you'll experience no change in sexual function.'

This is just not so! *The Hite Report* lists numerous comments from women describing uterine contractions during orgasm. Here are just a few:

'I feel vaginal contractions at the moment of release, and in a strong orgasm, uterine contractions also . . .'

'. . . There are definite contractions of the uterus and vagina, which were most apparent to me when I was a good deal pregnant . . .'

'A few times it has been so intense that I felt brief cramps in my uterus.'

The body may bend inward during orgasm which, according to Hite, reflects 'the uterine spasms that often accompany orgasm'.[17]

All of this goes to show that sexuality is an individual matter. One-third of all women become orgasmic during intercourse and a certain percentage of these women neither require nor desire any external stimulation of the clitoris or vaginal opening. Many women derive pleasure from uterine contraction alone and are not satisfied by clitoral stimulation. Others achieve an orgasmic response with stimulation of the vaginal walls. In these cases, the lack of a uterus and/or the shortening of the vaginal vault after hysterectomy would result in the lack of orgasm and sexual dysfunction. Yet others do not experience uterine sensation. Perhaps this is why hysterectomy does not result in sexual loss for every woman.[18]

A Japanese study of 171 women who had undergone hysterectomy (with ovaries left intact) makes this point:'

- 52 per cent of the women felt a loss of femininity.
- 39.2 per cent complained of deterioration of sexual desire.
- 27.1 *per cent experienced a loss of uterine sensation during coitus.*
- 69.2 per cent of those in that group, complained of a decrease in the ability to reach orgasm.

On the other hand, those who had not felt any loss of uterine sensation during inter-

course had no difficulty in achieving orgasm.[19]

How is it possible that some women continue to experience uterine sensations even after a hysterectomy? Although there is no clinical explanation, Masters and Johnson suggest that this may be a conditioned response.[20] Perhaps it is similar to the 'phantom limb' phenomenon known to occur when arms or legs are amputed.

In an informative article published in 1981, in the prestigious *American Journal of Obstetrics and Gynecology*, the late Dr Leon Zussman sums up the pertinent research about post-hysterectomy sexual responsiveness and the uterus.

For some women, the quality of the orgasm is related to the movement of cervix and uterus, and for these women the intensity of the orgasm is thus diminished when these structures are removed. For other women, orgasm is achieved mainly by clitoral stimulation so that the loss of the internal structures does not have a comparable effect. Evidence that women experience one or both types of orgasm, sometimes blended, has been reported over many years and conforms with our clinical observations. The percentage of women for whom the cervix and uterus are important is unknown . . .

Women and their doctors today may now jointly consider the possibility of sexual loss through hysterectomy with or without oöphorectomy, realizing the difficulties of predicting sexual outcome in individual cases . . .[21]

The risk factors

Truly, we are just now beginning to understand the complex importance of the uterus. Who knows how many more functions are still to be discovered? Yet you may not have been informed of the potential risks and losses you face with hysterectomy. Your questions may have been dismissed; your concerns minimized.

The following chapters will clarify how, in some cases of benign uterine disease, your uterus can be saved.

Update: hysterectomy as birth control

When Chrissy, twenty-nine years old, came in for a routine examination, I saw that she had had a hysterectomy. She explained that by the time she was twenty-six, she had had three children. Her religious beliefs forbade birth control. She loved her children but couldn't cope, financially or physically, with another one. Desperate, she begged her gynaecologist for a hysterectomy. He discouraged her, but she persisted, finally seeing the gynaecologist of a friend who had had a hysterectomy to limit childbearing. He told her he'd gladly do the surgery.

Chrissy had her hysterectomy; she was back to 'normal' in two months . . . looking forward to having intercourse with her husband. She discovered that the penetration of the penis hurt terribly; each thrust caused her intense pain and tears. She and her husband tried again and again . . . to no avail. Chrissy's sex life was over.

Chrissy's medical records revealed that her surgeon had performed an anterior and posterior repair along with her hysterectomy. Her vaginal opening was now so tight that it was difficult for her husband's penis to enter. And with a deficiency of oestrogen from having her ovaries removed, the vaginal mucosal cells failed to stretch or lubricate. Chrissy's vagina was numb where she used to feel intense pleasure. This 'G-spot' area was also where her anterior repair had been performed; coincidentally, this repair is often performed on women who are incontinent. But Chrissy had had no complaints of incontinence.

In early 1989 Dr Bart Masterson, an expert in urinary stress incontinence, stated, in a speech before the Southern California Assembly of Obstetrics and Gynecology, that 'abdominal hysterectomy has no place in the treatment of urinary stress incontinence'. Half the audience failed to acknowledge this important statement. The other half grimaced and frowned at the honesty of his remark.

I avoid removing tissue in this particularly sensitive area. All of us need to re-evaluate commonplace surgeries in light of our expanding knowledge about the female sexual response.

'In the private sector, women will sometimes seek out as many as three consultants until they get the hysterectomy they feel they need. There are no clinical protocols: all the consultant has to do is agree to do the operation—and send in his bill. The number of private operations in the UK for example, has risen by more than 25 per cent in the last four years.'

Private health sector business analyst

CHAPTER 8

Clarifying the mysteries of endometriosis and adenomyosis

'Women are being offered hysterectomy, with prophylactic removal of the ovaries, for endometriosis, one of the commonest female complaints. What they are not told is that hysterectomy does not completely eradicate endometriosis: as soon as they are put on HRT (hormone replacement therapy) their endometriosis comes back.'
Toni Belfield, Family Planning Association

Endometriosis is a major cause of hysterectomy. From 1965 to 1984, the number of hysterectomies performed for endometriosis has increased by 176 per cent, more than for any other diagnosis,[1] despite the fact that successful surgical techniques and drugs which can conserve organs have been developed during the last twenty years.

Endometriosis has been characterized as a 'mysterious' and 'frustrating' disease. Its causes are still the source of intense speculation and, until recently, its cures have seemed as elusive as the killing of the mythical Hydra—cut off one of the beast's nine heads and two more grow in its place. Even diagnosis can take months to achieve, because its symptoms mimic those of other problems. In fact, you may have extensive endometriosis but experience little or no discomfort, whereas your friend with only tiny endometrial growths suffers from exquisite pain.

What is endometriosis?

Endometriosis refers to the growth of small portions of the normal tissue that line the uterus (the *endometrium*) away from their normal location. These bits of misplaced tissue, called *endometrial implants*, survive within the pelvic cavity—on the fallopian tubes, ovaries, bowels and, in rare cases, as far away as the lungs, thighs, chest, and arms—in fact, anywhere in the body.

Endometrial growths are not malignant. When examined under an electron microscope, this tissue appears like the cells lining the uterus. It even responds to the monthly stimulation of hormones. Each month these foreign colonies of uterine tissue build up and then break down and bleed, as if they were still within the womb.

As you might expect, this presents a problem. The lining of your uterus goes through its monthly cycle and leaves your body through the vagina during menstruation. But the blood and tissue sloughed off by the endometrial implants have nowhere to go. The result is:

- Internal bleeding
- Degeneration of the blood and tissue
- Inflammation of the surrounding areas
- The formation of scar tissue and adhesions

In *very rare* cases intestinal bleeding and

obstruction, bladder difficulties, and kidney obstruction can occur.

Sometimes a colony of endometriosis develops so much scar tissue that it cuts off its own blood supply; it is no longer receptive to hormones. This is called a 'burned-out' *plaque* of endometriosis. In other cases, patches of tissue may rupture during menstruation, spreading more cells to other surfaces within your pelvis, causing new spots of endometriosis to grow. The condition can gradually worsen with time, although you may experience an ebb and flow of symptoms.

Left unchecked, endometriosis can cause internal organs to stick to one another and the pelvic cavity to be filled with adhesions. Endometriosis is a frequent cause of infertility.

What are the symptoms of endometriosis?

Because the symptoms of this condition often masquerade as other problems, a careful evaluation and frank discussion with your gynaecologist are necessary to help in the diagnosis.

Painful Periods (Dysmenorrhoea). Your doctor may be able to distinguish endometriosis from simple cramps by the timing and extent of your pain during menstruation. You may suspect endometriosis if your discomfort:

- Begins five to seven days before your period
- Peaks at the time of the maximum flow
- Persists throughout the period and beyond
- Is less cramp-like and more constant
- Occurs in other areas and not the uterus alone

- Is accompanied by heavy flow and blood clots

Pain During Intercourse (Dyspareunia). Midvaginal pain is almost never due to endometriosis. However, if you experience sharp pain during deep penile penetration (especially premenstrually), you can consider endometriosis. On deep thrust with intercourse, the penis moves the vaginal wall and cervix and puts pressure on the ligaments that hold up the uterus. These *uterosacral ligaments* are frequently the site of endometrial implants. In addition, ovaries scarred from endometriosis may adhere to the ligaments, as well. When this area is 'hit', the pain may be excruciating.

Chronic Pelvic Pain and Low Backache. The pain of endometriosis varies from woman to woman. Some doctors may throw up their hands in frustration, call their patients' complaints psychosomatic, and refer them to a psychiatrist for tranquillizers and treatment.

The discomfort does not depend on the size of the implants but, rather, on their location. One of my endometriosis patients was accused of wanting to avoid sex because her former doctor had difficulty pinpointing the source of her pain. She had small implants on the uterosacral ligaments, which left her in agony during intercourse. Another patient was 'lucky'. The endometrial growths on her ovaries reached 10 to 15 centimetres, but still did not cause much discomfort because her ovaries were relatively insensitive.

Endometrial implants can also grow on your appendix, causing chronic or sharp pain on the right side, which may imitate appendicitis. If the tissue has invaded your bowels and bladder, there may be blood in the stool and urine during menstruation. It may cause painful bowel movements. The symptoms may worsen before, during, and after your period and then subside until the next cycle.

Infertility. According to the Endometriosis Association, 30 to 40 per cent of women who suffer from endometriosis are infertile and, conversely, 30 per cent of *all* infertile women have endometriosis. Infertility is likely to result as the disease progresses. Endometrial implants may cause:

- Damage to your ovaries
- Damage to your fallopian tubes
- Adhesions that may block the descent of the egg into your uterus
- Irregular periods
- Painful sex resulting in less frequent intercourse
- Hormone imbalances
- Change in the body fluids that interferes with fertilization and implantation of the egg

Diagnosing endometriosis during your period

If your history of problems makes you and your doctor suspect endometriosis, you'll want to confirm its presence as soon as possible so that treatment can begin without delay. Because the symptoms of this condition can be so vague and changeable, your doctor will want to actually 'see' the endometrial growths. S(he) will begin with the usual medical history and pelvic examination. This time, however, you should be asked to *return during your period*, when the pain or symptoms are at their worst.

You may feel squeamish and embarrassed about having a pelvic examination at this time of the month, but the reasons for doing it then are obvious. During menstruation, your endometrial tissue swells, up to ten times larger than normal. Any endometrial growths in your vagina and pelvis will be detected much more easily at that time, and your doctor will be able to make a comparative evaluation.

Your gynaecologist may also perform a recto-vaginal examination. Again, this may cause some emotional discomfort, but it is essential in being able to locate the growths. If your doctor touches an implant behind your uterus, you are likely to recoil in pain. This would be another tip-off.

Laparoscopy to confirm the diagnosis

The best way for your doctor to visualize endometrial growths accurately is to perform a laparoscopy, again while you are menstruating or when your pain is most severe. During this outpatient surgery, your abdomen will be distended with carbon dioxide gas in order to separate the organs from the abdominal wall. A small lighted tube (*laparoscope*) will be inserted through a tiny cut right in your naval. Looking through this little periscope, your surgeon will be able to see where the implants are growing and how extensive the scar tissue and adhesions have become. These areas are removed by laser. The sites may also be bleeding actively. Some tissue may be sent to the pathologist to confirm the diagnosis.

Carla had been seen by numerous gynaecologists in Los Angeles. In fact, her last doctor performed a laparoscopy just nine months before she came in to see me. Despite all of the doctor visits, however, Carla's complaints remained the same: pain and swelling every month with her period.

I read the laparoscopy report and it showed that everything was normal in this woman. Why was she having such severe pain? The mystery began to clear up when I noted the timing of the laparoscopy. Despite the fact that Carla suffered most during her period, the procedure was performed between cycles.

Scheduling diagnostic laparoscopy when you aren't experiencing your worst symptoms is ill-advised, especially with a disease like endometriosis, which waxes and wanes with your menstrual clock. I performed a laparoscopy on Carla during her period. Not only did I find endometriosis, but I also discovered a fibroid tumour on the back of her uterus encrusted with endometrial growths. The fibroid had begun to degenerate. This might have been missed at other times during the month, when it could have appeared as a slight change in the uterine surface. During menstruation it was unmistakable.

Making sure of the diagnosis

It is essential that your doctor make a positive identification of the endometrial implants before any treatment is begun. This is made more difficult by the fact that endometriosis doesn't always appear the same. Although textbooks refer to it as 'gunpowder-like spots', it also appears as clear spots that change over time to white, yellow, blue, and red.[2] Thus, biopsy during laparoscopy is indispensable.

If you have endometriosis, you'll want to know:

● How bad is it?
● What are my chances for fertility?
● Should I try to get pregnant, wait, adopt?

But by no means should you agree to a hysterectomy before you are certain of the diagnosis and other, more conservative and corrective measures have been taken.

Rosa's was a tragic case in point. She was 26 years old and every month she had severe pain with her menstrual cycle. Her doctor told her that she had endometriosis and the only cure would be a hysterectomy with the removal of her ovaries. He held out the hope, however, that if one ovary was healthy, he would leave it behind.

At 26, Rosa lost her organs. The doctor never even performed a laparoscopy. Did he really know what was ailing this young woman? Did he treat it properly? Of course not. Following her hysterectomy, Rosa's pain did not subside. Her bladder and vagina fell, rendering her incapable of intercourse. The new problems were worse than Rosa's original difficulties.

In reviewing Rosa's medical records, pathology reports, and operative notes, I found absolutely no mention of endometriosis by either the surgeon or the pathologist. The ovaries, fallopian tubes, and uterus were normal. There was no endometriosis—or anything else wrong. She had been suffering from a urinary tract infection that had been missed.

How can abuses like these take place? And, perhaps more important, how can you protect yourself from being victimized? Education is the answer. When you know what endometriosis is and how it is diagnosed and treated, speak up. Ask for confirmation. You can make a difference in your own medical care. After all, it's your body.

Do I need a hysterectomy if I have endometriosis?

Traditional recommendations for treating endometriosis are often based on your age and desire to bear children. Every patient handbook and medical guide discusses the possibility of 'radical' surgery—that is, hysterectomy and oöphorectomy as the definitive answer to this condition if child-bearing is no longer an issue.

I am deeply opposed to this 'treatment'. It simply ignores the serious, long-term consequences of losing one's organs. Besides, the medical literature does include many cases where the endometriosis was not fully eradicated by hysterectomy. If microscopic implants lodge on other internal structures, they may continue to grow after hysterectomy (especially if the woman is on oestrogen replacement therapy). Hysterectomy should be your last option—after everything else has been tried.

Female reconstructive surgery can help

Whether or not you wish to become pregnant, I feel the best approach to controlling endometriosis is the coupling of Female Reconstructive Surgery with appropriate medication. Your endometrial growths can be successfully arrested using microsurgery, laser surgery, or electrocautery. I perform this procedure carefully through the laparoscope or, in more severe cases and where other problems exist, during abdominal surgery.

Laser surgery uses a light beam to excise or burn away the tissue, whereas electrocautery employs a high-heat electrical current. Although electrocautery can be adequate, I prefer the laser beam because it is more accurate.

During laser laparoscopy:

- A small section of suspicious tissue is removed.
- It is frozen and analyzed by the pathologist on the spot.
- If endometriosis is confirmed, the heat of the laser obliterates all of the endometrial tissue, starting at the surface and working more deeply into the tissue.

I'm certainly not the only surgeon advocating this therapy. Dr Harry Reich, a friend and colleague in Pennsylvania, reports successful laparoscopic laser treatment for 79 of his patients suffering from endometrial growths on their ovaries. He also uses laser laparoscopy to vaporize endometriosis on the rectum, especially in cases where it is firmly stuck to the back of the uterus and vagina. [3]

As I've mentioned earlier, the advantages of laser surgery include:

- Bloodless surgery
- Precision destruction of endometrial implants
- Precise cutting
- Ability to reach poorly accessible areas

During the surgical procedure it is essential to avoid the formation of future adhesions, so FRS incorporates the use of irrigations and the careful handling of the tissue. It's usually a good idea to take a second look with the laparoscope four to six weeks after the initial surgery, to check for adhesions and to loosen them. I laser adhesions if I find any. The only currently known additional surgical risk involved in the laser surgery is the possibility of an accidental burn.

Drug treatments

Surgery alone is often not sufficient to control endometriosis, because new implants may occur and microscopic growths might have been missed. Therefore, immediately following FRS, I often prescribe the drug Danazol. This drug, when taken from six months to a year, suppresses the oestrogen level while it raises the amount of testosterone in the bloodstream. It creates what some people like to call 'pseudo-menopause'.

If you're on Danazol therapy, your ovulation and menstruation may stop temporarily. The drug causes your uterine lining to shrink and the endometrial implants to degenerate and reabsorb. Your pain should be greatly lessened. This treatment is particularly effective in re-establishing fertility if you are unable to conceive as a result of endometriosis. Once therapy is completed, ovulation re-establishes itself, usually within six weeks.

Danazol is a synthetic, weakened male hormone analogue that contains neither oestrogen nor progesterone. It may create some side effects, including acne, water retention, hair growth, and deepening of the voice. Of course, because menopause is simulated, there may also be menopausal symptoms, such as depression, hot flushes, and insomnia.

In most cases of endometriosis I have treated, these symptoms have disappeared after the treatment is completed. And Danazol can now be administered in small doses to keep side effects to a minimum. The effective dose varies from woman to woman, depending on how much is needed to stop the menstrual cycle. Many women do well on Danazol and often feel much better.

One more note of importance: Danazol treatments should be begun during menstruation or when pregnancy tests are negative. This drug must not be taken during pregnancy because it may cause abnormalities. A few women continue to ovulate during the course of treatment, so non-hormonal contraceptive precautions (like condoms, diaphragm, and spermicide) should be taken.

Birth control pills also work

Oral contraceptives are another alternative. You'll need to take these continuously for six to nine months. Rather than simulating menopause, 'the pill' mimics pregnancy. The small constant doses of hormones contained in birth control pills create a much thinner than average endometrium. This shrinking effect carries over to endometrial implants in the pelvis and has controlled endometriosis in some women.

The controversial but widely used injectable contraceptive *Depo-Provera* has been proven effective against endometriosis. It suppresses ovulation and prevents the growth of the endometrium. Bothersome breakthrough bleeding can be controlled by the use of oral oestrogens.

Although Depo-Provera produces dramatic results in reducing endometriosis, this method has the drawback of creating prolonged *amenorrhoea* (no menstrual period) for many months following the end of therapy.

Alternate ways to help yourself

Clinically, I have found that certain vitamins and food supplements seem to control some of the symptoms of endometriosis. Presently, I prescribe certain materials for my patients with endometriosis, in the hope that these will alleviate some of their suffering. These include folic acid, vitamin B_6, essential fatty acids, oil of primrose, and other minerals and herbs.

Follow-ups

In order to establish that the endometriosis has been controlled, I perform a laparoscopy six months to one year following the initial surgical treatment. Small implants can be lasered through the laparoscope. Although we still await definitive studies into the long-range effectiveness of the drug therapies, it may be reassuring to know that if symptoms do recur, the drugs can be re-administered.

Pregnancy and breast-feeding also stop ovulation and can force endometriosis into remission. Of course, no sensible woman would become pregnant just to control its spread; after all, the creation of a child is a lifetime commitment, not a medical 'treatment'. On the other hand, if you wish to have a child, you should not delay, because you have a higher risk of infertility with endometriosis.

Am I at risk for endometriosis

Classically, endometriosis begins after the onset of menstruation and is most often diagnosed in women in their thirties and forties who have never had children, although I've seen it in many younger women, as well. Known as the 'career woman's disease', it was once thought that endometriosis afflicted only the upper middle class. This myth arose because 'career women' were better able to afford medical treatment for their pain and infertility, and thus were more likely to receive the proper diagnosis.

Experienced clinicians estimate that between 5 and 15 per cent of all pre-menopausal women have some degree of endometriosis. This disease afflicts black, Oriental, and Middle Eastern women in rates similar to whites.

Because pregnancy and breast-feeding may prevent the development of endometriosis or slow its progress, if you have delayed pregnancy, you may be at greater risk for the disease. However, it is difficult to set hard-and-fast rules with this ailment. I have even seen endometriosis coincide with pregnancy.

What causes endometriosis?

If you have endometriosis, you are probably curious to know where it comes from. Although there are no definitive answers yet, two dominant theories have emerged to explain how this mysterious disease occurs.

The Transformation Theory suggests that undifferentiated cells present at birth mutate into endometrium-like cells during adulthood. This could be caused by uterine abnormalities that prevent the outflow of menstrual blood. Such abnormalities have been correlated with extensive endometriosis in adolescent girls. There may be some genetic link that causes this to occur in some women and not others.

The Transportation Theory has received much credence lately. It suggests that endometrial tissue somehow leaves the uterus and finds its way into the pelvic cavity where it implants and grows. How do the cells get where they're going? The blood and lymphatic systems may carry them; prior surgery may have inadvertently caused the endometrial cells to be moved to other abdominal locations; or it could be the result of *retrograde bleeding.*

Retrograde bleeding

Jennifer came to my office complaining of severe monthly pelvic pain. It began about a day or two before her menstrual cycle, continued during menstruation, and tapered off two days after her bleeding ceased. This nine-day siege was chronic and disabling, often sending Jennifer to bed.

After taking a medical history, the only significant clue I found was an episode of cryosurgery, on the cervix. Upon performing a pelvic examination, I discovered that Jennifer's cervix was scarred to such an extent that the opening through which the menstrual blood should flow was blocked.

I asked Jennifer to come in for an examination during her period to see whether the cervix opened up more at that time. It was still so tight that little of the menstrual blood actually flowed out. I dilated the cervix and an astounding gush of 'old' blood that had been trapped in the uterus finally escaped. Jennifer's acute pain was relieved instantaneously.

The following months, however, she still experienced inner pelvic discomfort. Unless dilation was performed regularly, the pain was severe. I decided to take a closer look. During a diagnostic laparoscopy, I found endometriosis. And, because the cervix was blocked, the menstrual blood was backing up into the uterus and could actually be visualized as a blue distension of menstrual blood in the fallopian tubes.

This backward flow is called *retrograde bleeding*. The fallopian tubes seem to act like two-way streets. That is, they serve as the conduit for the egg to travel from the ovary to the uterus, but they can also transport tissue from the uterus back out into the pelvic cavity.

Retrograde bleeding may occur without the severe problems I encountered with Jennifer. A large proportion of women undergoing dialysis for kidney failure, for example, have bleeding within the pelvic cavity just before menstruation. In fact, studies confirm that 90 per cent of healthy women experiencing laparoscopy during menstruation also have bloody fluid within their pelvic cavity. This provides direct evidence that cells from within the uterus do find their way into the pelvis.[4]

Any problem that prevents the outflow of the menstrual blood can contribute to retrograde bleeding and should be considered as a risk factor for endometriosis. These include:

- Scarring and adhesions on the cervix from trauma or surgery (like conization or cryosurgery)
- A closed or stenotic cervix
- Severely tipped (*retroverted or retroflexed*) uterus
- Fibroids
- In theory, devices that block menstrual flow: cervical cap, diaphragm, and bulky tampons

The existence of endometrial tissue may not even be limited to the moment of menstruation—it can even be there during ovulation. The cells may enter the pelvic cavity during the previous menstrual cycle and remain alive. Experiments with primates have shown that endometrial tissue can survive in the pelvic fluid for up to four weeks.[5]

The menstrual cycle as a factor

The character of a woman's menstrual cycle may also have some influence on retrograde bleeding. Women with endometriosis:

- Tend to start menstruation at an earlier age
- Have shorter cycles (27 days instead of the average, 28 to 34 days)
- Have more frequent, longer, heavier, and more painful periods

Short cycles and heavy periods are conducive to the flushing out of excessive blood and tissue through the fallopian tubes. If you have intense cramps at the lower end of your uterus, they may cause severe contractions that force the blood to flow up and out.

Prostaglandins as a factor

Women suffering from painful menstruation

have significantly higher concentrations of the chemical *prostaglandin* in their bodies than women with normal menstrual cycles. Prostaglandins are substances produced by the endometrium (and, interestingly enough, are also found in great concentrations in semen), which promote uterine contraction during and after labour. They can be a potential lifesaver in the case of haemorrhage after birth or after gynaecological surgery.

If you have endometriosis, you may have two much prostaglandin. A hormonal imbalance can upset the production of this chemical so that some fraction or type of it is either not produced or overproduced. This may lead to changes in the uterus and tubes and create retrograde flow.

Excessive prostaglandins have also been implicated as a cause of endometriosis-related infertility. Because this substance creates contractions within the pelvic area, it is theorized that the tiny hair-like structures, or *cilia*, in the fallopian tubes of women with endometriosis work much harder than those in women without the disease. The cilia push the egg along on its journey from the ovary to the womb. The increased activity may cause the egg to pass too rapidly through the tube and reach the uterus too early in the cycle for proper implantation. Or, they may push the egg in the wrong direction!

Many drugs are prostaglandin inhibitors and may offer you pain relief. I also treat with D-phenylalamine, vitamins, and amino acids.

The danger of flushing the tubes during D & C

One medical practice may heighten the potential for endometrial cells to find their way into the pelvic cavity. While doing a diagnostic workup using a laparoscope, some gynaecologists perform a D & C to remove the uterine lining. Then, to check whether the tubes are open, they force fluid through them, flushing the fragmented pieces of lining from the D & C through the tubes and out into the body.

Because of its potential for initiating endometriosis, I disapprove of this practice. If you're prone to endometriosis, you are unnecessarily endangered. Besides, with retrograde bleeding, your body already has to contend with some uterine blood and tissue in the pelvic cavity monthly. Why add more?

Why me?

If most women experience retrograde bleeding, why does endometrial tissue implant and grow in your pelvic cavity and not your friends'? That's still the subject of intense speculation. Scientists have suggested:

● Defects in the immune system
● Genetic problems
● Uterine abnormalities
● Failure to ovulate
● Lack of certain hormones that could inhibit the growth of implants[6]

Menstrual variations and prostaglandins may be a factor. It's clear that despite what we do know, elements of this disease remain a mystery to us at this time.

Adenomyosis

Grace came to see me after having been hysterectomized. She was 49 and had ceased menstruating two years earlier. She hurried to see her doctor because she suffered pain on her right side—the famous cancer scare!

Grace's gynaecologist performed a hysterectomy. He discovered a big ovarian cyst, filled with blood. He took her uterus and ovaries to 'prevent future cancers'. But the pathology report came back with a diagnosis of *adenomyosis*. 'What's this?' Grace wanted to know. 'Is it dangerous? Is it cancerous? I never had any problems with my uterus—no pain or bleeding. Where did this come from?' Good questions!

What is adenomyosis?

Adenomyosis is not cancer and does not predispose one to or cause cancer. Only rarely is it associated with malignancy. It is a benign disease with little clinical significance for many women. A uterus affected with adenomyosis can become bulky or enlarged, although in one study of 161 adenomyosis specimens, uterine enlargement or tenderness were rarely observed.[7]

An alternative name for adenomyosis is 'internal endometriosis'—and for good reason. In adenomyosis, the endometrial tissue (the uterine lining including the glands and connective tissue) invades the deeper muscle layers of the uterus. In rare cases, the endometrial tissue can penetrate the uterine wall completely and emerge on the outer surface. When this occurs, the condition would look exactly like endometriosis during a laparoscopy.

Normally, there is a barrier between the endometrium and the deeper layers of the uterine wall. This barrier acts as a defence against invasion from endometrial tissue. For reasons that are still unclear, the protection breaks down in some women, causing adenomyosis to develop.

What are the symptoms?

Like its sister disease, endometriosis, adeno-myosis may or may not cause symptoms. If you have small, focused growths, you may have no pain, whereas others with more extensive invasions experience painful and heavy periods. Theoretically, the greater the proliferation of glands, the heavier the flow. The deeper the penetration into the uterine wall, the more severe the discomfort.

You should keep in mind, however, that up to 40 per cent of women with adenomyosis have no symptoms at all, whereas only approximately 20 per cent have the classic symptoms of both heavy bleeding and pain. Although women with adenomyosis may have symptoms, there are none that are peculiar to this disease alone, making detection difficult.[8]

How is adenomyosis diagnosed?

Classically, adenomyosis is diagnosed by a pathologist only *after* a hysterectomy. In fact, because adenomyosis often occurs in association with other common uterine conditions such as fibroids, many clinicians are reluctant to make a diagnosis before the hysterectomy. It is rarely diagnosed correctly before surgery. And often a suspected case of adenomyosis is not confirmed by the post-hysterectomy pathology report.

I would prefer to exercise every option at my disposal before resorting to hysterectomy. This may take some careful detective work. My first step, when a patient complains of heavy bleeding, chronic pelvic pain, and painful periods, is to discover the cause. I try ultrasound and medications. If these fail, I perform a laparoscopy. A D & C is ineffective for adenomyosis because it would not show the extent of the invasion. If, during the laparoscopy, no cancer, endometriosis, or fibroids are in evidence, I then suspect adenomyosis.

Next, I use a needle that can safely take small biopsy samples of unusual-looking uterine tissue, without causing damage to the uterus. A narrow column of tissue is extracted and sent off to the pathologist for an instant appraisal while the patient is still on the operating table. The pathologist can tell me if endometrial tissue has invaded the muscle layers of the uterus.

During surgery for fibroids, I have found some unusual growths of adenomyosis. One of my patients had adenomyosis growing inside a fibroid tumour. Another's adenomyosis formed into a tumour similar to a fibroid, whereas the rest of her uterus was normal.

Many of these adenomyotic tumours are found on the back wall of the uterus. They can be removed using the laser. And, interestingly, many of these women's uteruses were tipped, either *retroverted* and/or *retroflexed*. Other women have more extensive and diffuse invasion. The area of adenomyosis feels wooden and fibrous—not the usual soft of feeling of uterine muscle. Ultrasound cannot routinely distinguish between fibroids and adenomyosis.

In the future, the new scanning device, Magnetic Resonance Imaging, may help in the detection of adenomyosis.

If adenomyosis is suspected, must the uterus be removed?

The traditional treatment for suspected adenomyosis is hysterectomy, but I believe that adenomyosis functions much like endometriosis. If laparoscopy, laser surgery, and medication have been effective in treating endometriosis, perhaps these methods can be used to control this disease?

I prescribe Danazol, which can shrink

overgrown endometrial tissue outside the uterus and within. I've had patients with adenomyosis who were able to conceive after treatment with Danazol. In fact, there is some evidence that non-cyclic birth control pills used to thin the uterine lining can also be prescribed for adenomyosis. Natural progesterone may help other women.

What are my risks for developing adenomyosis?

Although adenomyosis has been recognized for over 120 years, to date little is known about how or why it develops. An enigmatic condition, there is still widespread disagreement as to how often adenomyosis occurs and what its symptoms and associated pathology are. Depending on how many samples of tissue from a single uterus are examined, and which research article you read, it is said to occur in as few as 8 per cent or as many as 67 per cent of the hysterectomized uteri studied.

We do know, however, that women in their forties and fifties who have given birth to at least one child are more likely to have the condition. Rather than reduce fertility, adenomyosis has been seen by some researchers as a consequence of pregnancy and delivery. Or, it may simply be a normal physiological development, to a certain degree, in all mothers. And there may be genetic factors that cause some women to develop it.

Evidence has been accumulating, indicating that perhaps a hormonal imbalance, like an excess of oestrogen or a defect in the gland tissue, may lessen the ability of the muscle layers to resist the aggressiveness of the endometrium. A tip-off to the oestrogen connection is the greater-than-chance association of other oestrogen-dependent lesions (like endometrial hyperplasia) with adenomyosis and the finding that women with adenomyosis had given birth to their last child more than ten years prior to their hysterectomy, and subsequent diagnosis. In that case, the action of oestrogen would be uninterrupted over many years.

Other scientists, however, refute the importance of oestrogen, pointing to the fact that synthetic progesterone treatments, which help alleviate endometrial hyperplasia (see Chapter 10), seem to do little for adenomyosis. Yet I have had good results with natural progesterone.

Why should these results vary? Perhaps a woman's response depends on the depth of invasion of the adenomyosis; the amount of adenomyosis relative to normal tissue; or whether or not the adenomyosis is diffuse or appears like a tumour. An Israeli researcher found that women with adenomyosis had an excess of certain enzymes.[9] Clearly, there remains much we do not know about this disease.

It is possible that you may develop adenomyosis if you have experienced:

- Pregnancy
- History of endometriosis
- History of fibroid tumours
- Endometrial hyperplasia
- Retroflexed or retroverted uterus

Whether or not we understand the causes of adenomyosis, however, my commitment is to save women's organs. It's easy to perform a hysterectomy and cry 'adenomyosis' later. The difficult task is finding a way to treat and cure so that the present quality of life can be maintained.

For women with severe and disabling bleeding problems who have not been helped by hormone therapy, D & C, and/or laparoscopy (to rule out degenerating fibroids or other problems), YAG laser burning of the endometrium can serve as an alternative. And the medical literature does carry reports by surgeons who have surgically removed focal tumours of adenomyosis. If even these treatments fail to alleviate the problem, hysterectomy may be the only solution.

CHAPTER 9

The case against monitoring fibroids

'Women don't realize how much they can do to help themselves. Both heavy bleeding and fibroids are oestrogen-dependent and oestrogen levels can be controlled by a healthy diet that contains essential minerals like iron and magnesium and essential fatty acids (from vegetable oils). Exercise helps reduce body fat which reduces oestrogen levels which again helps heavy bleeding.'
Arabella Melville, author of *Natural Hormone Health*

Fibroid tumours (also called *uterine myomas* or *leiomyomas*) are the most common tumours of female pelvic organs and the most frequent reason given for abdominal hysterectomy. Forty per cent of women over the age of 50 have them, as do 20 per cent of all women. From 1982 to 1984, 551,752 hysterectomies were performed to excise these benign growths.[1]

These figures are astounding. But what is even more astounding is the fact that many of these hysterectomies are carried out on women in their twenties and thirties who have no children. They are not told that they have options.

What is a fibroid

Fibroids are abnormal masses of muscle tissue with a whorling band pattern. They can be hard or soft, solid, or with a liquid interior. *They are almost always benign. Fewer than .2 per cent are ever found to be malignant.*[2] Fibroids range from microscopic to as large as a basketball. I removed one from my patient Arlene that weighed in at a hefty 3 pounds!

Fibroids can grow on all levels of your uterus:

- *Subserosal fibroids* protrude from the outer surface of the uterus.
- *Intramural fibroids* are buried within the uterine wall.
- *Submucosal fibroids* protrude from the endometrial lining into the uterine cavity.
- *Pedunculated fibroids* grow at the end of a stalk and are usually subserosal or submucosal (fig. 12).

Fibroids have also been found growing in other areas within the pelvis. *These are not cancerous and shouldn't be treated as such.* They do not require a hysterectomy, but, rather, can be removed surgically.

There is some evidence that fibroids are hereditary: three times as many black women suffer from them as white. If your mother has had this condition, you may also be at an increased risk.

What are the symptoms of fibroids?

Small fibroids often create no symptoms,

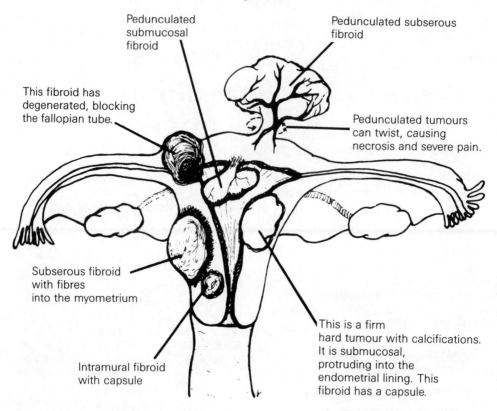

Pedunculated
submucosal
fibroid

Pedunculated subserous
fibroid

This fibroid has
degenerated, blocking
the fallopian tube.

Pedunculated tumours
can twist, causing
necrosis and severe pain.

Subserous fibroid
with fibres
into the myometrium

This is a firm
hard tumour with calcifications.
It is submucosal,
protruding into the
endometrial lining. This
fibroid has a capsule.

Intramural fibroid
with capsule

Fig. 12. The various types of fibroid tumours. Fibroids can grow anywhere, including on the ligaments of the uterus.

whereas large fibroids or groups of fibroids can cause more problems. If you are suffering from:

- Abdominal swelling
- Abdominal, pelvic, and/or back pain
- Infertility
- Heavy or irregular bleeding
- Painful periods
- Constipation
- Pressure on the bladder and frequent urination

you may suspect that fibroids are to blame.

Invasive fibroids

Most fibroids grow encapsulated by a membrane so that they are easily separated from the uterine wall. A clear border exists between fibroid and uterus—it's as if the surgeon is given a 'dotted line' to cut on!

In some cases, however, if your fibroid is allowed to grow over a period of time, it may not increase in size but may change the way in which it grows. These fibroids become *invasive*, embedding a fine network of microscopic fibres, like 'feeder' roots of a plant, deep within your normal uterine tissue (figs. 13, 14).

This type of fibroid lacks a 'capsule', so there is no clearly definable line between fibroid and uterus. The tissue in the uterus gradually changes from soft muscle to hard, with a density similar to wood or rubber. But because the change from normal to abnormal is so diffuse, surgical removal can be very tedious. I have removed such invasive fibroids, and in doing so, I realized how easily a surgeon can feel forced into performing a hysterectomy because of the complexity of the surgery.

How are fibroids diagnosed?

Bimanual Examination. Your gynaecologist performs a bimanual examination when s(he) places two fingers in your vagina and the other hand on your abdomen. S(he) elevates the cervix, bringing the uterus up close to the abdominal wall. Your doctor feels the shape and outline of the uterus between the two hands, making a rough estimate of its dimensions and shape. Large fibroids are often detected this way.

Ultrasound. Ultrasound is an extremely helpful tool for looking into your body for abnormalities and for measurement. Sound waves are sent through your pelvis and reflect back on a television monitor. A visual image of the body's interior can be created. With ultrasound, your doctor can measure, record, and monitor the size of your uterus. This device gives a clearer picture of the uterus than a bimanual examination.

Do I need a hysterectomy if I have fibroids?

If you have a small fibroid, you may have no symptoms or problems. If this small tumour can be visualized and is not located in an area that endangers you for future infertility or other risks, it can be re-evaluated over time.

I have found, however, that most fibroids do grow or degenerate, causing more serious difficulties. The common approach to treating fibroids is to monitor them and then perform a hysterectomy. In some cases, the fibroids don't grow at all, but as the woman ages, her doctor announces the existence of

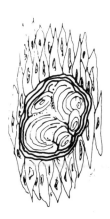

Fig. 13. Fibroid with capsule.

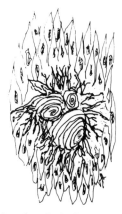

Fig. 14. Fibroid with 'feeder root' fibres growing into normal uterine muscle tissue.

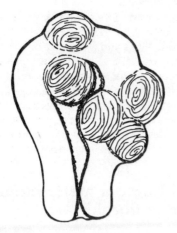

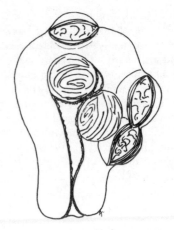

Fig. 15. FRS technique and myomectomy technique: a uterus with multiple fibroids.

Fig. 16. Traditional myomectomy: three incisions are made to remove serosal fibroids.

rapid growth suggestive of cancer. 'Now that you're older, and risking cancer, it should all come out'. Don't be intimidated into a hysterectomy with the old cancer scare! Even if the fibroids do grow rapidly, they usually are not malignant.

In relatively few cases, especially in younger women, the fibroids will be removed, using the surgical procedure called *myomectomy*. Monitoring/hysterectomy and myomectomy are less than ideal. I prefer to use Female Reconstructive Surgery (FRS) when fibroids are diagnosed.

Can I rely on myomectomy to remove my fibroids?

Traditionally, the only option to hysterectomy has been a surgical procedure called *myomectomy*—the simple removal of fibroid tumour, most often from the outer uterine wall. *Multiple myomectomy* may remove several tumours, but again they are often taken from the surface of the uterus. Pedunculated fibroids—those that grow on a stalk—can also be removed.

Myomectomy does not, however, routinely remove fibroids that grow within the uterine walls, cavity, or ligaments, or those difficult to reach because of their anatomical placement. Clinically today, few surgeons take the time to remove all the fibroids, although in the future more will.

An infertility specialist may suggest myomectomy to you if you are young and your fibroids are impeding attempts at becoming pregnant. The decision to perform this surgery is often based on your age, your desire to bear children, and your failure to conceive with a fibroid in the uterus.

When surgeons perform a myomectomy, they make incisions on the surface of the uterus at every tumour site, remove the growths, and then close the surface with large stitches (see figs. 15, 16). By operating in a traditional manner, there are numerous incisions; in fact, the uterus can bleed profusely at the removal sites of these tumours. Healing can be irregular and the structural integrity of the uterus does suffer.

Conventional myomectomy is not routinely offered to many women because of the fear of bleeding and the possibility of infection and complications. This is why women with very large or numerous fibroids are routinely referred for hysterectomy. It is not offered at all to older women—'older' being a relative term. Older simply means whatever age the doctor chooses as being 'older'.

Regrowth after myomectomy?

It is often said that a patient who undergoes a myomectomy faces the possible 'regrowth' of the excised fibroids. Actually, regrowth is rather rare—occurring 2 to 3 per cent of the time.[3] However, I have read operative reports indicating that often the surgeon cuts out only the fibroids on the uterine surface, leaving the deeper fibroids within the uterine body. *The fibroids left inside continue to grow after the myomectomy.*

Recently, I operated on Charlene, a young woman who had had a myomectomy. Two weeks after her surgery, Charlene's infertility specialist informed her that the fibroids had grown back. In truth, the large fibroids inside the uterus were never removed, as the operative report clearly showed. Only the small fibroids on the surface of Charlene's uterus had been excised. Charlene's is not an isolated case.

Advantages of female reconstructive surgery

With FRS, there is no need to lose your organs because of benign tumours. The fibroids can be removed safely, early on, and the uterus can be repaired. Furthermore, FRS does not limit the removal of the fibroids and the reconstruction of the uterus to young, reproductive women. You now have the opportunity for this option and the possibility to maintain fertility, should you choose to conceive 'later' in life. And if childbearing is no longer desired, you still have the choice to maintain the integrity and functioning of your body.

During FRS, the uterus is brought up onto the abdomen to be fully visualized and examined. Special medications are injected into the fibroid sites and the uterus *to prevent bleeding.* This technique, which I've used on hundreds of women with fibroids, causes the blood to leave the uterus and the fibroid, thereby reducing blood loss considerably during surgery. The effects last 15 to 30 minutes. (These drugs should not be used on women with a history of angina, heart attack, or chronic nephritis, because there can be side effects.)

The injection is placed between the fibroid and the normal muscle tissue. It helps to cut the fibroid free and closes off the blood supply to the tissue surrounding the growth. I remove all fibroids in this way, including the difficult ones that grow deep within the uterine wall and endometrial lining.

All this is possible because of innovative

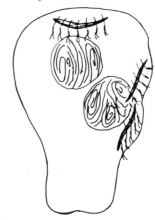

Fig. 17. Traditional myomectomy: three incisions on the uterus; two fibroids remain deep inside the uterus. They have not been removed.

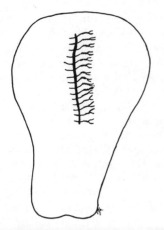

Fig. 18. FRS: one single incision and all fibroids are removed.

surgical approaches. Rather than making incisions at the various sites of the fibroids, I choose a surgical line on the surface of the uterus (see figs. 17, 18). All fibroids from the three levels of the uterine wall and at every site can then be removed often through a single incision site. This decreases the number of incisions, and the potential for bleeding and possible infection, while increasing the structural integrity of the uterus on healing.

I don't cut the fibroids with a scalpel. Rather, to discourage bleeding, I use laser surgery in the removal of the fibroids. The laser beam actually does the 'cutting'. And the heat of the beam closes the edges of the wound as I operate. As I've mentioned in previous chapters, laser can:

- Increase the surgeon's precision in destroying abnormal tissue
- Prevent blood loss
- Preserve more normal tissue than traditional surgery
- Decrease tissue injury
- Enhance the surgeon's ability to reach inaccessible areas

The final stage of FRS for fibroids is the reconstruction of the uterus. At this point, I bathe the uterus in a second solution to prevent further infection, scarring, and adhesions. Then, layer by layer, I reapproximate the uterus, bringing it back to its normal anatomical structure, moulding it to resemble the normal pre-fibroid organ. Where fibroids were removed from within the uterine wall, I make repairs, flaps, and modifications to accommodate for spaces and gaps left behind by the now absent growth. Then I re-suspend the uterus on its supporting ligaments and completely restore its position within the pelvis.

I have refined these techniques to such an extent that this surgery is nearly 'bloodless'. There is no reason why others cannot operate in the same way, or shouldn't be trying. They haven't been because of the beliefs that hysterectomy is easier, the uterus is useless, the fibroids can't be removed.

A word about the size of a uterus containing fibroids

It is an unwritten law among gynaecologists that once the fibroids cause the uterus to attain the size of a 12-week pregnancy, it is time for a hysterectomy. I find this rule rather arbitrary. In my opinion, a 12-week size uterus is relatively small—less than 3½ inches in diameter. The Female Reconstructive Surgery procedure needed to remove the fibroids is usually relatively simple at this stage. Indeed, I commonly see women with more complex cases, whose uteri have grown to an average size of a 16- to 20-week pregnancy, where the uterus extends up to the navel.

Why do fibroids grow?

No one knows for sure. Some researchers

theorize that fibroids are sensitive to oestrogen and are more likely to grow when that hormone is present. They point to the fact that fibroids grow during pregnancy and 'shrink' after menopause to support their theory.

These researchers use the existence of *oestrogen receptors* within the cells of the fibroids[4] to explain that hormone's role. What are oestrogen receptors? One pathologist with whom I work likens these to little locks on the cell. The keys? Oestrogen, which bonds to the receptor site, locking it up. The tissue is sensitive, absorbing the hormone that makes changes in the cells.

Will my fibroids shrink at menopause?

The promise of the shrinking fibroid is based on the theory that oestrogen causes these fibroids to grow. If you look forward to menopause as a way to avoid surgery, however, you should bear in mind that the oestrogen depletion, which may cause the fibroid to shrink, can also create severe problems for you in the form of osteoporosis, vaginal atrophy, hot flushes, and so on.

Oestrogen replacement therapy can alleviate these problems. But, if the oestrogen theory actually works, wouldn't the hormone encourage the further growth of the fibroids? 'Waiting for menopause' may become a vicious cycle.

Fibroids—a threat to fertility

Because fibroids occur so frequently among women of reproductive age, having them does not mean that you are automatically infertile. However, researchers have indicated that up to 40 per cent of married women with fibroids of appreciable size, are, in fact, unable to conceive.[5] The fibroids cause sterility because they can damage the tissue of your reproductive system. They may:

- Interfere with sperm transport
- Impinge on, distort, or destroy your fallopian tubes
- Compress your cervical canal or alter the position of your cervix
- Distort the internal shape of your uterus
- Compress and obstruct blood vessels within the uterus
- Create cell abnormalities in the endometrium

The removal of fibroids can re-establish fertility in many cases. Several studies show that fertility rates improve dramatically (over 60 per cent) when fibroids are removed.[6] You should keep in mind, however, that the pregnancy rate varies according to your age, the length of time that you're infertile, the size of the largest fibroid, and the number of fibroids removed. And, the removal of fibroids using FRS (which suppresses bleeding during surgery) is less risky than hysterectomy or traditional myomectomy— there are fewer operative complications, post-operative infections, and blood transfusions required.

Fibroids during pregnancy

Some women with fibroids can become pregnant and have normal deliveries, whereas others may not have normal labour and may require Caesarian section because of the fibroids. There is no hard-and-fast rule. Because fibroids may distort the normal uterine cavity, however, they can interfere with:

- Implantation of the fertilized egg

- Normal foetal development
- Normal foetal presentation during birth
- Normal uterine contractions

In addition, their presence during pregnancy can predispose you to bleeding, premature labour and contractions, and postpartum haemorrhage.

The risk of monitoring

Leslie was only 26 when her gynaecologist told her that she had fibroids. He advised her that surgery was drastic, and because the fibroids weren't causing her any problems, she should just 'sit tight' and do nothing. At 29, Leslie came in to see me. In the interim, she had got married and found herself unable to conceive.

This young woman's doctor hadn't (or perhaps couldn't have) determined three years earlier that the fibroids were growing right where the fallopian tubes entered the uterus. In fact, both of the openings that allow the eggs to descend from the ovaries into the uterus had been blocked.

Had Leslie undergone surgery to remove the fibroids earlier in their development, her tubes could have been saved. Now, we had to reimplant her tubes into another site on the uterus. This type of surgery is more complex and involves greater risk than the early removal of the fibroids.

The difficulty in monitoring fibroids

Have you heard your gynaecologist make the following statement?

'Since your fibroid isn't causing you any pain, I'll monitor it for you and check on its growth every six months. You don't need a hysterectomy yet.'

Doctors typically say this when they find evidence of fibroids. The words come as a stay of execution to a woman who envisions herself as being saved from hysterectomy. But is she? Is she really safe, or has she been promised a reprieve, only to be hysterectomized later, when her symptoms become unbearable or when she is told the fibroid is too big?

Despite great technological advances, there is no absolute way to monitor a fibroid tumour. The fibroid can grow into a fallopian tube or a uterine artery and cause damage by pushing on the ovaries or bowels without your doctor's ability to see what is happening. Therefore, any claim that your doctor makes, that he or she is 'monitoring' your condition, is somewhat misleading.

Problems with bimanual examination

In some cases, bimanual examination can be difficult, if not impossible. If you are very tense or in pain, your doctor cannot feel through the abdominal walls, especially if they are in spasm and will not relax. If you are overweight, fat deposits make examination unreliable.

In addition, even the most experienced gynaecologist can make a mistake. You need to understand this fact in order to be persistent when you feel something is wrong. If your doctor doesn't find your problem in the initial examination, you can insist on a re-evaluation. A second opinion may also be helpful.

Problems with ultrasound diagnosis

Although ultrasound is a wonderful tool, it is not the ultimate answer for diagnosing fibroids. Using ultrasound, we cannot determine accurately how many fibroids exist, where they are actually positioned, or how deeply they have invaded the uterus. Only surgery tells the full story.

I have seen several cases where doctors diagnosed and confirmed fibroids with ultrasound. The women in question had second ultrasound evaluations. In all cases, fibroids remained the diagnosis. Yet when the women went to surgery, no fibroids were found. Instead, the uterus had tilted back on itself (retroversion), giving the impression of a fibroid.

Patricia, who was experiencing chronic pelvic pain, had had four ultrasounds at four different facilities with a diagnosis of posterior pelvic tumour. When I examined her, I wasn't certain. I felt inadequate because I could not confirm what everyone else seemed so sure about. I thought that perhaps I was just feeling the uterus.

To further evaluate Patricia, I performed a diagnostic laparoscopy and discovered her problem: she had chronic appendicitis. In fact, her appendix was entwined in adhesions and inflamed. The condition must have existed for months! In addition, her uterus was tilted and its abnormal position caused it to rub against the appendix, creating more pain. Our team was able to help Patricia immediately by performing an appendectomy, removing the adhesions, and then resuspending the uterus off of her rectum. Patricia has suffered no pain since her surgery and continues to do well.

Elaine came to me with fibroids, again having been diagnosed as needing a hysterectomy. She was 39 and had had two children. She was losing a lot of blood each month with heavy periods and was anaemic.

The ultrasound that we obtained from the hospital showed that she had one large posterior fibroid. The ovaries were still visible and appeared normal. This gave me a rough idea of her condition. At surgery, however, I discovered that Elaine had a phenomenal number of fibroids: I removed over 100, which had clustered together. They ranged in size from a large orange, to grapes, to peanuts, to pinheads.

In another case, Jane flew in from Florida for surgery. Her scan showed that she had several fibroids. At the time of the operation, I actually found one large grapefruit-size fibroid that had begun to break down, bleed, and degenerate.

The ultrasound gives one a rough idea— but not the full picture. Just how the fibroids grow, where they are placed in the body, their invasiveness, and their true size can only be determined during surgery.

Monitoring: a practice that warrants re-evaluation

When your doctor tells you that your fibroid can be watched, you may be given a false sense of security. You may view your doctor as benevolent and may even feel grateful to him or her for letting you go so long with the fibroid. While your fibroid is being 'monitored', it can continue to grow. Just look at the damage it can do:

- Frieda began to bleed more often and more heavily. Eventually, she suffered from anaemia and even required blood transfusions.
- Monica's fibroid became so large, it pressed on her bladder and rectum, eventually causing kidney damage and bowel obstruction.
- Renee's fibroids invaded near the major uterine arteries, making their removal very difficult.
- Francine's fibroid changed from being encapsulated to invasive. It sent feeder roots, extensively damaging normal uterine tissue.

Now, there is panic and dismay. At this point, the fibroids have become too large or too diseased for traditional myomectomy. The ensuing destruction and heavy bleeding from the fibroid are too great. The doctor can't risk an alternative surgery. The monitoring stops and a hysterectomy must be performed.

The conspiracy against the uterus

When your doctor mollifies your fears with the 'monitoring' routine, (s)he is following the unwritten code of private practice. Your gynaecologist knows that while your fibroids are being 'monitored', (s)he can't define how the fibroids are affecting your uterus over time. As I've explained, diagnostic procedures are, at best, roughly accurate. But, chances are (s)he is likely to perform a hysterectomy once your uterus reaches the size of a 12-week pregnancy.

The manipulative second opinion

If you are told that you need a hysterectomy, you are likely to seek a second opinion. Monica had contacted another doctor but, unbeknown to her, he turned out to be a colleague of her current gynaecologist. He automatically concurred with the first assessment (since the unwritten 'good old boys' rules eschew open conflicts and disagreements) and sent her back to the original gynaecologist's office for surgery.

Frieda found a doctor unassociated with her current doctor and with whom he was in competition. Her new doctor ordered the reprieve she sought, and offered to monitor the fibroid for a while longer, knowing full well that the future held a hysterectomy

in store for his patient.

I must admit that these scenarios are bleak. The fear of surgery coupled with the false belief that women are destined to be hysterectomized have prevented many women from seeking alternatives. There are no benefits to monitoring, unless you have a small, single fibroid and have completed your family. (The small fibroid may never grow.) And, during the observation period, problems can multiply: the fibroid mass may grow, pushing on organs, creating fatigue, anaemia, pain, and PMS symptoms. The final outcome is unchanged. Everything must come out.

I do offer hope, however. I suggest that we break out of this cycle entirely. The first step is for you to educate yourself about the medical issues involved in fibroids. The second is to change your mind-set about surgery, from a negative to a positive experience. Fibroids that are causing you symptoms can be removed surgically.

FRS and fertility

Several of my patients who have undergone massive fibroid removal had been told earlier by numerous infertility specialists (who save organs) that they would never conceive because the fibroids were blocking the fallopian tubes. In fact, the surgeons informed them that even if the fibroids were removed by myomectomy, they would never be able to carry a foetus to term or labour.

But this is not so. In many cases I have had deliveries of healthy infants after FRS. In fact, when Deborah failed to progress during labour, her obstetrician performed a caesarean section. He noted that there *was no evidence* of prior surgery on the uterus itself. This means we have achieved complete and adequate healing, which allows us to maintain a functioning organ after the FRS procedure is done.

Joanne was given no hope of ever being able to conceive because a fibroid and endometriosis would prevent an egg from implanting in her uterus. Her doctor told her 'point-blank' that she would not be able to bear children and she was devastated.

Imagine her joy, then, in discovering Female Reconstructive Surgery. After surgery to remove the fibroid and several months of medication to treat the endometriosis, she became pregnant. She wrote:

My husband and I are very excited about this and cannot begin to thank you enough for what you have done and what you are doing to help other women save their uteri and become more aware of their health and their rights . . .

Other benefits of having those fibroids out

Some women complain that their fibroids produce many symptoms. But others have lived for years with their fibroids and voice no complaints. Why? One fortunate group may have neither symptoms nor problems and so may never require surgery. For others, the growth of the fibroids may occur so gradually and yet so insidiously that they become accustomed to the symptoms. And for some, the fear of hysterectomy may have kept them from seeking a remedy. As a consequence, they allow the fibroids to grow, filling up their abdomens with superfluous and damaging tissue.

Imagine the revelation of the FRS option for women who suffer from their fibroids. Suddenly, there is hope. And, beyond that, many of my patients have reported extraordinary benefits after their surgery is completed. For many, sex improves after fibroid removal. A good number of my patients report having 're-found' orgasm. I

believe that the fibroids interfere with the wave pattern of uterine contractions at orgasm. Once they are removed, the pattern can be re-established.

Even when fibroid growth has not resulted in anaemia, many women experience profound fatigue and weakness with their fibroids. this tiredness is relieved immediately after surgery. General body function improves with FRS, especially with the bladder and bowels. One patient described her post-surgical experience as 'finding the Fountain of Youth'. In fact, the majority of my patients report feeling healthier, more vital, and certainly sexier after surgery.

We are not completely sure why this is so. Because of their slow-growing nature, many women may not realize that the fibroids are creating changes in the body until they exert pressure on the bladder and rectum. The fibroids may be producing toxin-like substances that interfere with normal hormonal function. I believe that women who suffer from fibroids have severe hormone imbalances much like those found in premenstrual syndrome. These symptoms may persist for years and increase gradually as the fibroids grow.

The empowerment of female reconstructive surgery

On a psychological level, women who have undergone FRS to remove fibroids feel as if they have some control over their bodies. They have retained their organs and view themselves as having options, rather than feeling like victims. They no longer live with the fear that hysterectomy is inevitable. They resume their active lives, and are generally optimistic. They can still have a hysterectomy, if absolutely necessary, later.

Having the courage to go against the grain

We have all heard a multitude of stories about women needing to undergo hysterectomies for fibroids. We are prepared, as young girls, when we listen to tales told by our mothers and their friends, that our female heritage includes the loss of our uterus because of these pernicious but largely benign growths. It is therefore not surprising that when 'fibroids' is the diagnosis, the final chapter is already self-evident: hysterectomy.

Of course, the solution I offer you, FRS, is not the avoidance of surgery, but actually a more delicate and intricate operation than is traditionally expected. Would that I had the power to make those bothersome fibroids disappear with the wave of a magic wand—and without the use of my laser beam. Unfortunately, no one can do that today. Yet I do suggest an operation which, in the long run, may be beneficial. It saves and restores the uterus, rather than destroying it. It improves the quality of your life.

I have met women who will do anything to avoid surgery, whether FRS, myomectomy, or hysterectomy. They have spent thousands of dollars seeking an answer to their fibroid dilemma. They change doctors, seek holistic solutions, travel across the country to see psychic surgeons, wait until menopause for their fibroid to 'shrink'. Fasting, vitamin therapy, diets, acupuncture, acupressure, chiropractic manipulation, and massage have all been tried. I encourage alternatives and none of these treatments are harmful in and of themselves, but they don't solve the problem and they do cause delay.

Delay, of course, results in additional fibroid growth, which can destroy more normal tissue. This can contribute to the eventual loss of an otherwise healthy uterus. As the fibroid grows it becomes harder to ignore.

Instead, I offer you hope. Hope that your uterus can be preserved. Hope that your body can remain intact. Hope that your life will not be disrupted by hysterectomy, although some may still find a hysterectomy beneficial.

Female vivisection

Gynaecologists, at a recent teaching course, were given eight, normal, freshly removed female uteri to allow them to practice their skills. Whose organs were these? Why were they removed? Imagine my horror on hearing about this blatant form of female vivisection. Eight normal female uteri were removed so that gynaecologists could practice! The motive was not the advancement of science, the motive was the 'project'.

When uteri are removed like this as an everyday matter of fact, fibroids are dumped into the incinerator. Little effort has been put forward to find the cause for the formation of fibroid tissue. Hundreds of thousands of tumours that could have been studied are overlooked, because the uterus is unimportant in gynaecology, easily removed and dispensable. In the operating room, uteri with tumours are given to a pathologist who examines them, and then disposes of them. Fibroids are not part of any national or cooperative study to investigate some very basic questions about them. Why are they formed? Why do some have hard capsules and others not? What regulates their growth patterns? Answers, hopefully, will come with time.

CHAPTER 10

Endometrial hyperplasia and endometrial cancer

What is endometrial hyperplasia?

Marissa was 28. Though active and lively, she was obese (165 pounds on a 5'2" frame) and was plagued with excessive facial hair growth. Her periods were few and far between. I suspected and then confirmed that she suffered from polycystic ovary disease. She rarely ovulated and, thus, her system was flooded with an excess of oestrogen. She had endometrial hyperplasia.

Helene had been taking oestrogen shots to alleviate the hot flushes and nervousness of menopause. Now she was bleeding post-menopausally. She, too, had hyperplasia. Was her condition serious? Could it be reversed?

What is endometrial hyperplasia? The word *hyperplasia* comes from Greek. The prefix, *hyper-* means excessive, whereas the root, *-plasia* refers to development or growth. So, *endometrial hyperplasia* is a general term referring to the overgrowth of the uterine lining. This thickening may cause spotting or abnormal bleeding and generally occurs among women in their twenties and thirties who don't ovulate, and women approaching and concluding menopause. Hyperplasia is thought to be caused by too much oestrogen coupled with not enough progesterone.

Not all forms of endometrial hyperplasia are dangerous. Indeed, some are completely benign, almost never leading to cancer, whereas others do indicate a pre-cancerous state. This may not have been made clear to you. Mistakes in diagnosis and treatment are common.

As you take a closer look at the various forms of hyperplasia, keep in mind that these are not discrete diseases, but rather steps in a continuum. And do bear with me. The characteristics and terminology of the forms of endometrial hyperplasia can be confusing. It's important that you understand the distinctions between the various stages, because these can determine whether or not you are a candidate for a hysterectomy.

The hyperplasia continuum

Classification	Behaviour
Proliferative or bleeding-phase endometrium	Benign
Hyperplasia (also called cystic hyperplasia and adenomatous hyperplasia)	Benign but hyperstimulated
Atypical adenomatous hyperplasia (also called severe adenomatous hyperplasia atypical	Pre-malignant

hyperplasia, and cancer in situ (CIS)
Well-differentiated cancer   Malignant

Let's look at these stages individually.

Proliferative or bleeding-phase endometrium

This long term simply means that you are not ovulating and therefore may experience bleeding as a result of non-stop oestrogen stimulation. When you don't ovulate, your endometrial lining grows improperly and doesn't shed completely. You may bleed irregularly.

Cystic glandular or mild hyperplasia

This term is applied to the excessive growth of *normal* cells in the *normal* tissue arrangement of your endometrium. It is closely related to the bleeding-phase endometrium, but is a heightened endometrial response to persistent oestrogen stimulation.

Cystic endometrial hyperplasia is NOT cancer and rarely, if ever, leads to cancer. Cancer develops in fewer than 1 per cent of patients with this problem.[1] Your doctor should approach cystic hyperplasia initially at its root cause—your hormone imbalance. In most cases, this form of hyperplasia is easily reversed with proper medication and without surgery.

You should regard the diagnosis of cystic hyperplasia as both a warning sign and a blessing in disguise. The abnormal bleeding is your body's own red flag of danger. It tells you that you are producing too much oestrogen. You may be at higher risk for all female cancers—not just uterine cancer. Without treatment, you could go on for ten to twenty years, overstimulating your organs with excess oestrogen, and eventually producing a true cancer.

When cystic hyperplasia (stemming from too much oestrogen) is diagnosed, you can be placed on a cancer-screening and prevention programme to help eliminate future problems. You will need to be followed closely for the rest of your life.

Although cystic endometrial hyperplasia is not cancer, many doctors refer to it as a cancer that requires an immediate hysterectomy. I believe this inaccuracy can cost thousands of women their uteri.

Adenomatous hyperplasia, without atypical cells

If your endometrial cells continue to be stimulated by too much oestrogen, with no intervention on your doctor's part, the cells themselves may begin to change. The condition evolves from cystic endometrial hyperplasia to adenomatous hyperplasia. Despite the changes in the cells, however, this is still a benign condition and usually does not progress to a well-differentiated carcinoma.[2] It can be treated medically and monitored.

Atypical adenomatous hyperplasia or severe hyperplasia

The stage on the continuum that precedes cancer is called *atypical adenomatous hyperplasia, severe hyperplasia, or carcinoma in situ* (CIS). It may occur in small areas of your endometrium or as a general change in the entire lining of your uterus. This stage is dangerous, because a greater percentage of women with atypical hyperplasia progress to cancer than those with milder forms of the disorder.

The lesion is frequently reversible in young women by the administration of progesterone. If you have this form of adenomatous hyperplasia, you are at higher risk for developing endometrial cancer.[3] I will be covering treatments for all forms of hyperplasia at the end of this chapter.

Confusions and perplexities

If you feel bewildered by all of this terminology, you are not alone. Adenomatous hyperplasia is frequently misdiagnosed because the experts, themselves, can be confused by the various stages and the terminology. And, endometrial hyperplasia can be mistaken for other, less serious—or even normal—conditions. According to eminent pathologist Dr Robert Kurman, 'the diagnosis of so-called adenomatous hyperplasia has probably led to more unnecessary hysterectomies than any other'.[4]

Why is this so? It's difficult to tell the difference between a normal endometrium and hyperplasia in women who are menstruating or who have had recent bleeding. And, when oestrogen is withdrawn, the changes in the endometrium can also be confused with cancer.

Even more bewildering is the medical community's failure to define clearly the exact nature of adenomatous hyperplasia. Some pathologists use the term to describe a mild lesion, whereas others use it for a severe one. Over the years, gynaecologists reading the pathology reports have come to regard this condition as serious (no matter what criteria the pathologist uses), and a hysterectomy is performed once the diagnosis is made.

Atypical adenomatous (severe) hyperplasia and endometrial carcinoma in situ (CIS) are also often confused and lead to differing treatments. From the clinical point of view, severe hyperplasia and endometrial CIS are the same. It becomes very difficult to define when severe hyperplasia ends and carincoma begins. Yet a doctor who gets a pathology report reading CIS will feel that s(he) must do a hysterectomy, whereas the diagnosis of atypical adenomatous hyperplasia still may be treated with medications, especially in young women who wish to retain their ability to bear children.

Because of these confusions, I can't stress enough how important it is to seek a second opinion on your pathology report. Differing points of view and approaches to the same problem may make all the difference in the world.

Endometrial cancer

Endometrial cancer is a malignancy of the uterine lining, which occurs most often in women from 50 to 64 years of age. Each year approximately 54,000 women are afflicted by it, yet it is the least deadly of all female cancers with an estimated survival rate of between 75 and 90 per cent. *If you have endometrial cancer, a hysterectomy can save your life.*

What are the symptoms of endometrial cancer?

Symptoms of endometrial cancer include:

● Bleeding or watery, bloody discharge after menopause
● Bleeding between periods or increased bleeding during menses
● Unusual discharge or spotting

The stages of endometrial cancer

Like most cancers, endometrial cancer progresses in stages.

Stage 1: Your uterus remains the normal size. The cancer is confined to the body of the uterus (no cervical involvement). The tumour may be well differentiated or diffuse.

Stage 2: Your uterus is mildly enlarged and there are undifferentiated tumours or deep penetration of the tumour into the myometrial layer of the uterus.

Stage 3: Your uterus is quite enlarged and the cancer extends outside that organ but remains within the pelvis.

Stage 4: Adjacent organs as well as distant ones are involved.

Although the survival rates of cancers found in Stages 1 and 2 are good to excellent, depending on the grade and depth of invasion, Stages 3 and 4 are dangerous. *Early detection is essential.*

How are endometrial hyperplasia and cancer diagnosed?

Although the cervical smear is 90 per cent accurate in diagnosing cervical irregularities, it is only 50 per cent effective in finding endometrial cancer. To more accurately diagnose problems associated with the uterine lining, you should routinely undergo a series of studies. These provide your doctor with the maximum amount of information. Some exciting breakthroughs have been made, which may make it feasible to screen all perimenopausal and menopausal women easily, safely, and early.

The hysteroscope

The hysteroscope is a slender light-transmitting viewer that allows your gynaecologist to examine the inside of your uterus. S(he) can see any abnormal cells, growths, tumours, and scars on the endometrium. The length of the uterus is also measured. This can be videotaped for your information and discussion with your doctor.

The hysteroscope is helpful in allowing your gynaecologist to visualize and operate. A special small biopsy instrument is put into your cervix through the hysteroscope to remove any suspicious cells in the uterus, and even small submucosal fibroids.

Forceps are introduced through the hysteroscope to remove polyps and take biopsies. I like to use a soft plastic suction tube to remove the remaining tissue. In that way, I get adequate tissue samples without scraping with a sharp instrument.

The diagnostic D & C

The best ways to diagnose endometrial hyperplasia and endometrial cancer are a uterine biopsy or a *dilation and curettage* (commonly called a D & C), which is minor surgery. Prior to performing the D & C, your gynaecologist should culture for various organisms that may potentially live in the uterus. These include aerobic bacteria—those that need air such as 'gonnococcus', which causes gonorrhoea—and anerobic bacteria, which must live without air. Smaller, more difficult to culture bacteria (because they actually live inside the cells) like chlamydia, mycoplasma, and ureaplasma should also be looked for.

If you are suffering from a disease caused by these microbes, you should be treated for it, too. This would help avoid the possibility of spreading the infection, bleeding, and other complications following surgery.

Some women, however, have these infections but have no symptoms. Their gynaecologists wouldn't suspect the presence of disease. If that's the case, the cultures can be done, as a preventive measure, during the D & C. It's better to have this information late than not at all.

After the cultures are made, your cervix will be dilated to permit larger instruments. A *fractional curettage* involves the independent scraping of each separate sector of the uterus: first the endocervical canal—the juncture between the uterus and the cervix —and then each wall of the uterus and the fundus. This technique enables your gynaecologist to identify and evaluate any existing cancer, to discriminate between endocervical and endometrial cancer, and to assess its extent.

If major surgery is to be undertaken, and the D & C occurs in the hospital, the pathologist can and should be called into the operating room to examine the tissue samples with your surgeon. I routinely operate in this fashion.

Proliferating endometrial carcinoma can be recognized with the naked eye. It comes away in fragments that are greyish and dead, whereas normal endometrium tissue comes off in thinner or thicker strips. The tissue is examined microscopically to rule out or confirm cancer.

Having your D & C in the doctor's office

Most D & C operations routinely call for hospitalization, because of the use of general anaesthetics. I have been successful in performing many right in my office, however, using a local, or no anaesthetic at all. That avoids the attendant dangers of sedation and saves my patients hundreds of dollars in hospital costs.

Aspiration curettage uses a suction device or small pump to 'vacuum' the uterine lining, rather than the traditional scraping with a sharp metal device or *curette*. The aspiration curettage is performed with minimal discomfort or damage to the uterus. And it provides samples of tissue that are virtually the equivalent of those produced by the more expensive hospital-performed D & C. My patients can go home in just 15 minutes.

Not only is this procedure faster and easier, it is also far less damaging to the endometrial lining. Aggressive scraping can be dangerous; it may cause perforation of the uterus, adhesions, and scar tissue.

The importance of a second opinion

Because of the confusions inherent in diagnosing the various forms of hyperplasia, I feel that you should never sign a consent form for a D & C that includes the wording, 'and a possible hysterectomy'. You may want to get the results from the pathologist and send the slides for a second opinion before you take such a drastic step. Besides, you need time to prepare for any surgery.

That's one of the reasons why I advocate 'office' D & C—it's impossible to follow it up with an 'instant' hysterectomy. I have known some doctors to perform the surgery without ever waiting for the pathologist's report to come in. And whatever your condition, the three-day to one-week wait for results will not endanger you as much as an unwarranted hysterectomy.

When I receive a report that indicates a possible cancer, I always ask the hospital pathologist to send my patient's slides for an outside opinion. Second opinions on pathology specimens have changed diagnoses for many women. Interpretations on slides may vary greatly.

Kathleen was a teacher who had been told that she had endometrial cancer after her D & C. We sent her slides to a lab that dealt only with female diseases and the report came back negative. No cancer. We resubmitted it, and, again, it was negative, much to everyone's great relief. Although Kathleen needed to be monitored closely and placed on medication to reverse her cystic hyperplasia, the second and third opinions did help to save her organs.

While I'm on the subject of second opinions, I would advise you to seek *independent* corroboration of your medical problems at all levels. I have seen women needlessly lose their organs because they were afraid to offend their doctor of many years by asking for a second opinion from another gynaecologist. If you are hesitant, I must ask you, *what's more important*—your doctor's fragile ego or your own body's health and well-being? In fact, I would be wary of any doctor who opposes your search for outside evaluation.

Reading your pathology report

One of the ways in which you can empower yourself is to request a copy of the pathology report following your D & C. Remember, if the report reads cystic or adenomatous endometrial hyperplasia, this is not cancer and does not require a hysterectomy. If the cells are *atypical*, you'll want to send it to a second pathologist for evaluation.

In the US, my own organization the Institute for Reproductive Rights (Appendix 1), and others, are striving to make women aware that their records are legally 'their records'. All citizens in the US by law have direct access to their own medical records: operative report, pathology report, anaesthetist's and operating room record. All of these reports are essential to provide you with knowledge about what took place. Consumers in the US, however, are not educated to understand these rights. They do not routinely ask questions of their surgeons and they rarely ask to read their reports. It is surely a basic human right that the individual should have access to these reports. Moreover, in my opinion, it should become a matter of routine practice to give copies of these reports to patients.

In the UK the Data Protection Act requires that a patient has access to automatically stored data. This 'freedom of information' may in the future be extended to manually stored data. At the moment there is nothing in UK law that requires a doctor to furnish a woman with a copy of her pathology report although it is considered good practice to do so and if a woman asks there is no real reason for a doctor to refuse. So a woman has a right to ask for her pathology report, but as yet no inherent right to be given it except through a court order. The UK Department of Health is currently consulting on a non-statutory Code of Practice that would give patients right of access to their medical records.

Am I at risk for endometrial hyperplasia and cancer?

Endometrial hyperplasia and cancer essentially are caused by hormonal imbalances. Although this area is still under active investigation, I believe at least three factors contribute to the development of these diseases.

Overabundance of Oestrogen. Your body can make too much of this hormone (called *endogenous* oestrogen), or an excess can be introduced from outside sources (called *exogenous* oestrogen). Where does the extra oestrogen come from?

Oestrogen sources within your own body:
- Body fat/obesity
- Overproduction by ovaries or adrenal glands
- Genetic factors: women with a family history of female cancer secrete more oestrogen

Oestrogen from external sources
- Herbs like ginseng and cohash
- Hormone-fed meats and poultry
- Cosmetics made with hormones
- Prescribed 'unopposed' oestrogen medication

Excess oestrogen causes the endometrium to be stimulated constantly. The lining of the uterus isn't being shed in its regular cyclic manner, and this may lead to an increase in the number of cells. If, for example, you normally have three layers of endometrial cells, six layers may develop. The stimulation of your endometrium by oestrogen may allow the endometrium to use the majority of its energy for growth, which can lead to hyperplasia and cancer.

Deficiency in Sex Hormone Binding Globulin (SHBG). SHBG regulates the amount of free, active hormones—especially oestrogen and testosterone—in the body. When enough SHBG exists, it keeps oestrogen bound up, as if under lock and key, so it cannot be used by the body. When there is not enough SHBG, abnormal amounts of oestrogen are set free, causing overstimulation of the female organs that can eventually create hyperplasia and cancer.

Deficiency in Progesterone. Extremely low *progesterone* levels may be as important as high circulating oestrogen levels. Progesterone 'antagonizes' oestrogen's effects on the body. Normal amounts of progesterone in the blood stop negative effects of oestrogen by causing the endometrium to shed during menstruation.

Am I likely to develop endometrial hyperplasia?

The most efficient way to avoid endometrial cancer with all of its attendant dangers, is to recognize whether you are at risk for developing adenomatous hyperplasia. Early treatment and reversal of abnormal cells can minimize this disease, if not eradicate it entirely. This would eliminate the need for a hysterectomy. Study the following factors, and talk them over with your doctor.

Unopposed Oestrogen Therapy. Cancer of the endometrium has been found among women who received 'unopposed' oestrogen —that is, oestrogen without progesterone— without a pretreatment biopsy and periodic follow-up by their doctor, including a sampling of the endometrial tissue.

If you need oestrogen replacement to combat menopausal symptoms, it must be prescribed with the appropriate dose of progesterone at regular intervals. When progesterone is lacking, your uterine lining is not given a rest from the constancy of oestrogen stimulation. There may be breakthrough bleeding and a degeneration of the blood vessels and tissue within the endometrium. None of the normal phases of menstrual cycle are stimulated when your doctor prescribes oestrogen alone.

The highest incidence of endometrial cancer occurs among women treated with oestrogen alone and the lowest among women treated with a combination of the two hormones. In fact, women who take the oestrogen/progesterone therapy have the lowest cancer rate of all—lower even than untreated post-menopausal women.[5]

Rushing to your doctor for an oestrogen shot whenever you feel depressed can be damaging to your endometrium (and other oestrogen-sensitive areas of your body, such as your breasts and gastrointestinal tract). Your doctor should regulate the dosage and frequency of your hormone replacement therapy very carefully. The indiscriminate and haphazard prescribing of 'unopposed' oestrogen can lead to cancer and has given oestrogen a bad name! If you have been taking this form of hormone replacement, an endometrial biopsy is essential.

Irregular Menstrual Cycles. Since puberty, Lois has had very long cycles (over 35 days). Now, at 31, she sometimes even missed a period or two, every few months. She failed to make mention of these irregularities to her previous doctor because the cycle seemed normal to her. All abnormalities in your cycle should be discussed, especially because too long a time between menses may cause the endometrium to receive too much stimulation.

Lois had polycystic ovary disease (PCO). Her ovaries didn't ovulate regularly but created many nonrupturing follicles, which sent excess oestrogen through her body without the benefit of the natural suppressing action of progesterone. Given the causes of hyperplasia, you can see why this would be of concern. I made a tentative diagnosis of Lois's problem by taking a careful menstrual history.

However, if you report a menstrual abnormality, don't assume your gynaecologist will automatically do something about it, unless you insist. Doctors often don't see the importance of regulating the menses, particularly in women 20 to 30 years old who

experience *amenorrhoea* (no menstrual periods) or *oligomenorrhoea* (infrequent, light periods) and make no complaints because they don't want children.

In the long run, this attitude can raise your future cancer risk and lower your fertility. If you have these problems, your cycles should be evaluated and regulated with hormones.

Ovarian Cyst. Occasionally an ovarian cyst will continue to produce excess oestrogen if it fails to rupture at the normal time.

Long Menstrual History and/or No Pregnancies. The following factors appear frequently in the reproductive histories of patients with endometrial cancer. They are responsible for a more prolonged exposure of the uterus and other female organs to oestrogens.

● Early onset of menstruation
● Late menopause
● Irregular periods
● No pregnancy

Post-menopausal Bleeding. Esther was post-menopausal, yet she continued to spot. She had twice the oestogen level in her blood than women who are not menstruating. This put her at greater risk for endometrial problems.

Oestrogen in the post-menopausal phase of life comes not only from the ovaries (which continue manufacturing lessened amounts of oestrogen after menopause), but also from 'peripheral' sources (body fat). The ovary also produces androgens such as *testosterone*, which are converted in the fat cells of the body into oestrogen. If you are menopausal, you should have a diagnostic D & C or other uterine sample before receiving treatment for any menstrual abnormality.

Obesity. Obesity has been associated with

an enhanced susceptibility to oestrogen-linked diseases. In fact, there is a threefold increase in the risk of endometrial hyperplasia for women 25 to 50 pounds overweight and a ninefold increase in women more than 50 pounds overweight. If you are obese, you have higher levels of oestrogens circulating in your blood.[6]

Hypertension and Diabetes. The correlation of these diseases with hyperplasia may be consistent with the fact that they are also often present in obese women.[7]

Smoking. Pre-menopausal women who smoke place themselves at risk for endometrial cancer.[8]

Endometrial hyperplasia and cancer checklist

Use this list to help evaluate your risks for developing hyperplasia:

● Caucasian
● Upper income
● Obese/diet with high meat and fat content
● Family history of uterine hyperplasia or female cancer (mother, sister, grandmother, etc.)
● Unopposed oestrogen therapy
● Diabetes
● Hypertension
● Polycystic ovarian disease
● Irregular or anovulatory menstrual cycles (where menstrual flow is not preceded by ovulation)
● Long history of menstrual cycle or no pregnancy
● Smoking

Any of these factors requires a discussion with your doctor.

Medical treatments for hyperplasia

Your endometrial hyperplasia must be treated in order to prevent cell irregularities from becoming cancerous. Your case is unique, and treatment should be individualized. No matter what the circumstances, however, your doctor will need to stop the constant stimulation of oestrogen. Here are some guidelines that I find useful:

1. *If you are menopausal and have been on oestrogen therapy only*: switch to oestrogen with progesterone for the rest of your life. The post-menopausal endometrium has a remarkable ability to return to normal when treated with this combination. It can mimic the menstrual cycle and prevent endometrial hyperplasia and cancer.

Progestogens (such as progesterone) physically shed the uterine lining each month. Once this occurs, fewer glands and cells are left to continue growth, which might eventually lead to hyperplasia and cancer. Oestrogen/progesterone can reverse as much as 96.8 per cent of all hyperplasia cases. The majority of women who elect to take progesterone have the lining of their uterus return to normal within six months.[9]

I recommend a follow-up D & C to make sure that the endometrial cells have normalized. As a precaution, I also advise a yearly endometrial biopsy. Even if you have had a hysterectomy, I recommend oestrogen with progesterone. These hormones in combination block oestrogen receptors in the breasts and ovary and possibly prevent the development of cancer sites outside the uterus.

2. *If you have adenomatous hyperplasia or atypical adenomatous hyperplasia from oestrogen replacement therapy*: oestrogen replacement can be stopped for one to two months. At that point, I would repeat the D & C to

see whether the endometrium has returned to normal.

Of course, you need the oestrogen to protect against osteoporosis, hot flushes, and other menopausal symptoms. In addition, your adenomatous or atypical hyperplasia may not be cured simply by stopping oestrogen replacement. In that case, I would continue with the oestrogen therapy but also give progesterone daily for three months and then follow up with a D & C.

In most cases, you will have withdrawal bleeding and your endometrium will revert to normal; the progesterone will have suppressed the hyperplasia. However, you may have to stay on this regimen for the rest of your life to prevent the hyperplasia from recurring.[10]

The choice of treatment will depend on your body. If the atypical cells result solely from the externally provided oestrogen, then stopping the administration of that hormone may be enough to reverse the proliferation. If, on the other hand, you are an oestrogen secretor, then I feel that the progesterone is necessary. You may or may not need a repeat biopsy six months to a year following the start of this treatment.

3. *If your atypical adenomatous hyperplasia does not resolve*: the risk of developing cancer is too great. A hysterectomy should be performed if:

● You are an older woman
● You continue to bleed during the medical therapy
● Your repeat biopsy shows persistence of atypical cells

A hysterectomy is lifesaving in these cases.

4. *If your hyperplasia results from polycystic ovary disease*: you should be treated with drugs like clomiphene citrate to induce ovulation. If you don't want to get pregnant, 'progesterone', Provera, or birth control pills are also effective. You should be monitored carefully with repeat biopsies every six months to a year to make sure that the hyperplasia has disappeared. The use of combination oral contraceptives protects against the development of epithelial endometrial cancer. The protection can last up to fifteen years after you stop taking the pill.[11]

The life sentence

It may be frightening to realize that you must stay on drugs for the rest of your life to prevent cancer. This 'life sentence' may have some far-reaching implications. I have known women who resist taking long-term drugs. 'It's easier to just have the hysterectomy', they reason. 'No fuss, no bother'.

These women are unconsciously and erroneously blaming the uterus for a problem originating elsewhere (the ovaries, fat tissue, external sources). Besides, the uterus is not the only organ reacting to the effects of oestrogen overstimulation. If you accept their reasoning, shouldn't the breasts, the gastrointestinal tract, and ovaries be removed, too, as a precaution, or because it's 'easier' than a lifetime of pill-taking?

By using progesterone, you may be protecting other organs from cancer. Long-term progesterone use reduces the risk of breast cancer in post-menopausal women, and oestrogen can fight osteoporosis by promoting the formation of new bone mass.

Oestrogen/progesterone for the rest of your life makes enormous sense. Yet many women are likely to shy away. Why?

The trouble with hormones

Perhaps no women's health issue is as fraught with myth, misinformation, and fear as hormone treatment. In a misguided attempt to explain the delicate balance of hormones to their patients, many doctors have referred to oestrogen as the 'female' hormone, whereas progesterone plays the role of the heavy—the 'male' hormone.

This has caused some women to fear that they will become masculinized with progesterone treatments. They imagine growing fat and hairy and cultivating a voice to rival Caruso's. Nothing could be further from the truth. The ovary naturally produces progesterone. It is an integral part of our female endocrine system, providing a conservative force that enhances the strength of the glands, cells, and blood vessels within the uterus. It does, however, need to be balanced correctly with the oestrogen in our bodies, much like the oriental concept of *yin and yang*.

Christine was 52 when she came to see me for a second opinion. She suffered from severe back pain and didn't lubricate in the vagina. At 49, she had experienced bleeding in the middle of her cycle. Her gynaecologist performed a D & C and found cystic hyperplasia. He had offered her progesterone and she flatly refused. She was convinced that progesterone would turn her into a man. She had read a lot about it in women's magazines.

Christine had a hysterectomy with oöphorectomy to treat her hyperplasia. After surgery, she refused hormone replacement therapy. Now, three years later, she had developed osteoporosis. Christine's unwarranted fears and media exploitation imperiled her more than the original condition. I find it tragic and dangerous that fear of hormone-induced cancer is so well inculcated that women have refused oestrogen with progesterone—the only correct treatment for endometrial hyperplasia—when that option is offered by their doctor.

And now I'll get back on my soapbox! I believe that the media has sensationalized the effects of *improperly dispensed* female hormones to such an extent that many women would rather have a hysterectomy than suffer the dubious fate that awaits them with 'deadly' oestrogen/progesterone—even if these hormones are prescribed in the correct dosage. Many women view hysterectomy as their only option. But they are wrong. It is their last resort.

'Women are not told that having a hysterectomy does not affect their menopause. They still produce hormones, they still cycle, all that happens is that they don't bleed. It may be less easy to try to cope with symptoms of PMS or the menopause when you no longer have periods to date them by.'
Dr Prudence Tunnadine

Most hyperplasias will not progress to cancer. They can be reversed. And hysterectomy does not correct the body's hormone imbalance.

What if I have endometrial cancer?

Because this disease is life-threatening, usually the best treatment available is hysterectomy. It cures most endometrial cancer. The scope of the surgery will depend on the extent of the malignancy. The hysterectomy may include removal of the ovaries and fallopian tubes because these are the first to be involved if the cancer spreads. In some cases, surgery may be combined with radiation treatment.

Stage 1: Treatment is hysterectomy/oöphorectomy without pre-operative radiation. Well-differentiated tumours in small uteri have a cure rate of 90 per cent.

Stage 2: During hysterectomy, lymph nodes are examined for spread of disease.

Stage 3: The recommended treatment is pre-operative radium followed by a radical hysterectomy and removal of the lymph nodes.

Stage 4: Because other organs may be involved, the treatment is individualized for each case.

It is rare that endometrial cancer strikes younger women, say, those aged 15 to 25. A recent study has found that in selected young patients with well-differentiated endometrial carcinoma limited to the uterine lining only, conservative hormone therapy with progesterone and a D & C may be adequate treatment.[12]

Future treatments

I can foresee the day when laser surgery will be used to treat small, localized cancer lesions within the uterus, just as it is used today to vaporize cervical lesions. Of course, this doesn't mean that one should burn the entire endometrial lining. Such a 'YAG laser hysterectomy' for abnormal bleeding, as recently touted in the press, would scar the interior of the uterus, permanently interfering with normal reproduction, hormone receptor exchange, the production of hormones, and other chemicals in the female organ system. It has its place, especially in cases of uncontrollable bleeding, but it is not a cure-all, replacing hysterectomy.

One day perhaps, medical treatments coupled with the careful use of laser therapy will eliminate endometrial cancer as a threat to women's reproductive organs and lives.

Update: 'Rollerball' surgery and laser ablation

She is beautiful, strong, self-willed, intelligent, famous, and rich enough to buy the best medical care. The star of the movie *Rollerball* made the choice to have 'Rollerball' surgery—very likely to avoid a hysterectomy.

Rollerball surgery may not be the saving operation that women across the nation were told it was. 'Rollerball' surgery is the use of an electrocautery unit that sends a burning, searing heat to the lining of the uterus. If there are small fibroid tumours directly in contact with the endometrium, the rollerball will burn them as well as the endometrium. This is *not* the laser technique mentioned earlier, but rather a burning technique that causes scarring of the tissue and actually destroys the normal endometrium of the uterus.

As we have seen, the endometrium is a very important part of the uterus. Rollerball surgery removes the endometrium, causing scarring and adhesions. This increases a woman's chances for infertility. When the rollerball is applied to the entire surface of the lining of the uterus, it destroys the entire endometrium and a woman no longer menstruates. In addition, rollerball surgery only treats the *symptoms* of bleeding; it may not have cured all of the diseased states that caused abnormal bleeding.

Rollerball, along with laser ablation, has been sold by the media as the *ultimate alternative* to hysterectomy, a safe, out-patient procedure that is low in cost and without complications. Informed only by the media, women may have been misinformed of the irreversible side effects that may occur. The loss of the receptors from the lining of the uterus, the loss of certain specialized substance production, the increased risk of Asherman's Syndrome, severe scarring which could result in loss of uterine orgasm, the development of pulmonary oedema, death from the procedure itself, burning beyond the uterus into the bowel or bladder, and the failure to treat the fibroid tumours that lie within the uterus itself are the risks of rollerball or laser ablation surgery. Ablation *is* an important technique, but you, as the consumer, have to do research before consenting to undergo the procedure.

Certainly the ability to destroy the endometrium with a laser has specific uses that can be very beneficial. Endometriosis may be identified in the uterine cavity and be lasered. The stalk of a polyp that has been removed can be lasered to assist in prevention of regrowth. A woman may have a single small fibroid tumour in her uterine cavity that can be removed by ablation. In cases where the cause of the uterine bleeding can not be found, laser ablation has an important place—not as the first choice of treatment but rather as a last restort. Most uterine bleeding has a specific cause (i.e., hormone imbalance, polyp, fibroid, etc.), which can be treated by medical treatment or conservative surgery.

In the future, lasers may be used to ablate small areas of abnormal cells and even non-invasive carcinoma—but this is for our future.

CHAPTER 11

Prolapse

'If there is prolapse of the vault of the pelvis (vaginal vault) due to weakening of the supports, the surgeon will as part of the procedure to tighten up the tissues of the vault, remove the uterus. It must be carefully explained to the patient that she'll lose her uterus. Removing the uterus, however, is only a means to try to prevent a recurrence of the prolapse and this it has to be admitted is one of medicine's "grey areas".'
Consultant gynaecologist

Gina, a recent immigrant, was unfamiliar with the kind of care she should expect from America's system of medicine. Although an educated woman, she was naïve and frightened about giving birth to her first child in a strange country.

Gina's progress was followed at a community clinic, where she received little instruction on nutrition, exercise, or anything else concerning pregnancy. There was no genetic counselling. Her visits to the clinic consisted of basic tests such as urine analysis and blood pressure. As a first-time mother-to-be separated from more experienced family and friends, she had no way to judge the kind of care she was receiving.

On the day Gina went into labour, the situation worsened. The nurses took forever admitting her to the hospital. She was in great pain and extremely fearful, but was left alone in the labour room. Neither she nor her foetus's status were monitored. She begged for a doctor, but no one came. She was told she was in early labour and her concerns were dismissed.

But the intensity and rapidity of Gina's contractions were highly unusual. She was experiencing a *precipitous labour*. In such cases, the baby is shot out of the uterus, like a bullet from a gun. Yet no one was monitoring her progress.

Finally, screaming out in pain, Gina attracted a nurse who discovered that the baby's head was already emerging. Gina was taken for an emergency delivery. During the ordeal, Gina's pelvic tissue suffered great damage. Her uterus, cervix, and vagina were traumatized. The delicate tissues of the vaginal vault were lacerated and blood vessels torn. Nevertheless, Gina felt grateful that the baby was healthy and the affliction was over.

But was it? Indeed, Gina's nightmare only began with the delivery. When she arrived home with her new baby daughter, she urinated constantly; she couldn't control her bowel movements; her vaginal area was bruised, bloody, and sore. She was told this was normal healing.

When days turned into weeks, Gina realized her body was not as it should be. In addition to her other complaints, her uterus hung down, filling her vagina. Her bladder had fallen completely. The trauma of the dleivery had been so great that Gina suffered a total prolapse.

The poor woman had just had her first child, and she could no longer be sexually active. Although she was only in her twenties, she felt ugly and deformed. She soiled her bed in her sleep. Her husband was afraid to touch her. She cried constantly.

Back Gina went to the clinic. Her doctor reassured her, saying, 'Gina, when we remove your uterus, all of your problems will be gone.'

'But I want more than one child,' Gina objected.

'I'm sorry, I can't help you with that,' he replied. 'This sort of thing happens to women who have children.'

There was no admission that her labour hadn't been controlled and that all of the tissue damage was caused by the lack of care. And now, she was being made to feel that the pregnancy was to blame for the problem. There shouldn't be any reason for her to want another child or to even keep her uterus. She was foolish for considering it.

As Gina sat in my office telling her story, tears streamed down her face. The trauma that she had sustained was immense. But worse, perhaps, was the psychological damage. Fear and anxiety surrounded her. She could no longer share the bed with her husband. Gina had suffered a breakdown of her function as a woman.

What exactly is prolapse?

Prolapse is the term used to describe the falling or sinking of an organ. Every organ has a 'normal' position in your body related to your overall anatomy. Your uterus, for example, sits in a certain place, at a certain 'suspension' level. The bladder has its own designated position, as does the rectum. All of the organs are held in place by various sheets of tissues called *fascia*, *ligaments*, and *muscles*.

Over time, the position of your organs can change, to the right or to the left of centre and forward or backward. Frequently, the organs fall or descend. When they do, you experience prolapse.

What are the symptoms of prolapse?

Common complaints that indicate possible prolapse or relaxation of the pelvic organs include:

- The uneasy feeling that 'something is falling out'
- A dragging sensation or heaviness in your lower abdomen
- Constant lower back pain or pressure
- Tired achiness akin to mild menstrual cramps, which worsen after long periods of standing
- Difficulty achieving penetration during intercourse
- The frequent urge to urinate even after your bladder has been emptied; urinary incontinence
- Constipation, difficulty in defecation, and the need to bear down

To understand why these complaints occur, let's look at the consequences of the descent of the organs involved.

The different forms prolapse can take

The descent of the uterus is called *uterine prolapse*. When your uterus descends in a straight line, it can come down one-third, two-thirds, or the entire length of the vagina (see figs. 19, 20, 21, 22). In the most severe cases, like Gina's, the cervix will protrude from between the labia. In this situation, intercourse is impossible because the whole vagina is filled with uterus, which entirely obstructs the penis's entry. When this occurs, your tissue can be traumatized and damaged from leaving its protected environment. And, even worse, the cervix is exposed to urination and defecation and can become infected.

The uterus can also descend at an angle: forward, pressing on your bladder, or backward, pressing on your bowels and rectum. The constant pressure of the uterus pushing these organs can cause physiological dysfunction such as continual urination and chronic constipation. Finally, as a result of the pressure, uterine prolapse can contribute to the falling of other internal organs (or they can fall as a result of their own tissue weakness). These related conditions are as follows:

Cystocele. Marcia's bladder fell from its normal position, making it difficult for her to empty it completely. She experienced frequent, recurrent urinary tract infections.

Fig. 19. Some of the support ligaments that hold the uterus in place.

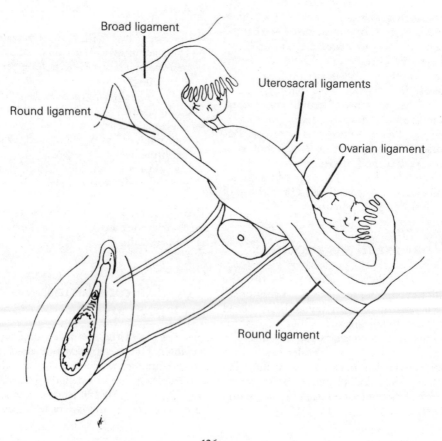

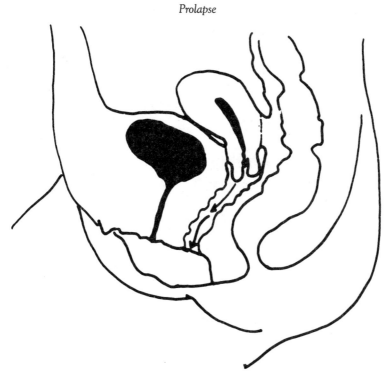

Fig. 20. A side view of prolapse: the uterus begins its descent.

With a large cystocele, urine may remain in your bladder after urinating, causing it to overfill and leak during coughing, sneezing, walking, and even laughing.

Urethrocele. The muscles supporting Barbara's urethra separated, causing her urethra to sag into the vaginal wall. Like Marcia, she experienced involuntary loss of urine when pressure was increased in her abdomen. Urethrocele can occur with cystocele.

Rectocele. Adelle's rectum bulged into her vagina, rendering her bowel movements more difficult. She had a condition called *rectocele*. When this happens, severe constipation occurs because the stool packs into the pouch formed by the bulging rectum.

Enterocele. A portion of Phyllis's small intestine bulged into the back wall of her vagina. She had enterocele. With enterocele the sensation of pressure occurs higher than in rectocele.

Prolapse in historical perspective

Over the centuries, many treatments have been used to 'correct' uterine prolapse. An Egyptian papyrus written in about 1550 BC prescribed a paste of honey and other ingredients to be smeared on the fallen womb before its replacement in the vagina. To facilitate repositioning, it was also recommended that an 'ibis of wax be heated on coals, and that the fumes be permitted to

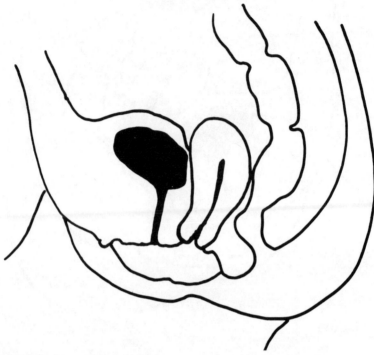

Fig. 21. Second degree of prolapse: uterus at entrance to vagina.

penetrate into the woman's sex organs'.[1] It was believed that the uterus was an animal that responded to pleasing and fetid odours by coming forward or retracting.

Later, other techniques were tried, including manual reposition, vaginal tamponade, the wearing of utero-abdominal supporters, the insertion of pessaries (devices introduced into the vagina to support or reposition the uterus) of countless shapes, the application of astringents, cold sitz baths, seawater douches, postural exercises, and leeching. By the late nineteenth and early twentieth centuries, surgical treatment for prolapse included scarification of the vagina (making numerous superficial incisions), sewing together of the labia majora, cervical amputation, and vaginal and abdominal hysterectomy.

Hysterectomy: the imperfect solution

Today, hysterectomy is the standard treatment recommended for prolapse. Yet I find a few doctors singularly insensitive and unsympathetic to the needs of women suffering from this problem. There is a genuine lack of interest in treating these patients or discussing their sexual and hygienic problems.

Most often, prolapse occurs in women who have already had children, women whose bodies are worn by the passage of time or the strain of obesity, or women who may have chronic complaints of urinary or faecal incontinence or constipation. The male-dominated medical community has an easy answer: 'Let's cut out that uterus!' I find such a solution appalling—especially because all

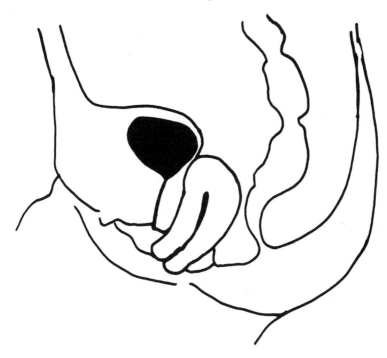

Fig. 22. Third degree of prolapse: the uterus emerges from between the labia.

women eventually may have to face these same problems—including me. Besides, the prolapsed uteri are otherwise absolutely healthy. They can be re-positioned and repaired, not removed.

When hysterectomy itself causes secondary prolapse

The uterus occupies a central position within the pelvis, holding many of the other organs in place. It is small and round, like a cup, but it is surrounded by relatively large sheets of ligaments. Once these sheets are cut or repaired during hysterectomy, inadequately suspended organs (the bladder, rectum, and vagina) may fall.

I have treated many women with prolapse after hysterectomy because the surgery did not repair the ligaments. The remaining tissue itself may have been weak. In one unusual case, Lynne's vagina was sewn directly on top of her bladder. It was not free to move about as it should, but was simply fastened there. This, as you can imagine, played havoc with Lynne's sex life. Intercourse was painful and penetration caused her to urinate immediately. Her bladder went into spasms from the trauma.

Many women experience post-hysterectomy prolapse less than two years after their surgeries. This early recurrence can mean that the hysterectomy was improperly done, the tissue didn't hold, or some other unknown factor intervened. Indeed, even if the hysterectomy is performed with excellent technique, prolapse still can occur.

The tragedy of vaginal prolapse after hysterectomy

One of the most difficult and least discussed forms of prolapse is *vaginal prolapse*. This condition decreases sexual desire and responsiveness. When the vaginal muscles are overstretched, the accompanying motion of intercourse is minimal. Because of their laxity, the muscles can no longer grasp and hold the penis tightly, or even make contact, thereby reducing you and your partner's stimulation.

In severe cases, the walls of the vagina cave in from the sides, the top, or the bottom. This blocks the tissue from moving in its normal manner during intercourse and prevents you from receiving stimulation of the clitoris or the inner part of the vagina.

Several procedures have been developed to prevent complete vaginal prolapse. In one, the vagina can be suspended from a piece of umbilical tape, which is a strip of cloth sewn onto the vagina and stretched to a band of tough, fibrous tissue lying right above the spine. You should be aware, however, that this procedure sometimes fails.[2] And, your vaginal canal, having lost its anchor, can—in the worse cases—actually fall out of your body, much like a sock that has been pulled inside out (see fig. 23).

When this happened to Eva, a 68-year-old widow, she simply could not function sexually or as a woman. The vagina is a mucous membrane, like the inside of your mouth. It must be bathed and protected by its own lubricants. When it turns inside out, it becomes dry, cracked, and irritated. It is urinated upon and is prone to infection.

This is a horrifying prospect, and one that is rarely discussed, even among women. But perhaps more horrifying is the traditional 'cure' for this condition, a cure that Eva's doctor used on her. Eva's vagina was summarily sewn closed, thus putting an abrupt end to her sex life and creating further

Fig. 23. Vaginal prolapse.

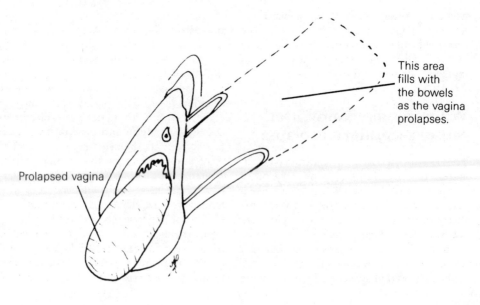

This area fills with the bowels as the vagina prolapses.

Prolapsed vagina

problems, including urinary incontinence.[3]

Eva's doctor didn't believe he was acting cruelly. He simply followed the prevailing attitude among gynaecologists. The sexual lives of elderly women who are widowed or whose spouses are ill with prostate or cardiac problems are often considered inconsequential. One study in the treatment of this problem concludes that, 'when it is no longer essential to preserve sexual function, we believe that a tightly 'coned-down' vagina of one-finger depth and diameter, rather than a total vaginectomy, should be provided . . .'[4]

What can this mean? Who is to determine when another human being has lost her sexuality? Was there not still the possibility that Eva could have met another man? Remember, this problem is a direct result of a prior hysterectomy. In my opinion, we need to keep women healthy and functioning even at 100 years of age!

The limited help of Kegel Exercises

Now I'm going to let you in on a little medical school hearsay told to me in my student years. The famous Dr Kegel was married when he supposedly had an illicit love affair with a Scandinavian beauty. As the story goes, poor Mrs Kegel had one of those lax vaginas that was singularly unstimulating, but the blond beauty knew how to tighten her vaginal muscles in order to pull on Dr Kegel's penis. What a thrill.

Ever after, Dr Kegel devoted himself to teaching women how to exercise their vaginal muscles and develop the muscles of the pelvic floor. The 'Kegel Exercises' became an institution.

The Kegel Exercises were actually suggested as a replacement for surgery in many so-called cases of prolapse. But how could

they be effective? Although the exercises may strengthen the pelvis and vaginal vault, surgical reconstruction is necessary for women with severe tissue damage and prolapse. Many women require hormone replacement.

In fact, women with these conditions often feel like failures when they do the exercises to no avail. Some contract and release 200 times a day, and still suffer from urinary incontinence and constipation. Their doctors may accuse them of neglecting their exercises and label them frigid, implying that they really didn't want to improve their sexual responsiveness.

In truth, there may be little relationship between muscle strength and orgasmic ability.[5] And all the Kegels in the world can't raise a completely fallen bladder or put your uterus back in its proper place. Severe prolapse requires correction—FRS.

How female reconstruction surgery corrects prolapse

FRS restructures all of the ligaments and organs in your pelvic cavity and lifts them, with complete resuspension and correction of the prolapse. FRS can be used on all degrees of the condition, without the usual residual side effects of hysterectomy. The major benefits of FRS over hysterectomy in the case of prolapse are:

- You experience no loss of the vaginal vault.
- There is no shortening and no impediment to normal sexual relations.
- All organs remain in the body so that your normal menstrual cycling and hormone functions continue.
- Hospitalization and post-operative recovery time are markedly shorter due to the delicacy of reconstructive surgery versus hysterectomy. You can resume

normal activities and return to work usually within four to six days.

You should bear in mind, however, that if the prolapse is quite severe, FRS may not be able to achieve a 100 per cent restoration. Sometimes the correction of prolapse is 80 per cent successful. And, there are few guarantees in life. Prolapse can recur after FRS and all women consenting to have this procedure should be told that prolapse of the uterus and other organs may re-occur after any surgical procedure to correct or improve the original condition.

New surgeries for vaginal prolapse

I feel great empathy for the post-hysterectomy patient suffering from vaginal prolapse. Because I am so upset with the prospect of sewing closed the vagina, I am working to develop new ways to correct this problem. I believe it possible to create an artificial pelvic floor or diaphragm by fashioning synthetic materials to reapproximate the lost ligaments and fascia within the pelvis. The vagina can be sewn onto material in the proper place, as can the other pelvic organs like the bladder and the rectum. If this surgery is successful, it may save many women from the horror of sewing closed the vagina.

A word about the 'tipped' or 'tilted' uterus

You may have a mild degree of *retroflection* or *retroversion* when your uterus tilts backward into the rectum. If severe, it may cause you to experience a dull pain that radiates to your back and intensifies with your period.

FRS can change the position of your uterus, relieving all symptoms and avoiding the loss of your organs. You may have been frightened by a statement like, 'your uterus is so tilted, you'll never get pregnant'. This simply is not true. Having a tilted uterus is normal and rarely causes problems. But if difficulties do exist, they can be resolved. Each case is individual. If there is pain, the uterus can be lifted, without sacrificing it.

Why does prolapse occur?

Many theories have been advanced as to why some women suffer from this condition. In the nineteenth century, some doctors blamed 'singing, dancing, riding on horseback, and skating',[6] for prolapse as well as sexual abuse and tight lacings! We now know otherwise.

Pregnancy

It is thought that in the majority of cases, prolapse results from pregnancy and childbirth. When your uterus and surrounding support tissues expand to accommodate pregnancy and delivery, they may lose their ability to contract back to their normal position and elasticity.

Muscle tissue normally has the flexibility needed for this expansion and contraction. Sometimes, during the process of labour, the muscle tissue in the vagina and perineum is torn. Non-muscle tissue, like the ligaments and fascia, may not have the resiliency needed to return to the normal position or shape.

I have seen severe prolapse and loss of tissue integrity in women who have given birth to ten or twelve children. Many never received adequate obstetrical care; these women often suffer from internal tearing and other birth problems that destroy the integrity of their pelvic configuration. In addition, the walls of the vagina collapse on themselves and the vaginal tissue is toneless and flabby. Weak tissue, after being chronically damaged, is easily injured, doesn't heal properly, and can become infected. Such tissue is difficult to repair and may not hold.

Obesity

Marian was 5'3" and weighed 220 pounds. She suffered from severe prolapse, as do many obese women. The effects of poor nutrition are evident throughout the bodies of overweight women. Their tissue is not fed with adequate blood supply or nutrients, resulting in a loss of tissue integrity surrounding the female organs. Marion's tissue lacked resiliency and was characteristically unhealthy.

You may think that fat exists only on the outer, visible areas of your body. In reality, however, we all have protective areas of yellow fat inside our bodies. This is part of the *omentum*, a double fold of fat-containing membrane which covers the intestines, surrounding them on each side.

Marion had enormous amounts of internal fat. The omentum and the *pendulous*—an external overlay of fat, like an extra organ hanging from the abdomen—pushed directly on the pelvic area, pressing down her uterus and other female organs and structures. The weight of the fat can also exert pressure on the bowels, pushing the intestines deeper into the pelvis, slowing normal bowel function.

The constant pressure is like a perpetual pregnancy bearing down on the organs. It tears tissues and damages elasticity. Unhealthy tissue, along with the lack of muscle tone and the weight of the fat, took its toll on Marion's pelvic organs, eventually causing prolapse.

Hormone deprivation

The tissue of the female system—the mucosa, fascia, and muscles—may atrophy for some women who eschew hormone replacement during menopause. Losing strength and elasticity, the ligaments, fascia, and mucosal tissue become thin, stretched, and weakened. Prolapse can result. The obvious solution to this problem is the maintenance of adequate hormone levels after menopause, a good diet, and exercise.

Fibroid tumours

The constant weight and mass of a fibroid growing in the uterus can stretch out the musculature of the uterus and surrounding ligamentous tissues, putting pressure on all of the female organs, and directing everything toward the angle in which the tumour is growing.[7] In fact, I have seen fibroids leave an impression or mould of their shape on the bladder and rectum, and the spine create an impression on a fibroid.

A large fibroid in the front of Loretta's uterus, for example, caused multiple problems. The growth pushed down the uterus and the vaginal wall, stretching and extruding them outward. The fibroid exerted direct pressure on her bladder, chronically stretching its tissues, making them flaccid. This created urinary incontinence. Eventually, the bladder also fell.

In such a complex case, the removal of the fibroid alone will not correct the problem. During surgery, I had to bring the uterus back out of the vagina and reinstate the bladder to its normal position. The permutations of this type of problem are endless, given the random placement of fibroid growths within the uterus.

Other speculations

Although doctors are taught that prolapse is most often caused by childbirth, in my practice I have encountered women suffering from this condition who have never been pregnant. Neither obesity nor fibroids were in evidence. In such cases, I surmise the passage of time, hormone deprivation, the long-term effects of gravity (after all, we are the only species that spends much of its life in an erect state), and perhaps a genetic predisposition to having less collagen and elastin in the tissue are to blame.

Complicating factors

Sometimes prolapse occurs in conjunction with other female problems (I mentioned fibroids earlier), which makes diagnosis a careful stripping away of symptom after symptom. I think it is well worth the time and effort to save a woman's uterus, even when the presentation is complex.

In one such case, Marilyn, a 33-year-old woman, drove in to see me from Phoenix. She had heard of the surgery I performed. Marilyn was the mother of three children. Shortly before she came to my office, a profound tragedy had struck her life: her husband and children had been killed in a car accident.

Despite her tragic loss, however, this courageous woman displayed a strong will and youthful outlook. She had managed to pull herself together and, to her credit, continued to look upon life as a positive experience. She was determined to put aside the tragedy and create some happiness for herself.

That effort was being disrupted, however, by female problems. Marilyn had been experiencing heavy, irregular bleeding and pain in her pelvic area for some time. Her gynaecologist told her that this was caused by her fallen uterus—the result of her pregnancies. He had scheduled Marilyn for a hysterectomy.

This doctor had not placed Marilyn on hormone therapy or any other medical treatment. He never even suggested a D & C to diagnose the possible reasons for the excessive bleeding. There had been no discussion of fixing the prolapse of her uterus. Marilyn was still devastated from her incredible loss and was now facing hysterectomy as a 'cure' for her physical difficulties.

When I completed my physical examination, I noted that Marilyn's uterus had fallen. I could feel that her uterus was pushing back toward her rectum and because of the stretching of the ligaments, that position had created the pain and discomfort. As for the abnormal bleeding, I thought that with Marilyn's recent history of severe emotional stress it was possible that her hormones were not cycling in the normal manner.

I performed an extensive hormone evaluation and D & C and found that Marilyn wasn't ovulating normally. She skipped cycles and then bled heavily. I had to find out what was going on inside her body. During FRS I discovered that her uterus was normal (except for the position, back deep in the pelvis) and her fallopian tubes were healthy.

The ovaries, however, were abnormal. Functional cysts had formed, causing them to enlarge and become heavy. With their extra weight and the space created by the prolapsed uterus, the ovaries had fallen onto the back of Marilyn's vagina, creating the pain in her back and deep within the vaginal vault.

I drained the cysts and then resuspended the ovaries. Next, I repositioned Marilyn's fallen uterus off the pelvic bone and pushed the rectum back into its midline position. I reconstructed all the ligaments in order to get the organs back in place.

On Marilyn's post-operative visit, I was pleased to see that the prolapse had been eliminated. I placed her on hormone therapy for a few months to regulate her cycles until she was in a more stable situation and under less stress, at which time her own hormones could kick in. I also emphasized the importance of good nutrition.

With one operation, Marilyn's problems were reversed. She retained her ability to have children as well as to function normally. Her hospitalization lasted only three days. Yet this woman had been told her only alternative was hysterectomy. What if Marilyn had taken the advice of her original gynaecologist? Any man in her future would have found her unable to have a family. And she would suffer the lifelong consequences that hysterectomy can bring.

Marilyn's case is instructive. Prolapse is a difficult problem. Yet alternatives to hysterectomy can be found if we actively seek them out. No woman should face the certainty of hysterectomy when the diagnosis is prolapse.

CHAPTER 12

Cervical cancer

What is cervical cancer?

Your skin is a living organism. Every day it sheds dead cells while new cells are being produced. This is a perpetual process. The same holds true for the cells of the uterus and cervix; they are in a constant state of flux.

Cervical cancer is the abnormal growth of cells of the cervix. These abnormalities usually are first apparent in the endocervix —the narrow canal that leads from inside the uterus out to the vagina (see fig. 24). The endocervical canal is particularly vulnerable to cancer because it is an area of cellular transition and constant change.

What constitutes this change? The cells lining your uterus are called *cuboidal*. They make up the glands of the endometrium and shed every month. These cells have a different structure than those covering the cervix. The cervical cells are *squamous* and are similar to the cells of your skin (see fig. 25). The endocervical canal is the point at which the two cell types meet. Here, cuboidal cells actually transform into squamous cells. The intense cellular activity leaves this area susceptible to abnormalities.

The progression from abnormal cells to cancer

Cancer is often diagnosed when abnormal changes occur in the surface cells (*epi-*

thelium) of this transition zone. Early cell abnormalities may not cause symptoms. Over time, cervical cells may undergo a series of changes from normal to cervical dysplasia to carcinoma in situ to invasive cancer.

Cervical Dysplasia. Cervical dysplasia is an early form of cell abnormality that occurs most often in women between the ages of 25 and 35, although it has been found in some women in their late teens. Dysplasia refers to microscopic changes in the cells of the cervical epithelium. These rarely cause symptoms and *may or may not* become cancerous. In some women, however, the dysplasia goes through a series of permu-

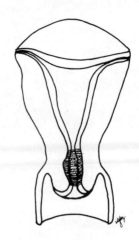

Fig. 24. Endocervical canal: the transition zone.

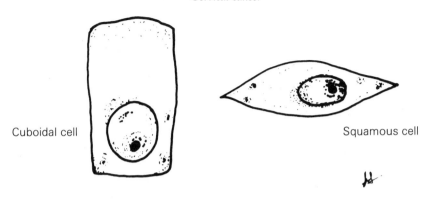

Cuboidal cell

Squamous cell

Fig. 25. Squamous and cuboidal cells.

tations that can then develop into cancer if left untreated.

In the past, we were correct in saying that cervical cancer is a slow-growing cancer: it could take twenty years for cells to make the changes from dysplasia to invasive cancer. The disease was found primarily in older women. In the last decade, however, with the dramatic changes in our society's sexual habits, the age at which women have been diagnosed as having dysplasia is much younger than we were accustomed to seeing previously. Indeed, the cellular changes from dysplasia to invasive carcinoma in these women take place with alarming rapidity.

Carcinoma In Situ (CIS). Non-invasive cervical cancer or carcinoma in situ (CIS) develops most often in women between the ages of 30 and 40. The growth of cancer cells involves only the top layer of the epithelium —the layer above the 'basement membrane'. It seldom causes symptoms and is almost 100 per cent curable if treatment is started at the time of diagnosis.

Carcinoma in situ (CIS) means that abnormal cells have not invaded beneath the surface epithelium of the cervix. Left unchecked, it may take from three to fifteen years for CIS to become 'invasive'. The American Cancer Society estimates that in 1987, 45,000 new cases of in situ carcinoma will have been diagnosed, as opposed to 13,000 cases of invasive cancer. Early detection and treatment of CIS are absolutely essential to preventing its spread.

Invasive Cancer. Invasive cancer is diagnosed when cancer cells grow into the deeper layers of the cervix. The cancer crosses the 'basement membrane' where it comes in contact with blood vessels and the lymphatic system. This form of cervical cancer occurs most often in women between the ages of 40 and 60, although 25 per cent of all cases occur in women over 65. Some cervical cancer can be very aggressive, becoming invasive and spreading rapidly, especially in younger women. The National Cancer Institute estimates that in 1987 there were 12,800 new cases of invasive cervical cancer and 6,800 deaths from this disease in the United States.

What are the symptoms of cervical cancer?

Cervical dysplasia and CIS may have no symptoms at all. *Pain is not an early sign of cervical cancer.* There may be bleeding only when the disease has begun to destroy the tissue of your cervix. Early symptoms may be absent. However, the most common symptoms—if they do occur—are:

- Bleeding between menstrual periods
- Bleeding after menopause
- Bleeding after intercourse
- Bleeding after a pelvic examination or douching
- Increased, unusual, or foul-smelling vaginal discharge

These symptoms may occur with other, less serious ailments, but you should not ignore them. Consider them reminders to see your doctor at once. Untreated invasive cervical cancer will continue to grow and may spread to other parts of your body.

Diagnosing cancer—the importance of a yearly Pap smear

Because there are few warning signs of cervical cancer, early detection of this disease through regular screening is most important. Papanicolaou (Pap) smears (also known as cervical smears) have done more to save women's lives in the last fifty years than any other screening programme. The test is quick, relatively inexpensive, and painless. It is 95 per cent accurate in detecting changes in the cervix long before cell abnormalities advance to cancer.

Named after George Papanicolaou, the doctor who developed it, the Pap smear consists of the gentle scraping of cells normally shed from your cervix and uterus. A sample of tissue is taken from the cervical canal (because of its vulnerability) as well as the surface of the cervix. The tissue is spread on slides and analyzed under a microscope in the lab.

Understanding your cervical smear test

In order to participate actively with your doctor in choices made for your continuing health care, you should have a basic understanding of the terminology on your cervical smear. In that way, you'll be able to ask intelligent questions about your condition. And you will have some insight into whether or not your situation warrants a hysterectomy or other more conservative treatments. *All abnormal cervical smears need further investigation, either by repeat cervical smears, re-evaluation from a different laboratory, or further medical observation and tests.*

When you read your test results, you may find different designations for your condition. As scientists learned more about cervical cancer, they found their original classification system inadequate to identify all the gradations of change. Now there are two distinct classification systems for cell irregularities. These parallel systems may cause some confusion for patients. But both systems are based on the understanding that cells taken from your cervix fall into a continuum ranging from normal to malignant.

The 'class' system

The 'class' system is used to name the *kind* of cells found in your cervix. There are five major classifications, from normal cells to invasive carcinoma.

Class I: Normal smear; no abnormal cells
Class II: Atypical cells present, but no cancer

Class III: Abnormal cells showing mild to moderate dysplasia

Class IV: Abnormal cells showing severe dysplasia; includes carcinoma in situ

Class V: Invasive carcinoma

The 'CIN' system

CIN is an abbreviation for *cervical intraepithelial neoplasia*. *Intraepithelial* means within or among the epithelial cells. *Neoplasia* literally means the formation and growth of 'new' tissue. *Differentiation* in the diagnosis refers to the structure of the cells themselves. As the cells change, their components, like the nucleus, look more abnormal. They lose their typical appearance of 'differentiation'. The less well-differentiated the cells, the worse the prognosis (see fig. 26).

You will be able to determine, from your CIN screening, how deeply the abnormal cells have invaded the epithelium. Here are the medical terms you might find:

CIN 1: Mild dysplasia. A well-differentiated lesion. Abnormal cells occupy the lower third of the epithelial tissue.

CIN 2: Moderate dysplasia. Less well-differentiated lesion. Abnormal cells occupy the lower two-thirds of the epithelial tissue.

CIN 3: Undifferentiated intraepithelial lesion.

With a diagnosis of CIN 3, you may strongly suspect cancer in situ. Abnormal cells occupy the entire epithelium.

With a Class III cervical smear, it is possible to have a CIN 1 assessment: abnormal cells exist, but the depth of invasion is mild. And conversely, a reading of CIN 2 could mean inflammation—not cancer—that affects the epithelium to some depth. If these symptoms have not been adequately explained to you, you might believe that you have invasive cancer, when your tissue is showing only irregular cells.

Should your report read *koilocytotic atypia*, it means you probably have venereal warts. These flat warts are often invisible to the naked eye, but are detected with a cervical smear and by other microscopic investigations like colposcopy and biopsy. As many as 80 per cent of diagnosed mild dysplasias are actually cases of flat venereal warts. I will explain the significance of venereal warts later in this chapter.

How often should I have a Cervical smear?

The current (1980) American Cancer Society guidelines for cervical cancer recom-

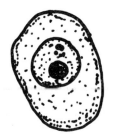 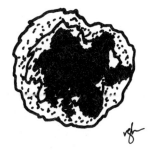

Fig. 26. Well-differentiated cell and an undifferentiated cell.

mend that smears need to be performed only once every three years in low-risk women. Their reasoning is based upon the slow-growing nature of cervical cancer. I disagree. Although it may take up to twenty years for malignant cells to appear, I think it best to diagnose abnormalities as soon as possible in order to take action that will halt malignant transformations. This is especially true because some forms of cervical cancer are fast growing. One of my patients had a normal smear and a perfectly normal-appearing cervix. One year later, however, I found invasive cancer on her routine examination. In the UK women over 35 years can obtain a cervical smear test every 5 years. If a woman is worried, however, or has reason to believe she has been at risk, the test can be done more often and the doctor will still be reimbursed.

False-negative results to the smear can mislead you into thinking that there is no cause for worry. Yet in a study of nearly a million smear test samples, it was found that 20 per cent of the study patients in whom invasive cervical cancer later developed had had at least two negative smear tests within three years of the cancer diagnosis.[1]

Why is this so? Either the cancer was of the rapid onset type, or the analysis of the original smears was inaccurate. *The Wall Street Journal* recently reported that many labs that perform smears are overworked[2] and similar incidences have been reported in the UK. If the volume is excessive, too many slides are examined per hour, and the cancer can be missed. California is the only state in the US which by law limits the number of slides a lab can examine per hour. The potential for failure in the system renders yearly examinations and re-evaluation mandatory.

The American College of Obstetricians and Gynecologists recommends that all women should have an annual examination.

Women at higher risk should have cervical smears more often. If you have had atypical cells, dysplasia, exposure to herpes, chlamydia or venereal warts, and/or numerous sex partners, especially partners with sexually transmitted disease, you must allow your gynaecologist to keep a close watch on potential changes in the cells of your cervix. I suggest smear tests every six to twelve months, and more often when irregularities are found.

When can I stop having a cervical smear?

Never, as far as I'm concerned. Forty-one per cent of all cervical cancer deaths occur in the age group of 65 and older. Surprisingly, elderly women are the least served by this test. Nearly half have never had a cervical smear:[3] they may have left their child-bearing years just as the test was introduced, they may have stopped seeking gynaecological care after menopause, or they may think they don't need it because they are no longer having sex. Are you one of this group? Is your mother?

The American Cancer Society suggests regular smears for women between the ages of 20 and 65 only. However, that recommendation is based on the assumption that a woman of 65 would have had many prior screenings during her lifetime.[4] Clearly, this assumption can be dangerous. Don't let the medical establishment abandon you and don't abandon it.

If you are over 65 and no longer consulting a gynaecologist, your family doctor can perform the test. Some cervical cancers are more aggressive in older women than in younger women, progressing from non-invasive to invasive stages as much as four times faster.

Even if you'd had a prior hysterectomy,

you should undergo yearly cervical smears. Your cervix may still be intact if you've had a partial hysterectomy. And hysterectomy does not protect you against other cancers. If you've had a hysterectomy for cervical cancer, there is a 1 per cent risk that cancer will reappear in your vagina.[5] Women who never get checked after hysterectomy run an unnecessary risk. The cervical smear is a lifesaver and it also brings you into the doctor's office to be checked for other problems such as breast or vulvar cancer.

If I have an abnormal cervical smear, must I have a hysterectomy?

That's an important and complex question. I will be answering it throughout this chapter. You may have been told that you have 'a premalignancy', 'a touch of cancer', or 'the beginnings of cancer'. And, indeed, the changes in your cervix may one day lead to cancer. This is frightening. If your cervical smear is abnormal, however, what you need *first* is an accurate diagnosis.

Whether or not you need a hysterectomy depends on the causes of the irregularities and how advanced they are when discovered. Earlier lesions (pathological changes in tissue) are, on average, smaller than the more advanced lesions and, consequently, are easier to treat without hysterectomy.

In addition, make sure to seek a second opinion if your report shows abnormal cells. Laboratories do make errors. Many cases of 'mild cervical dysplasia' are reclassified as venereal warts when re-evaluated.[6] I routinely have repeat cervical smears sent to labs that specialize in cervical cancer. It takes less than a week to receive confirmation of cell irregularities before undertaking surgery.

If you have venereal warts, dysplasia, or CIS, many treatments are available to help arrest the cell changes. *If you have invasive cervical cancer, a radical hysterectomy is required. It may save your life.*

What's next, if my cervical smear is atypical or abnormal?

Your gynaecologist has many tests available to determine exactly what the problem is and how to treat it if your cervical smear report shows some atypical or pre-cancerous cells. Hysterectomy should be *last* on the list.

Culturing for infection

Minor abnormalities in your cervical cells can be caused by inflammation from untreated chronic infections like herpes, chlamydia, gardinerella, trichomoniasis, or yeast. Routinely, on abnormal smears, I take samples of tissue and 'culture' (grow) the cells in my lab, in order to detect infection. Often, the vagina and cervix have been chronically infected and irritated by several organisms at once. These infections can produce cellular irregularities that mimic more serious disorders.

Conversely, sometimes an inflammation caused by infection can mask an underlying carcinoma.[7] This may present a dangerous situation, because the cancer can continue to grow without detection. Such was the case for Helen. She assumed that her Class II smear result merely meant that she had an infection. The dysplastic cells were not treated until she had invasive cancer. Her life was saved by a radical hysterectomy.

If your smear shows Class II, III, or IV cells, you should discuss with your gynaecologist the option of having a workup done for sexually transmitted disease, including venereal warts. It may save you grief and a possible hysterectomy in the future.

Has there been trauma?

When I get an abnormal smear result, I also look for 'mechanical' problems. I've seen abrasions and lesions on the cervix from:

● IUD strings
● Cervical caps
● Cervical sponges
● Diaphragms
● Tampons

When such problems are apparent, I ask my patients to avoid further irritation to the cervix.

Looking at your cervix

During your routine pelvic examination, your doctor can look directly at your vagina and cervix. If, from this visual inspection, or your smear report (s)he detects an abnormality, (s)he may stain the tissue using iodine and/or acetic acid (diluted plain white vinegar) and may remove or biopsy a tiny amount of tissue for microscopic examination. This can cause some minor pain and may be followed by a small amount of bleeding. These discomforts can be controlled with a local anaesthetic and anti-prostaglandins.

A *colposcope*, an instrument that magnifies the surface of the vagina and cervix, can pinpoint suspicious areas for biopsy. It is an excellent tool in helping to diagnose flat venereal warts and cancerous changes.

During colposcopy, your cervix is coated with vinegar. The solution draws out mucus

and accentuates the rough surface and vascular pattern changes that are found in neoplasia. This helps your gynaecologist differentiate between normal and abnormal tissue and aids in taking a biopsy, because (s)he can see what is abnormal and sample it. The biopsy is then sent to a pathologist for microscopic analysis.

Treatments for non-invasive changes in cervical cells

As with diagnostic procedures, many treatments are available for non-invasive changes in your cervical cells. The treatment that your gynaecologist chooses may depend on the depth and location of involvement and the surgical tools he or she has available.

Cryosurgery

Cryosurgery is the freezing of tissue, and it is frequently used to treat cervical dysplasia (CIN 1 and CIN 2). The dysplastic cells are literally frozen to death. I prefer to use laser surgery.

Laser surgery for dysplasia

Depending on the depth of invasion and your surgeon's ability to see the lesion, (s)he may be able to use laser surgery to vaporize the irregular cells in CIN. I scrape the endocervical canal (*endocervical curettage*) and biopsy for diagnosis and then use laser surgery to destroy the CIN leaving the cervix intact. Laser surgery's advantages are numerous:

● Your surgeon has constant visual control of the extent and depth of surgical destruction of abnormal areas.

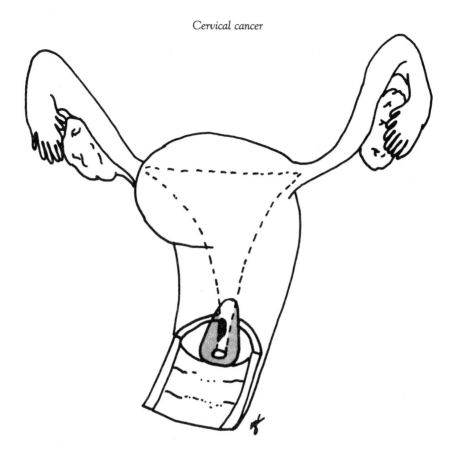

Fig. 27. Conization can eradicate in situ cancer.

- Surgery is more precise.
- You lose little blood.
- Your endocervical canal is preserved.
- You heal rapidly.
- You may feel virtually no pain.
- The discharge after laser is not troublesome.

Laser gives excellent post-operative results. Complete healing occurs within six weeks and the cure rate is 80 to 90 per cent for dysplasia and venereal warts. [8] You will need follow-up examinations because laser's cure rate is not 100 per cent.

Conization or cone biopsy to diagnose and treat CIS

A *cone biopsy* or *conization* is performed if your doctor suspects carcinoma in situ or especially to rule out possible invasive cancer. In this procedure, a cone-shaped chunk of tissue is removed from your cervix. Your surgeon will try to take all of the abnormal tissue and the surrounding healthy tissue, called the *margins*. In many cases, conization can completely eradicate in situ cancer (see fig. 27).

The success of a cone biopsy rests on your

surgeon's technical skill in excising the lesion's perimeters and on your ability to heal. If too much tissue is destroyed or if your tissue doesn't heal well, the cervix may no longer be able to sustain a pregnancy (*incompetent cervix*) or it can be scarred closed (*stenotic cervix*).

I prefer cone biopsy for CIS using laser

Cone biopsy with the laser is a relatively new treatment that has been highly successful.[9] The laser beam acts like a knife, cutting out the abnormal tissue. If a 'cold-knife' conization is absolutely necessary for diagnostic purposes, I have used the laser to heal the edges of the incision. I do this after taking the tissue sample and making sure that the margins are cancer-free. Laser technology has improved the outcome dramatically, leaving healthy cervices that are capable of sustaining pregnancies.

Despite the fact that all of these successful alternative treatments exist, total abdominal hysterectomy is the most commonly used form of treatment for carcinoma in situ.[10] Perhaps one day this will change, as lasers become more available and women learn more about their bodies.

Follow-up treatments are crucial

Treatment with antibiotics (for infections) and cryosurgery, cone biopsy, or laser (for venereal warts, dysplasia, and CIS) often return the cells to normal. But close follow-up is still necessary because the cell abnormalities do recur in a small number of cases.

In my own practice, I have seen women who have refused examinations and follow-up care for abnormal findings. Karen's

screenings went from CIN 3 to CIN 1 after antibiotic treatment for bacterial infections. Insisting that nothing was wrong, she refused further studies and a biopsy.

Such a non-compliant attitude is dangerous and can lead to invasive disease and a hysterectomy in the future. Many of my medical school professors reinforced a 'take it all out' approach for difficult patients like Karen as a means of protecting them. This belief is commonly held today. But, what's worse is the fact that some women *are* noncompliant, simply refusing to follow preventive measures. You must be responsible. Follow-up is important for all women and should include repeat cervical smears, endocervical curettage, repeat culturings, biopsy, and a possible D & C. Denial of problems can be deadly in the long run.

Follow-up D & C and Endocervical Curettage. If dysplasia was previously suspected but infection found, or if you are reinfected repeatedly over a long period of time by your partner(s), your gynaecologist should perform an endocervical curettage, colposcopy with biopsies, and a possible D & C no later than three months following a normal cervical smear. The D & C or hysteroscopy would make doubly sure that abnormal cells hadn't invaded higher up in the uterus where they weren't detected earlier (see fig. 28).

If you have dysplasia or CIS, you should have a repeat cervical smear three to four months following the conization or laser surgery. This wait is necessary because the cells of your cervix will be repairing themselves for several months following treatment. With all of the old tissue shedding, it is common to receive a falsepositive smear evaluation before this time.[11]

Sharon's so-called cancer was remedied using antibiotics, but she refused the followup biopsy and D & C. We wrote, explaining

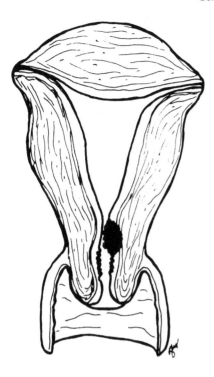

Fig. 28. Invasive cancer high in the cervical canal may require a D & C, endocervical curettage, or hysteroscopy for detection.

provide these for yourself, and thus your body is working harder with less support. Stressful situations may weaken the immune system and allow abnormal cells to be created and to proliferate. The cervix has been shown to respond to deficiencies of:

- Vitamin A
- Vitamin C in conjunction with folic acid (which plays a key role in the maturation and differentiation of cells)
- Vitamin E [12]

As part of normal follow-up treatment, I correct vitamin and mineral deficiencies with both oral medications and topical vaginal applications, especially after laser surgery for CIN and CIS. However, I do not advocate megavitamin therapy. In *Fit For Life* by Harvey and Marilyn Diamond, I was quoted as saying the overuse and abuse of vitamins can result in toxic reactions.

Hysterectomy is the answer for invasive cancer

Many women with carcinoma in situ are cured with cone biopsy and regular follow-up care. [13] Remember, this is not invasive cancer. If antibiotics, vitamins, laser cone, and other preparations fail to arrest the formation of abnormal cells, however, you should proceed with a hysterectomy.

Invasive Cervical Cancer Requires a Hysterectomy. This is a terrible disease that should be treated immediately. There are no options. Hysterectomy can save your life. If you have cervical cancer, it is possible that your ovaries can be preserved. There is no direct correlation between cervical cancer and ovarian cancer. If the original cancer has reached the ovaries, however, everything must come out.

her risk and urging her to come in to be re-checked, but she refused. She only wanted to hear that she didn't need a hysterectomy. She didn't want any surgery. Sharon's new doctor, after doing a cervical smear and getting a normal reading, did not believe that this woman had ever had a diagnosis of carcinoma in situ. A cancer higher up in the canal could be missed by the cervical smear and a follow-up D & C would have been reassuring.

Vitamins and Nutrition as Part of Your Follow-up Care. When you undergo stress, you need more nutrients. You may neglect to

Creating a surgical team

Should you have invasive cervical cancer, I highly recommend seeking out a gynae-cological oncologist to work with your gynaecologist. An oncologist is trained in the treatment of female cancers, whereas your gynaecologist has both your medical history and a rapport with you. That's the best of both worlds.

The risk factors

Now that you know the facts about what cervical cancer is and how it is detected and treated, you may be curious about its genesis. What are your risks for developing this disease? Of course, the origins of cervical cancer are complex, and not easily reduced to a simple cause and effect. Yet you may be surprised to discover that new research links sexual activity and cervical cancer.

Cervical cancer is probably a venereal disease

Startling research has brought to light information that strongly suggests a con-nection between sexual activity and cervical cancer. This disease may be the result of the interaction of many different external factors, together with venereal warts and the susceptibility of the cervix at certain times in your life.[14]

Venereal warts (Condyloma acuminatum)

If you recall, I mentioned earlier that venereal warts could show up on your cervical smear report. Warts, in general, are called *human papillomavirus* (HPV). There

are at least 46 different wart viruses that affect humans. Two of the viruses, HPV-16, and -18, are most often associated with cervical cancer. *The warts are sexually trans-missible.* In other words, they pass between men and women during intercourse. And they are quite common.

Men carry the warts on and inside the penis, in the urethra and bladder. The wart within the penis may be invisible, yet at the time of ejaculation the wart viruses can be passed into the vagina via sperm. Studies have shown an increased risk for cervical cancer in women whose sexual partners have penile venereal warts.[15]

You may not be aware of these warts, especially if they are on your cervix. They can be shaped like tiny cauliflowers or they can be flat. Many cervical abnormalities, including abnormal smear results and cervical cancer, are strongly associated with venereal warts. Although it's still too early to make a definitive statement, research has shown that the atypical cells seen in cases of venereal warts have been associated with cell abnormalities and carcinoma in a significant number of patients.[16]

The existence of these viruses has been the cause of many a mis-diagnosis. Errors occur because the wart infection causes abnormal-ities in the superficial cells of the cervix. Upon occasion the warts penetrate deeper into glandular cells, mimicking more serious, invasive forms of dysplasia and cancer.[17]

Despite the fact that the HPV infection is biologically distinct from cervical neoplasia, abundant evidence from many recent studies indicates that it may develop into that disease. HPV-16 and -18 are found most exclusively in severe dysplasia, carcinoma in situ, and invasive carcinoma. Scientists are now finding DNA from these two viruses within invasive tumours of the cervix.

It is still unclear just how venereal warts interrelate with the cervical tissue to create cancer. Many possibilities have been suggested. What *is* clear, however, is that the venereal wart virus is related to cervical cancer.[18] In the past these warts were treated as an inconvenience rather than as a potential cause for cancer in women. They should be taken seriously by your gynaecologist and your partner(s). In performing a colposcopy for an abnormal cervical smear, your gynaecologist should actively look for venereal wart lesions.

Treatments for venereal warts

If you have venereal warts, laser surgery is an excellent treatment. After the warts have been vaporized and the cervix has healed, I usually prescribe medications to be used directly on the cervix; *5-fluorouracil* cream (5-FU cream) is an effective drug. It weakens the bonds between the abnormal cells so that they can slough off. This 5-FU cream can be used in a maintenance programme to help stop abnormal changes on a cellular level, and may reduce the risk of future growths.[19]

Because of the danger of cancerous changes, you should be followed regularly with repeat smear tests and colposcopy to make sure that the warts do not recur. And your partner(s) need to be thoroughly examined (this may include *cystoscopy*, a look into the urethra and bladder) and treated. Otherwise you may re-infect each other.

Other sexual connections

In most cases, we do know that sexual intercourse is somehow related to the incidence of cervical cancer. Virgins almost never develop the disease, whereas all women who are sexually active are at some risk. Different answers have been sought to explain this.

Women who began having sexual intercourse before the age of 18 as do those who have numerous sex partners have a higher incidence of cervical cancer. In the United States and the United Kingdom, there has been a dramatic rise—up to 100 per cent—in carcinoma in situ in women aged 15 to 35. Alarmingly, significant numbers of younger women have been found to have invasive disease at the time of diagnosis (without a long pre-invasive phase) despite a recent benign smear. Women whose cell abnormalities are associated with venereal warts tend to be younger than women whose problems arise from other sources.[20] This is probably due to their increased sexual exposure.

In addition, there is a threefold increase in cervical cancer in second marriages where the husbands' previous wives also had the disease. Epidemiological studies also show a higher incidence of cervical cancer in wives of penile cancer patients. Some suggest that penile and cervical cancer have a common origin.[21] If your partner falls into one of these categories, he should be checked and you should opt for more frequent smear tests as a precaution.

Promiscuous male partners increase the risk as well. I had been treating Mary with antibiotics for months to arrest a dangerous infection, to no avail. She insisted that she remained faithful to her husband. We found out later, however, that he had had several affairs. He blithely continued to re-infect his wife. Any medical treatment would have proven useless against his habits. Mary has since left him.

Surprisingly, sperm has also been proposed as a factor.[22] Each sperm contains potent agents that can literally eat through cell walls. This is natural, because in order for fertilization to occur, the sperm needs the ability to break into the egg's nucleus, to contribute the male's vital DNA material to the female's.

These agents also have the capacity to split RNA and DNA, the proteins that contribute to the genetic code of each cell. Once the RNA and DNA are split, they can recombine to form new particles of genetic information. We don't have the answers yet, but it seems that the proteins may recombine with the virus in the cells or carry virus particles into the cells to create precancerous lesions.

Sperm might also become a source of cellular mutation, not because of its own qualities, but because at certain times in your life—early adolescence and first pregnancy—the tissue of the cervix is more susceptible to agents that cause mutation. This may help to explain why women who have been promiscuous at an early age are more likely to develop cervical cancer. To protect against sperm, venereal warts, and other infections, you should use latex condoms.

Complex infections

I believe that venereal warts, co-existing with other infections, such as herpes, mycoplasma, and ureaplasma, are contributors to cervical dysplasia. Let's take a look at some of these other infections.

Herpes Simplex Virus-Type 2 (HSV-2). The incidence of herpes has reached epidemic proportions in the United States. The number of visits to private doctors for genital herpes has risen from 30,000 in 1966 to 295,000 in 1981.[23] It is estimated that more than 20 million people have the disease. Herpes infections can be insidious. You may shed the virus even if you don't have symptoms. Lesions on the cervix may go unnoticed.

Since 1968, Herpes Simplex Virus-Type 2 (HSV-2) has been associated with cervical cancer. In some studies, over 90 per cent of women with invasive carcinoma were found to carry HSV-2 antibodies. And women with HSV-2 antibodies have a higher incidence of cervical dysplasia, carcinoma in situ, and invasive cancer. Herpes virus DNA has been found in malignant cells.[24] Genital herpes is thought to be a catalyst for the cancerous changes seen with venereal warts.[24]

Mycoplasma, Ureaplasma, and Chlamydia. Norma came to see me, complaining of chronic pelvic pain and discharge. Her problem had been diagnosed as a 'stubborn' yeast infection that would not clear up even after many months of medication. Because her cervical smear was abnormal, she had been scheduled for a hysterectomy. I decided further tests were necessary, so I obtained a cervical culture. What I found was that Norma had a severe chlamydia infection.

Mycoplasma, ureaplasma, and chlamydia are bacteria that act like viruses. They can cause pelvic inflammatory disease and sterility. These bacteria are unusual in that they don't live on the cell wall but actually live within the cell. This is probably how they trigger the abnormalities seen in cervical cells on the cervical smear.

These infections are passed between men and women like ping-pong balls. In fact, they are so prevalent that 40 to 50 per cent of the population carry them. If you have one of these infections, you may have *no symptoms* at all or you may experience:

● Abnormal smear test results
● Thick discharge
● Itching and irritation
● Bladder or urethral pain

- Pain in the vagina, cervix, uterus, tubes, and/or ovaries

Men can be asymptomatic or have non-specific urethritis and prostatitis, which produce pain on urination and defecation.

Because these agents live in the cells of your tissue, special laboratory procedures are required to grow and identify them. And, because they cause inflammation, your cervical smears may report abnormal cell development. This, of course, can lead to a misdiagnosis of a pre-cancerous condition with the recommendation of hysterectomy.

Treatment for these infections is prolonged antibiotic medication with tetracycline or erythromycin—often up to 30 days and longer. I have created vaginal suppositories to help in the treatment of these and other cervical infections. A follow-up visit is necessary to make sure the bacteria are gone and to see whether dysplastic cells were underneath the infected cells.

Trichomoniasis. 'Trich', as it is often nick-named, has been treated as an annoyance that does nothing but create a malodorous vagina. Yet I've seen this so-called simple infection cause many serious problems, including severe pelvic infection and miscarriage.

Trichomoniasis is transmitted sexually. It has been associated with atypical cervical cells and in some cases with invasive carcinoma. This is a treatable disease, and the cervical dysplasia associated with it can be corrected with medication.[25]

Gardnerella Vaginalis. This is a common bacteria that lives in the digestive tract and can be introduced into the vagina during coitus. It co-exists with other organisms and contributes significantly to pelvic pathology and inflammation. It can be transmitted by your sexual partner.

Other risk factors

Poor hygiene (see 'Safe Sex *Don'ts*' later in this chapter) increases your risk for cervical cancer. Women living on low incomes often suffer from inadequate hygiene, medical care and nutrition, and more infections, and venereal warts. Whatever your socioeconomic status, you need to keep yourself clean, use condoms and protect yourself from sexually-transmitted diseases.

Heredity. Many studies have shown that black and Hispanic women are considered to be at high risk for cervical cancer. It is possible that socioeconomic factors may come into play. Whether this problem is environmental, hereditary, or a combination of the two is still under investigation.[26]

Although cervical cancer is not as readily traceable to family groups as are other cancers (such as those of the breast or colon), a small number of cases have been reported of mothers and daughters or groups of sisters suffering from it.[27] I have seen a mother-daughter case in my own practice.

Research has not yet established why this disease should occur in certain families. If your mother or sister has had cervical cancer, however, it would be wise to alert your doctor and take extra precautions: cervical smears and colposcopy every six months, with an endocervical curettage yearly, vitamins and supplements, and decreased sexual exposure.

Interestingly, other family members of cervical cancer patients have a significantly heavy excess of skin cancer. I advise a consultation with a geneticist to discuss your risks and those of the other women in your family.

Smoking. If you smoke, you put yourself at risk for cervical cancer. In a study originating at the National Cancer Institute, researchers found that long-term smokers (more than 40 years), heavy smokers (two packs a day, or more), and those who use unfiltered cigarettes increase their chances of developing cervical cancer by 50 per cent over women who never smoke.[28]

How does smoking activate cancer cells? We are not quite sure yet. We do know that recent laboratory studies have detected the by-products of cigarette smoking—nicotine and cotinine—in cervical mucus. Those agents may cause mutations in the cells (as in the case of lung cancer) regardless of sexual activity. It's also possible that cigarette smoke lowers your resistance to pre-existing viruses, creating an environment conducive to malignant changes.

An orchestration of effects

When your body's immune system has been weakened by vitamin deficiencies, poor hygiene, stress, smoking, and/or inherited factors, it is less able to fight off infections that are associated with cancer. A whole tumour may originate from a single, altered cell,[29] which may lay dormant until the immune system is damaged by these other confounding factors.

Here is a summary of the risk factors for cervical cancer. Evaluate your own situation:

- Early sexual activity
- Multiple partners and unprotected sex
- Partner with penile cancer or prior wife with cervical cancer
- Poverty
- Vitamin deficiency
- Smoking
- Heredity
- Venereal warts
- Herpes-Simplex II
- Chronic infections (chlamydia, myco-

plasma, ureaplasma, yeast, gardnerella, trichomoniasis)

If any of these issues is a factor for you, it warrants discussion with your gynaecologist. Together you can create a preventive programme for you.

When it's infection all along

Laura was a vivacious, intelligent woman of 26. For four years she had been monitored by doctors because of abnormal cervical smears, which alternated between Class III and Class IV. When she came into my office, Laura was anxious and distraught. Her vaginal area and cervix were tender. She hardly permitted me to carry out a routine pelvic examination. She experienced pain during intercourse and backaches before her period.

In my discussions with her and my review of her prior medical records, I learned that Laura's cervical cells had never been cultured for all sexually transmitted disease agents. She had not been adequately treated for her numerous vaginal discharges. Despite this, biopsies, repeated cervical smears, cryosurgeries, and laser surgeries had been carried out.

Laura's last surgeon suggested hysterectomy because of the persistence of abnormal smear results. Her most recent cervical smear showed numerous atypical cells consistent with carcinoma in situ. No wonder she was frightened. Aside from the normal terror that the threat of cancer induces, Laura was still single and had not yet had children.

Before rushing to hysterectomy, I decided to have a closer look. I cultured Laura's cervix. Sure enough, she had a vast array of complex infections, ranging from ureaplasma and mycoplasma to gardnerella vaginalis and venereal warts.

I performed a D & C on Laura and biopsied her cervix. The first procedure showed that the lining of her uterus was absolutely normal. I suspected that the unusual cells in her cervix were the result of the irritation and inflammation, which the many chronic infections had produced. The biopsy of the cervix showed no cancer, so I treated the infections first in the hope that the cervical cells would return to normal.

It stands to reason that if the cell irregularities are associated with inflammation caused by sexually transmitted diseases, the microbes causing those diseases might respond to antibiotics. With treatment, the irregularities could resolve themselves. It was worth a try. The hysterectomy could be performed, if necessary, two weeks later.

I proceeded to treat Laura with antibiotics. And to everyone's great pleasure and surprise (including that of her prior gynaecologist), Laura's next cervical smear and colposcopy were completely normal. It took a while to clear up the infections, but Laura continues to have normal smears. I repeated her biopsies and endocervical curettage three months later and, again, she was normal. I check her every six months now because the inflammation could have masked a true cancer. We are both delighted with the outcome.

Because of my success in treating Laura and several other patients, I have come to realize that some cases of 'cervical dysplasia' are actually cells inflamed from infection. Chronic infections can lead to cellular changes that look like cancer but are not cancer. Conversely, cancer can appear as an infection. A biopsy is necessary to determine the seriousness of the cellular changes.

Prevention: cervical cancer is the avoidable cancer

Today, I tell all my patients that it's OK to postpone sex until marriage. There's something to be said for old-fashioned virginity and chastity. Why? For one thing, the many sexually transmitted infections I've discussed can contribute to infertility and tubal (*ectopic*) pregnancy in young women. And, equally important, I believe that the sexual revolution (especially multiple sex partners and early age at first intercourse) has contributed to the increase in the incidence of *rapid onset* cervical cancer that we see today.

Sexual habits and beliefs are hard to change. Some years ago, as a young and naïve doctor, I fell in love with the scion of a rich and powerful family. Promising years of matrimonial bliss, my fiancé asked me to overlook his herpes, and to participate in intercourse without benefit of condoms. He told me that he would know when his infection was active, and that we'd abstain then. But after all, he reasoned, I would probably catch it from him eventually, in our years together, so why lessen the pleasure now?

Well, the relationship didn't work out, and I was left with the legacy of herpes. How could I have been taken in? After all, I'm a doctor and should know better. Yet when it comes to sexually transmitted diseases, I, too, fell victim to myths and denial that we perpetuate.

One of my patients, Nancy, a single professional in her thirties, came in after experiencing a vaginal discharge two weeks after having intercourse with her 'new love'. She insisted she couldn't have caught anything from him. He was clean and professional—a lawyer, to boot. I asked if she had interviewed him about his prior sexual activity.

'Oh no,' she said. 'After all, this was our

first date and I didn't want to get too intimate. I want to go out with him again . . . and that would never happen if I asked such personal questions.'

I wondered how much more intimate one could get beyond having sexual intercourse and why those 'personal' questions should not be asked when one's health and even life may be at risk. Need I mention AIDS? *Today, there is no safe sex.* Meanwhile, and despite her protestations to the contrary, Nancy's lab report came back showing that she had contracted both chlamydia and venereal warts.

We perpetuate the myth that social status, profession, income, race, religion, physical attractiveness, and education keep people free from these problems. But only abstinence, monogamy, and condoms can help to do that. You should have a commitment when you're sharing your body with someone else.

Protecting yourself

I believe cervical cancer and infections may be avoided in most cases—but ultimately it becomes a question of your willingness to alter your life style. You can protect yourself if you:

- *Stop smoking.*
- Change your sexual behaviour (see below).
- See your doctor promptly if you are experiencing vaginal itching, burning, unusual discharge, pain during intercourse, pelvic pain, skin changes near the genitals, sores, or if you discover that you have been exposed to a sexually transmitted disease. In fact, I would make it a practice to get checked routinely for these diseases.
- Educate your sex partner about the

seriousness of venereal warts and sexually transmitted diseases for both of you.

Actually, my best advice is NEVER HAVE UNPROTECTED SEX—ALWAYS INSIST ON CONDOMS! Condoms are better than nothing, but in many cases of promiscuous sex, *nothing* is better, altogether. Although there is no absolutely 'safe sex', here are some tips to help you avoid sexually transmitted diseases, especially since cervical cancer is linked to them.

Do

- Reconsider the many virtues of virginity and monogamy. Changing your sexual habits could save your life.
- Have the courage to ask potential new sex partners about previous experience, prior diseases, and homosexual contact. Have they had problems, pain, discharge?
- Make sure your gynaecologist has any unusual discharges cultured for disease and takes a yearly cervical smear.
- Always insist on condoms. Condoms and spermicides help prevent sperm from coming into contact with vulnerable cervical tissue.
- Insist that your partner(s) also seek treatment if you are being treated for a sexually transmitted disease. Otherwise, you will re-infect each other.
- Wash after sex. This may flush away some bacteria.
- Urinate after sex. This may rinse away bacteria in the urethra and bladder.
- Wear cotton crotch underwear that allows for air circulation.
- Educate yourself about the signs and symptoms of sexually transmitted diseases and get cultures and blood tests routinely.
- If you are young and have never experienced sexual intercourse, don't submit to cultural pressure to do so until you are fully informed and ready.

- If you are a parent, encourage your sons and daughters to avoid promiscuity throughout their lives.

Don't
- Don't have sex with many people. You have no control over your partners' partners and their partners.
- Don't engage in sex while you're being treated for a sexually transmitted disease.
- Don't engage in sex during a herpes flare-up and do use a condom between episodes.

- Don't touch herpes sores, or, if you do, wash your hands well before touching your face, eyes, or partner.
- Never place anything that has been in the rectum in the vagina (this includes the penis, fingers, or objects).
- Don't have rectal intercourse.

With these safety hints in mind, you may be working to reduce your risk of cervical cancer. And that's a worthwhile goal—especially if it means preserving your reproductive capacity and avoiding a hysterectomy!

PART III
The ovaries

CHAPTER 13

Understanding your ovaries

'If you are keen to have your ovaries preserved you should state this since the "expressed wish" of the patient must be taken into account. This will be recorded in your records. Your specialist may, however, tell you that he feels he cannot have his clinical judgement limited in this way and suggest that you seek a second opinion. You should know that hysterectomy (removal of the womb) is one thing; preservation of the ovaries is quite another: it is a specialist task not always capable of being tackled by general surgeons. When the uterus is removed, the ovaries are no longer suspended in the pelvic cavity and there is a tendency for them to retract, reducing or even cutting off their blood supply. Many doctors, therefore, unless they use specialist techniques, prefer to remove them.'
Ex-gynaecologist

In order to make reasoned, well-educated decisions about your body, it is essential that you understand how your ovaries work and what role they play in your well-being. You need to know what constitutes a benign situation, how your cycles function, and which abnormalities in your cycle could lead to cancer.

As happens so often in the field of women's health, a myriad of myths and beliefs have clouded our understanding of our ovaries and malignancy. Only 100 years ago, doctors were advocating the routine removal of the ovaries for the relief of oöphoro-mania, oöphoro-epilepsy, oöphor-algia, nymphomania, invalidism, severe headache, neurosis, and psychosis.[1] The unfortunate consequences of these myths have caused the loss of untold numbers of ovaries over the last century and have perpetrated much suffering on the part of unsuspecting women.

Modern myths we perpetuate about ovaries

How many of these do you ascribe to?

- After childbearing years, women no longer need their reproductive organs.
- The ovaries stop producing hormones at menopause.
- All women over 40 should have their ovaries removed in order to avoid ovarian cancer.
- A cystic ovary *may* burst, haemorrhage, or become cancerous in the future and should be removed as a precaution.
- A woman who has had a hysterectomy but whose ovaries have been 'saved' will not suffer from the loss of her hormones.
- Birth control pills cause cancer.

How the myths can cause panic

Marsha came to me after her female gynaecologist had informed her that she needed an immediate hysterectomy, including an oöphorectomy (the removal of her ovaries). An ovarian cyst was causing her to experience deep internal pain on her left side. Marsha was 52 years old. Her gynaecologist told her that at her age the only thing she could have was *cancer*. She was frantic!

I performed an ultrasound and discovered a small cyst—about an inch in diameter—on her ovary. It was a 'simple cyst', made up primarily of fluid. Marsha's blood test came back showing that she was still ovulating and that her ovaries were functioning well.

Had Marsha been better informed about the anatomy and function of her ovary, she might not have been as alarmed about her doctor's diagnosis of an ovarian cyst. And she might even have questioned the mention of cancer—for ovarian cysts and cancer are *not* synonymous.

Fortunately for everyone concerned, we did not jump to hysterectomy. I viewed the ovary with a pathologist during laparoscopy. We found a 'functional' cyst (see Chapter 14) and I suctioned off the fluid within. The cyst collapsed. A biopsy of the ovary was taken to confirm the diagnosis.

What a great relief for Marsha. Not only was she cancer-free, but she also avoided major surgery. And, she delighted in learning that her biological clock was still ticking! It made her feel youthful—almost reborn.

The myth of the ovarian cyst

Every day terrified women like Marsha come into my office, having been referred by their doctors for a second opinion, because they have an ovarian cyst. Their panic knows no bounds. 'Please take the ovary out,' they cry. 'I don't want to die!'

I understand their fear. *It's cancer!* They know that millions of women have had their ovaries removed. Ovarian cysts are viewed as dangerous tissue formations likely to cause grave damage to the body. In fact, I believe a *basic misconception* about the nature of ovarian cysts is partially responsible for the numbers of hysterectomies done today.

Why do I say misconception? *Because every month women develop ovarian cysts as part of their normal menstrual cycle.* When you appreciate the anatomy of the ovary, you will understand why ovarian cysts—although possibly painful—are rarely as dangerous as they are made out to be. Functional cysts are not cancerous.

The anatomy of the ovary

The foetal ovary at 20 weeks contains two million *graafian follicles*. These are microscopic 'containers' holding potential eggs. At birth, the cortex area, or the outer surface of each ovary, is covered with approximately 400,000 follicles. (This number may vary from woman to woman and even from ovary to ovary within the same woman.) By age 40, you may only have a few thousand follicles left.

Your lifetime supply of eggs is enclosed in these primordial follicles. They are a progressively depleted genetic bank from which growing follicles continuously develop. Probably less than 0.1 per cent of all the follicles formed in the foetal ovary ever attain ovulation.

When you reach puberty and begin to have menstrual cycles, the oestrogen in your blood stimulates the pituitary gland to produce *follicle stimulating hormone* (FSH). This, in turn, further increases oestrogen production to a high level, causing one egg per month to begin the maturation process. By the middle of your cycle, a microscopic 'follicular cyst' develops, holding this single

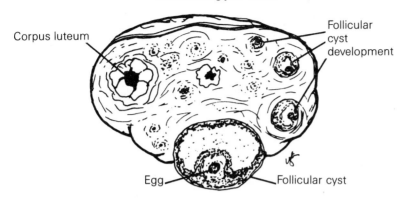

Fig. 29. The development of the follicular cyst of ovulation.

egg within.

The follicular cyst balloons out of your ovary, growing to about 0.8 inch in diameter. It is filled with a fluid rich in hormones and is fed by its own set of tiny blood vessels (see fig. 29). At just the right moment, when the egg is nearly mature, your pituitary gland secretes *luteinizing hormone* (LH), which triggers the follicular cyst to burst and spill the 'ripened' egg into your abdominal cavity. This may cause the release of a small amount of blood or mid-cycle spotting (the uterus may lose some lining), and we say that ovulation has occurred. (This egg finds its way into the adjacent fallopian tube where it may be fertilized.)

After the rupture, the tissue left behind on your ovary begins to shrink. The residual cells, at the base of the follicle, produce the second ovarian hormone, progesterone, as well as continuing production of oestrogen during the second half of the menstrual cycle. This is called the *luteal phase* (see fig. 30).

You naturally develop ovarian cysts monthly

Your fear-inducing ovarian cyst turns out to be nothing more than a normal part of your basic female physiology. In fact, it is abnormal *not* to have ovarian 'cysts' regularly. When you are not ovulating, eggs are not being manufactured and your ovaries are malfunctioning. This may occur premenopausally, when the number of healthy eggs has diminished. Or, the egg may be defective and thus unavailable for development because of genetic problems, infection, diet, hormone imbalances, stress, and immunological abnormalities.

Then why the panic when the doctor diagnoses an ovarian cyst? Any mass in the pelvis is suspect and should be investigated. And sometimes the cyst goes haywire and grows to the size of a grapefruit because of a failure in the ovulation cycle. Such a large cyst can cause a good deal of acute and alarming pain. Of course, this situation warrants evaluation by your gynaecologist (see Chapter 14), but it does not require a hysterectomy or oöphorectomy.

Why you shouldn't lose your ovaries needlessly

In 1984, 88.5 per cent of all bilateral oöphorectomies were performed in conjunction

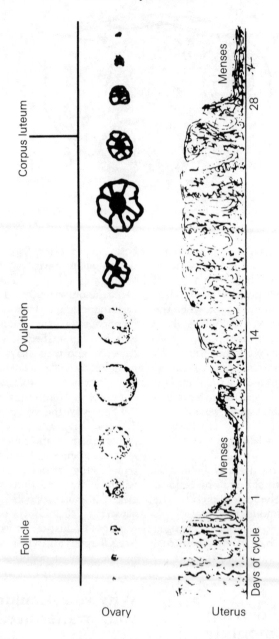

Fig. 30. Normal ovulation: these are the changes that normally occur during your menstrual cycle.

with a hysterectomy. In fact, 20 to 30 per cent of all women undergo an oöphorectomy routinely at the time of hysterectomy.[2]

Yet your ovaries are vital! They are virtual factories, manufacturing eggs and, in the process, producing many hormones. These are the body's natural messengers: the word *hormone* comes from the Greek *horman* meaning 'to stir up or arouse to activity'. Your hormones stimulate your organs, tissues, and body functions in specific ways. The interactions are complex and may take some effort to comprehend. But it's worth the effort. In learning about how ovarian hormones function, you will see why they are essential to your health and well-being.

How the glands interact with the ovaries

Several organs are closely involved, through interaction of their secretions, with your reproductive system. The *pituitary*, a 'master gland' located at the base of your brain, produces two major hormones essential for reproduction—follicle stimulating hormone (FSH) and *luteinizing hormone* (LH)—and many others, some of which are still unidentified.

Your *adrenal glands*, which are found above each kidney, produce hormones that break down into oestrogen and testosterone in varying amounts throughout your life. The *hypothalamus*, located at the base of the brain, acts as a control centre for the hormone messages.

You may be aware that the *ovaries* produce the 'female' hormone, oestrogen. In truth, these important organs produce a host of hormones, some traditionally characterized as being 'male', like progesterone and testosterone.

Hormones and the endocrine system

Oestrogen. Your body began producing oestrogen long before you were born—when you were a foetus of only 15 to 20 weeks. At birth, oestrogen had already caused an additional layer of fat to develop and to make your skin ultrasoft. By puberty, the increased production of oestrogen sparked the development of your breasts and the rounded contours of feminine hips and thighs, as well as pubic and underarm hair. Your sexuality became apparent and your reproductive organs matured and began to function in their monthly cycles.

From puberty to menopause, oestrogen stimulates your pituitary gland to produce Follicle Stimulating Hormone (FSH), which further increases oestrogen production to a high level and usually causes one egg cell to ripen each month. Oestrogen causes your uterine lining to thicken, in preparation for implantation of the fertilized egg.

Oestrogen's effects manifest themselves throughout your life. Acting on all the structures and organs of your body, this hormone helps to determine your height, weight, bone density, skin tone, muscle strength, digestion, heart rate, blood proteins and fats, and emotional reactions. Its presence protects you from arthritis and heart disease.[3]

At menopause, your ovaries produce less oestrogen. However, your post-menopausal ovary is not a dead or dying organ. It continues to produce oestrogen, albeit at diminished levels for at least twelve years following the onset of menopause.[4] Because of the decline in oestrogen levels, you may now begin to notice changes in your body and its functioning. It is my belief that this is a 'deficiency' state unique to humans because of our extraordinary longevity.

However, not all oestrogen is lost even

when the ovaries eventually do turn off. The conversion of adrenal gland hormones into oestrogen (which had little importance before menopause) increases. This oestrogen conversion occurs primarily in fat tissues. Because of this process, oestrogen production appears to continue at a slower rate for at least ten to twenty years after menopause. This can be quite variable from woman to woman, which helps to explain why some women age more rapidly than others.

Testosterone. Both the ovaries and the adrenal glands produce testosterone, yet studies have demonstrated that the ovary is probably a more important source of this androgen than the adrenal glands.[5] Although a major hormone for men, testosterone, you may be surprised to learn, is also of great importance to women. It helps determine secondary sexual characteristics such as muscle mass and hair growth patterns. It also increases your sexual desire, activity, and responsiveness.

Clinically, I have seen women who have lost their ovaries to the scalpel, or whose ageing organs produce diminished amounts of testosterone, complain of a decrease in their sexual desire. Many studies have charted the effects of testosterone on sexuality. In one, women given implants of oestrogen and testosterone enjoyed increased frequency and intensity of orgasm.[6]

There is a belief today that women neither make nor need testosterone. And women fear the 'male' hormones. The misuse of these labels frightens us needlessly, for *all* the hormones produced in a woman's body are 'female'. They are all necessary for normal cyclic functioning and the integrity of our other organs. It's the balance that's important.

Time after time, I've administered minute amounts of testosterone to women complaining of loss of libido after menopause, surgical removal of the ovaries, or hyster-

ectomy, and watched these patients spring back to life. Their energies and sexual activities returned to normal, and their marriages were saved.

Sarah, a young marathon runner, came to see me. She had lost one of her ovaries to a freak occurrence called *torsion*. Prior to her oöphorectomy, Sarah was capable of running 10 miles a day with ease. Emotionally she felt satisfied—she was in tip-top shape and loved her body and her running. Like most female athletes, she was lean and muscular. She was told that nothing would change as a result of the loss of the ovary.

After the surgery, however, Sarah fell into a deep depression. She felt lethargic, asexual, irritable. Her doctor thought she had become neurotic because she still had one remaining ovary. The problem was, this ovary was not ovulating regularly. When I administered a blood test to determine Sarah's hormone production, I discovered that her level of testosterone had dropped far below normal.

I implanted a testosterone pellet under Sarah's skin. This pellet slowly released just enough testosterone to replace her loss without causing the hair growth, deepened voice, and loss of breast body tissue that occurs when there is an excess of testosterone. In fact, many women do quite well on testosterone—just like Sarah.

Progesterone. One of the major functions of progesterone is the preparation of the uterine lining for the implantation of a fertilized egg. If conception occurs, this lining will sustain an embryo. Increasing amounts of progesterone will help maintain the pregnancy by quieting the muscles of the uterus. If conception does not occur, however, the production of oestrogen and progesterone falls sharply. The decline in progesterone triggers other reactions within the uterus, which cause the capillaries to burst, the uterine lining to shed, and the menstrual flow to start. Then, a new cycle begins.

Proceed with caution

I am saddened by the fact that a woman could lose her ovaries based on myths and irrational fears. These organs produce eggs and make a major contribution to her vital hormone balance. As you will see in the following chapter, many steps can be taken before resorting to oöphorectomy (the removal of the ovaries) when treating ovarian cysts.

CHAPTER 14

The ovarian cyst:
is it time for surgery?

A World Health Organization (WHO) study found that women are loathe to report 'minor' menstrual problems and cautioned that women *should* report any change in period pattern, unexplained bleeding, pain or 'dragging' sensation (perhaps due to the presence of an ovarian cyst) in order to avoid possible greater problems later.[1]

There was a time when ovarian cysts were considered universally fatal. Tapping the rapidly reaccumulating fluid offered the poor suffering woman only temporary relief. One case, prior to the nineteenth century, told of a patient whose cyst was tapped 299 times for the removal of 9,867 pounds of fluid![2] That seems extraordinary, if not commically exaggerated, yet old medical texts show illustrations of women with grotesquely distended abdomens. Benign ovarian cysts did kill.

Today, contrary to popular belief, having a cyst on your ovary does not mean that you have to lose your ovary or die. In fact, many ovarian cysts do not require surgery and can just be observed. It's essential to keep in mind that cysts are not cancer. There are several types of cysts, and each requires a different approach.

Follicular cysts

If you are in your twenties or thirties and have an ovarian cyst, it's likely that yours is *follicular*. In this case, an egg has failed to ovulate or rupture from your ovary, and fluid continues to accumulate in the intact follicle, fed by an ovary rich in hormones (see figs. 30, 31).

Some women are simply 'cyst formers'. Several times a year they are plagued by large, painful, benign cysts. If unlucky, they have repeated surgeries that can result in the eventual loss of the ovary.

What are the symptoms of benign follicular cysts?

- A delay in menstruation
- Breakthrough bleeding
- Pelvic pain—a constant dull ache or sharp jabbing
- Cramping

The pain comes from the stretching and pulling of the ovary tissue to accommodate for the enlargement. I have treated functional ovarian cysts the size of lemons, grapefruits—even melons!

How are follicular cysts diagnosed?

Your case will need to be evaluated individually to determine who best to handle your situation. Yet there are certain guidelines that you and your doctor can follow to help determine what's wrong and which course of

The ovarian cyst is it time for surgery?

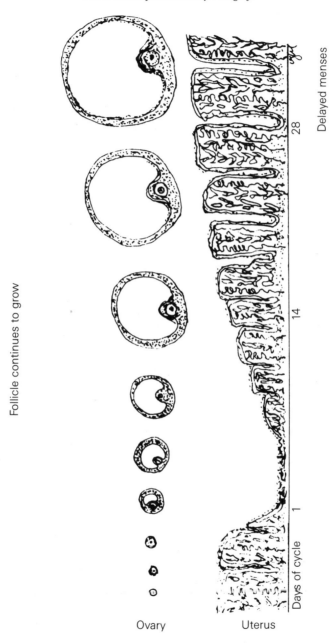

Fig. 31. How a large ovarian cyst develops.

action should be taken. Here is the safest and the most thorough protocol. Your doctor should:

1. Feel the ovary during pelvic examination to determine size. Any ovary over 2 inches should be investigated.
2. Order a blood test to see how well your ovaries are producing hormones.
3. Perform ultrasound scan to determine more accurately the size and composition of the ovary (if fluid and/or solid elements are present). CAT scan and nuclear magnetic resonance scan can be performed.

Waiting out the cyst

In most cases, I prefer to 'wait out' a small follicular cyst, remembering that follicles normally grow, rupture, and regress as part of the ovulation cycle. Follicular cysts usually shrink by themselves in a matter of weeks. If you're impatient, regression can be encouraged by taking proper dosages of oral contraceptives (provided you're under 40) or natural progesterone. These cysts are benign and pose little risk.

Circumstances can arise that warrant immediate action, however, especially if you're experiencing severe pain or if the cyst proves to be unusually large and appears solid. If you suspect a cyst, you must seek immediate medical attention—don't attempt to wait it out alone.

Re-evaluation

Once a follicular cyst has been diagnosed, and you've 'waited it out', you should be re-evaluated to confirm that everything has returned to normal. The following guidelines are helpful. If you're:

- Under 30 years old you can be re-evaluated in eight to ten weeks.

- Between 30 and 40 you should wait one menstrual cycle or six weeks for re-evaluation.
- Over 40 and have an enlarged ovary, you need an immediate medical evaluation.

Surgical treatments for follicular cysts

If, after you have waited the suggested time, the cyst remains, your doctor should perform a laparoscopy to better visualize your ovary. (S)he will want to know if it has a smooth surface or the rough, abnormal texture of cancer.

If the growth is smooth, your doctor will weigh other risk factors for ovarian cancer. (S)he will sample the fluid in your pelvic cavity to make sure no cancerous cells exist. Then (s)he will consider the cyst's appearance, your age, and family history to determine whether it is safe to drain the cyst. If so, a needle can be inserted through your abdomen and the fluid suctioned off or *aspirated* while using the laparoscope. Utmost care must be taken not to spill any of the contents of the cyst into the pelvic cavity.

In most cases, after aspiration, the cyst will collapse like a deflated balloon and the ovary will shrink immediately. You will be cured without major surgery.

If your ovary is unusually large, or if a more serious problem is suspected, a laparotomy (opening of the abdomen) may be performed. Your ovary will be biopsied and the cyst excised, depending on what is found. A pathologist should be present in the operating room.

Large, heavy, or polycystic ovaries (PCO)

I recently treated Cindy, a 25-year-old single woman with no children. She came to me from Oregon, having been told by her gynaecologist that she had severe endometriosis. Cindy's right ovary had been removed previously because of that disease. When she continued to have pain, her doctor said, 'Since we're now going to have to take out your left ovary, we might as well do a hysterectomy. Besides, you must be scarred up inside because of all of this endometriosis.'

Cindy asked me to clean up her endometriosis and reconstruct the remaining ovary during surgery. Imagine the utter shock that the pathologist and I experienced when I opened Cindy up. This young woman had no endometriosis—not one spot of it in her body! When we finally received the pathology reports from her original operation, it showed the removed ovary had had a functional cyst only.

But this does not mean that Cindy didn't have problems. She had polycystic ovary disease (PCO). Her remaining ovary had many immature cysts (see fig. 32). Because of her previous operation and scarring, the cysts had become encapsulated and were bound down to her ovary with adhesions, creating pain.

But more than that, Cindy's ovary swelled up to ten times its normal size. It was so large that it dwarfed her uterus. The ligament that

held it had stretched because of the excess weight, and the large, heavy ovary twisted and fell on top of Cindy's vagina, near the rectum. Whenever she sat or walked, she experienced pain. Normal intercourse was impossible.

This is not unusual. If you have PCO, you may experience:

- Large, painful ovaries
- Pain in the pelvis, back, and vagina
- Infrequent menstruation
- Obesity and facial hair growth
- Discomfort during intercourse

During Cindy's surgery, I removed the dense adhesions and drained the cysts. Then, I reapproximated her normal anatomy by shortening the stretched ligament and lifting the ovary back in position, securing it with permanent sutures. To prevent future problems, I placed Cindy on birth control pills.

Some non-surgical treatments for ovarian cysts

If you tend to have recurrent cysts, you may be suffering from a hormone imbalance resulting from stress, immunological abnormalities, a change in environment, nutrition, or genetic diseases. A failure in the

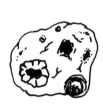
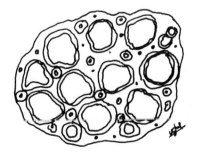

Fig. 32. Normal ovary compared to polycystic ovary. The latter is larger and shows no sign of ovulation although full of cysts.

release of cyclic hormones can cause the overgrowth of follicular cysts and their inability to rupture.

As in Cindy's case, natural progesterone or oral contraceptives can be prescribed to diminish ovarian size. Oral contraceptives appear to suppress the development of functional ovarian cysts and cause their rapid regression by inhibiting ovulation.[3] The follicles do not mature because the pill suppresses FSH and LH from the pituitary.

Oral contraceptive therapy has the added advantage of helping to diagnose ovarian cancer. In a survey of 286 women with ovarian masses treated with oral contraceptives, 5 were found to have cancer. Although the pill suppressed all of the cases of functional ovarian cysts within six weeks, it had no effect on the malignancies. This helped the doctor to decide more quickly to perform exploratory surgery, and consequently reduced the time that the cancers grew without surgical intervention.[4]

The size of your ovaries should also be followed closely. Your gynaecologist can measure them on ultrasound after the treatment programme has been begun. If there are no new cysts, then the condition is relatively controlled.

If you suffer from recurrent ovarian cysts, you can also take danocrine, bromocriptine, vitamins, and amino acids. Many options are available.

The fear of birth control pills

Your fear of hormone therapy may cause you to reject this relatively safe treatment and may put you at greater risk surgically. You are not alone in this. Many women have lost confidence in the pill.[5] It is perceived as a killer, but in reality it can be a saviour. You can be monitored with ultrasound or urine tests for ovulation to find the lowest level of medication that works for you.

Mara refused to take birth control pills, even though she was a chronic cyst former: she was operated on six times for ovarian cysts. Each successive surgeon became alarmed at the multiple surgeries. Despite the fact that these functional cysts were normal but had only failed to rupture, this childless young woman was only in her twenties when she had both ovaries removed and a hysterectomy.

In truth, none of this was necessary. The cysts could easily have been drained during laparoscopy and the condition controlled with hormone therapy, which would have prevented future cyst formation.

Mara's tragedy compounded itself. She went on to an early menopause with complications. She lost height due to osteoporosis and her vagina atrophied from lack of oestrogen. Eventually she agreed to hormone replacement therapy, but only after the disease processes had become severe.

If you make large, symptomatic cysts, you need to protect your ovaries. Responsible use of birth control pills can be an option. You should remember, however, that smoking while taking oral contraceptives can create new dangers. In fact, whether or not you are on the pill, you should avoid cigarettes.

The corpus luteum cyst

This cyst differs from the follicular cyst. It occurs after the follicle has ruputured and has released the egg.

Normally, during the regression phase of the menstrual cycle, the follicular sac shrinks back onto the surface of the ovary and eventually disappears. A corpus luteum cyst is a follicular sac that fails to shrink. Rather, the tiny blood vessels that feed the follicular sac and bleed during the rupture of ovulation do not close down. They continue to bleed into the cyst, causing it to collect blood. This is also called a *haemorrhagic cyst of ovulation*.

As dangerous as they may sound, corpus luteum cysts are very common. Most often, they stop bleeding and regress naturally. The majority of the cysts that fail to regress can be diagnosed and drained safely under laparoscopy. During the procedure, while the doctor holds the ovary and looks at it, (s)he can place a needle through the abdomen and aspirate the collected blood. This may suffice and prevent major surgery.

In some instances, however, the ovary may be too large or the bleeding so profuse that one cannot stop it without actually opening the abdomen, finding the bleeding vessel, and tying it off or coagulating it.

Bonnie had such a stubborn corpus luteum cyst. She was in her mid-twenties when she came into my office, complaining of severe left side pain. Her period had been on time but she had been bleeding two days longer than usual.

An ultrasound diagnosis showed her left ovary to be 'complex'—it had both solid and fluid components. It was about the size of an orange.

After waiting several weeks with no change, I used the laparoscope and found that the surface of the ovary was normal but the colour was not. It appeared purplish and darker than it should have been. I pierced the ovary with a needle and, indeed, blood poured forth. I removed 300 ml—about a cupful—in all. The ovary shrank immediately, and Bonnie felt much better.

I followed up one week later and found that the ovary still felt enlarged during a pelvic examination. It had decreased in size, but not as much as it should after being deflated. I performed an ultrasound and confirmed that the ovary was somewhat smaller, but it had enlarged since surgery. Bonnie continued to complain of pain.

After two more weeks of medical treatment with no improvement, we went into surgery. I opened Bonnie's abdomen, located the ovary, and operated on the cyst. Cutting into it, I found a small blood vessel that had continued to trickle blood, keeping the cyst enlarged. I tied it and the bleeding stopped. The ovary was left intact, and I was able to reconstruct the stretched ovarian tissue back to normal.

More complex problems

Some freaks of nature are inherent in ovarian cysts, which come not from the cysts themselves, but from complications that sometimes arise as a result of the cyst's existence. These tragedies are unexplainable. Often we don't know why they occur, how we can prevent them, or what went wrong to create them.

In rare cases, a large cyst causes the ovary itself to twist on its ligament. The *torsion* cuts off the blood supply to the ovary (like a tourniquet) and often to the fallopian tube. The ovary and the affected tube frequently die and must be removed.

Such an accident happened to Lori, a patient and close friend. Lori had been experiencing intermittent pain for two or three months, but she had not sought medical care because of a demanding career with a film production company. She was too busy.

One morning, however, she awakened in agony. Unable to stand or walk, she had to ask her mother to drive her to my office. As soon as I examined her, I felt an enormous mass in her pelvis. What could this be? I had performed a routine examination only six months earlier and everything was absolutely normal in this otherwise healthy young woman. Yet now, her pain was so excruciating and the mass so huge, I feared the worst—tubal pregnancy or torsion. When the pregnancy test came back negative, I had no choice but to look inside.

At surgery, I discovered that the ovary appeared to have enlarged with a functional cyst and had twisted on its ligament. The fallopian tube twisted with it. Both the ovary and tube had strangulated, appearing purple and necrotic. There was no saving the tissue. It had already begun to decay and I couldn't make it come alive again. How long had it been this way? No one knew. I felt stricken. I save the organs of hundreds of women every year, but I was powerless to help my dear friend. I had no choice but to amputate the ovary and tube. It was a humbling experience.

On even rarer occasions, other freak accidents may occur. When a cyst ruptures spontaneously at ovulation, a major blood vessel may also rupture. If the blood vessel fails to contract, bleeding continues. If this is left untreated, one can actually haemorrhage to death—a frightening prospect indeed. That is why I recommend that your cyst be monitored by your doctor.

Dermoid tumours

Dermoid tumours make up about 10 per cent of all ovarian tumours and are most commonly seen in young women. They can occur throughout your reproductive life and may produce minor complaints or abdominal pain. Dermoids are also the most bizarre tumours, growing hair, teeth, cartilage, and fat, as if one of the eggs produced by the ovary began to develop without ever having been fertilized! They look terrible to the surgeon, but because of their solid components they can be diagnosed using ultrasound and/or X-ray.

When a dermoid cyst enlarges, it can stretch the normal ovarian tissue extensively,

disfiguring it. The mass can grow to the size of grapefruits and even melons, and can rupture, causing damage to the organs. What's worse, malignant changes can occur in approximately 1 per cent of dermoid cysts, so once diagnosed, these strange growths should be removed. [6]

Dermoids are encapsulated by thick tissue, which enables the surgeon to separate them easily from normal ovarian tissue. Few doctors attempt to save the ovary, as I firmly believe they should.

Raquella came to see me with dermoid cysts on both ovaries. This 29-year-old, single woman was told by three prior surgeons that the ovaries could not be saved. They were badly affected and very enlarged. She was told that there was too much destruction—no functional tissue would be left. Raquella's current gynaecologist suggested hysterectomy because, in his words, 'What good is your uterus if both of your ovaries have to go?'

I did an ultrasound and CAT scan and the tests confirmed that, indeed, both ovaries had dermoids. I detected teeth in the scan. At surgery I removed from Raquella's ovaries large ugly cysts filled with hair, fatty material, and teeth. I reconstructed the ovaries. Three months later, I re-checked with a laparoscope and found beautiful, normal ovaries. I put Raquella on birth control pills to retard future cyst formation. I hope this will protect her ovaries until she decides to have a baby. Such surgical reconstruction of the ovary happily leaves women with functioning ovaries. What was once a massive tumour-filled ovary involutes (curves naturally inward) with time to return to its normal size.

Conserving the ovary with female reconstructive surgery

Ovarian cysts often make themselves

evident by pain and tenderness due to enlargement. When the mass is discovered during a pelvic examination, you fear cancer. Your gynaecologist performs surgery and discovers a large, distended, *but non-cancerous* ovary. The initial response? This ovary needs to be taken out: it's disease ridden and unrepairable.

This just isn't the case. One area of your ovary may contain a cyst, but the rest can be completely normal. If your surgeon carefully opens the ovary in the area of the cyst, (s)he can actually remove the affected tissue and keep the rest of the ovary intact. Endometriosis in the ovaries can cause expansion, as well. But these endometrial cysts can be opened, lasered, and the ovary repaired.

Time and time again, I have reduced the ovarian mass by opening the cyst, draining it, or surgically removing it by whatever means possible, and then reconstructing it. My goal is to have all my patients leave the hospital with functioning, healthy ovaries after FRS. Ovaries are removed only in cases like Lori's, where the entire ovary has abscessed or died and no healthy tissue is left to save.

Why have doctors routinely removed the ovary? Many surgeons feel that if the ovary is so enlarged, repairs can't be done. They believe that the pathology that has occurred has expanded and destroyed the organ. They are so impressed with how misshapen and disfigured the ovary looks, they may never attempt to conserve it.

If you take any organ and enlarge it, it will look grotesque. But actually, given the disease processes that can occur, *it's usually only one section of the ovary that is inflated like a balloon.* Once that area is deflated, the rest of the ovary can return to normal. The whole ovary can be saved.

I have seen ovaries removed needlessly for functional follicular and corpus luteum cysts, for dermoid tumours and endometri-

osis. Much like hysterectomy, oöphorectomy is quick and easy to perform. Surgically, the ovary can be amputated simply in a few seconds. I prefer to find a way to conserve the tissue.

Sculpting the ovary

As we all know from childhood, when you blow up a balloon and let go of it, it will expel all of the air within and return to the pre-inflation size. Human tissue doesn't function as conveniently, however. When you remove the material that causes the ovary to be expanded, you are still left with the stretched ovarian tissue that covered the problem area.

Of those surgeons inclined to save the ovary, most cut that 'excess' tissue off and leave a smaller portion of the ovary behind. The so-called excess, however, is all normal ovarian tissue. It's just misshapen. I want to leave a woman with as much functioning ovary as possible, so I try not to cut off any tissue.

Instead, I surgically reconstruct or sculpt the ovary by folding in the excess tissue on its surface into a reapproximation of its previous shape and size. This saves all the tissues and restores the ovary to normal function. It's a wonderful technique that is effective.

Infected ovaries

Even if you have a partially infected ovary, the dead area can be removed, leaving the remainder of healthy tissue behind. The whole ovary does not have to be cut out and discarded. You have the chance to maintain your hormone function by using antibiotics, special therapies, and irrigations.

I personally would rather be at risk for a second surgery than to lose my organs right off the bat. It's my body and I would like to have the option.

CHAPTER 15

Ovarian cancer—detecting the silent killer

'Removing healthy ovaries, especially before the time of the menopause, is entirely un-justified in my opinion. Some doctors remove these to try and prevent ovarian cancer. But we can check the ovaries at the time of the operation and thereafter we can do an annual scan using ultrasound. Of course surgeons must know what they're doing: once the uterus is removed there is a tendency for the ovaries to retract and this may affect the blood supply.'
Consultant surgeon

The magical age of 40

I can remember it clearly, as if it were just yesterday. Throughout my medical training I was told that when performing a hyster-ectomy for *any* reason on *any* woman 40 or older, it was my responsibility to persuade her to have her ovaries removed, along with her uterus. Some doctors use the age of 35 as the watershed.

A bona fide member of a medical crusade to save all women from ovarian cancer, I operated from the belief that our fortieth birthdays automatically predisposed ovaries to developing cancerous cells. So, during my residency, I dutifully explained to each of my patients that since she was 40, and wouldn't be needing her ovaries any-way, it was prudent to spare herself the future risk and grief of ovarian cancer.

Out those ovaries must come!

My entreaties were met with fear on the part of my patients. 'Won't I get fat?' they asked. 'Won't I become manly and grow hair?' 'How about my sex life?' These are, of course, reasonable doubts, given what we know today about the function of the ovary. But I (and many other doctors trained in the United States) was taught that these con-cerns were unfounded, hysterical fears of women who stupidly would risk their lives for the sake of organs that had already exhausted their usefulness.

The truth is, not all women are at the same risk level for ovarian cancer as they age. You will see, from the risk factors I cite later in this chapter, that ovarian cancer is a relatively rare disease when compared with the num-bers of ovaries removed. But it is a killer. If you are to keep your ovaries beyond the not-so-ripe age of 35 or 40, you need to educate yourself about your risks.

Menopause does not usually occur until the mid-fifties. The ovary itself, however, still continues to make hormones even after complete menopause has taken place. As far as the ovary being a target for cancer is concerned, only a few women are at risk and certainly the routine removal of normal ovaries for the possible later development of a cancer cannot be justified by any existing reliable data. Yet prophylactic removal—removal to prevent possible disease—does occur. In a survey of members of the British

Royal College of Obstetricians and Gynae-cologists, it was found that in 35-to-39-year-old women, only .4 per cent of British surgeons would routinely remove the ovaries. At the age of around 49, however, this figure rose to 51.2 per cent and when women were considered 'post-menopausal' the figure rose to 85.3 per cent. So in Britain at least there is more chance of women holding on to their ovaries until they are in their 50s. In the US surgeons begin prophylactic removal of the ovaries ten years earlier; the common cut-off age is 40. However, on both continents, the meno-pausal woman's ovaries tend to be removed with the same degree of eagerness. Old ovaries simply must come out and this can be seen as a kind of 'doctor's tale'. The idea of removing a man's testicles, just because he's somewhat aged, is entirely unthinkable.

The silent killer

None of this is to say that you should be lax in your vigilance for the diagnosis of ovarian cancer. On the contrary! Of all the female reproductive cancers, ovarian cancer is the most pernicious, killing more women than cervical and endometrial cancer combined. *Even if you've had a hysterectomy, you should continue with regular examinations of your ovaries, because ovarian cancer can be fatal.*

Ovarian cancer is so dangerous because it is rarely diagnosed before it has done enormous destruction to your body. It is, however, one of the least common of female cancers. Here are some facts you should know:

- Although ovarian cancer accounts for only 4 per cent of all cancers found in women, it is responsible for *half* of all genital cancer deaths.
- *Two-thirds of all ovarian cancers are detected after the cancer has already spread.*

- One of every 70 newborn girls (1.4 per cent) will develop this disease.
- It usually occurs after menopause in women between the ages of 55 and 64.
- Five to 10 per cent of ovarian cancer originates from the breast, bowel, or uterus.

What are the stages of ovarian cancer?

Stage 1: Growth limited to ovaries
Stage 2: Growth involving one or both ovaries with pelvic extension
Stage 3: Growth involving one or both ovaries with metastases outside the pelvis, into the bowel and abdominal cavity
Stage 4: Growth involving one or both ovaries with distant metastases (ie to the lungs).

A Stage 1 cancer has an 80 to 85 per cent cure rate. A Stage 4 cancer drops down to a 4 per cent cure rate. Although these statistics ar dismal, please don't consider them as a prediction of your own situation if you have ovarian cancer. As Dr Carl Simonton's and other psychosocial programmes for cancer patients (such as the Wellness Community in Santa Monica) have taught us, there is no predicting whether you, individually, are among the 4 per cent that survive. There is always hope with cancer.

What are the symptoms of ovarian cancer?

The symptoms of ovarian cancer are rarely as alarming as those for the much less serious ovarian cyst. Women with ovarian cancer complain of:

- Vague pressure in the pelvis or abdomen

Fig. 33. Bimanual examination: the ovary is the normal size and the patient is thin.

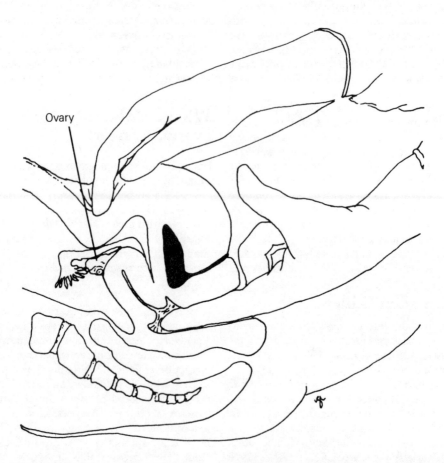

Ovary

- Uneasy feeling in the stomach area
- Gas or distension, bloating
- An enlarged abdomen or increased dress size
- Abnormal vaginal bleeding
- Chest problems, coughing, pressure, difficulty in breathing, flu-like symptoms

As you can see, the symptoms can indicate any number of problems, and often the pain is not acute until the cancer is quite advanced. In fact, many women with ovarian cancer medicate themselves with antacids, assuming that their discomfort is merely digestive in origin.

Even more frightening is the fact that approximately one-third of women with ovarian cancer have no symptoms at all. Seventy-five per cent of the remainder, including those with extensive metastases, have experienced symptoms for less than six months. Many seem in good health. *Any change in a general body function that becomes chronic needs immediate medical evaluation.*

Obesity makes early detection more difficult

The earlier your doctor detects and eradicates a cancer, the better the outcome for you. The key to diagnosing ovarian cancer early is finding an increase in the size of your ovary, usually using bimanual examination.

If you are overweight, you may have so much fat in the pelvic area that it is impossible for your gynaecologist to feel your ovaries until they are huge from cancer (figs. 33, 34). Early detection becomes even more difficult after menopause because your ovary normally decreases in size once ovulation ceases. Of all the reasons I've given you to maintain a healthy body weight, I can't think of a better one.

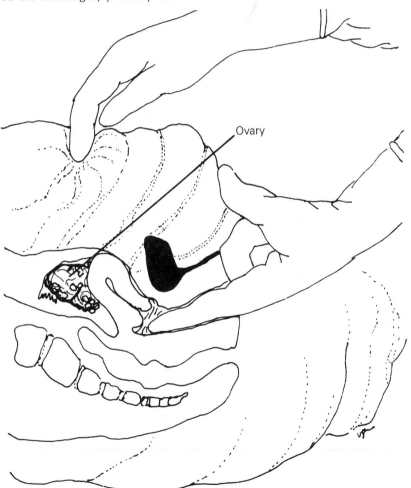

Ovary

Fig. 34. Pelvic examination on an obese woman. The ovary is enlarged with cancer. It cannot be adequately palpated.

What's a doctor to do?

As distressing as the facts are about ovarian cancer, for many years they were worsened by the lack of a technological screening method to detect this silent killer. By the time your gynaecologist can feel an ovarian malignancy, the cancer may be far beyond his or her abilities as a surgeon to cure it completely.

We have developed safe methods for screening other cancers: cervical smears for cervical cancer, D & C for uterine cancer, and low-dosage mammography for breast cancer. But what about ovarian cancer? Nothing exists. The medical profession needs to develop new ways to screen for this silent killer.

The miracle of ultrasound

Ultrasound may be a helpful breakthrough. It can help avoid unnecessary oöphorectomies while providing safe, effective *early detection* for ovarian cancer. Ultrasound is the passing of sound waves through your body, which reflect back, producing a picture on a monitor. It was originally used by submarines (sonar) to bounce back information about the shape of the sea floor or the location of enemy vessels in the vicinity. Today many obstetricians use this technological marvel to chart the growth and development of the foetus in utero. So far, it has been proven to be relatively safe and gives off no radiation.

It occurred to me that I could actually measure women's ovaries individually by ultrasound. I could take a picture of the monitor and keep a visual record of changes in the ovaries' size and shape, following my patients' progress from one year to the next—especially those who were obese or otherwise at risk. All this, without exposure to X-ray radiation.

I presented the concepts of ultrasound screening for ovarian cancer at the annual meeting of the American College of Obstetrics and Gynecology in 1982 and at other conferences. Here are the steps I suggest to help reduce the risk of undetected ovarian cancer:

1. If you are over 50, you should have an initial pelvic ultrasound to measure and evaluate the size of your ovaries, even if you have no uterus.
2. Your doctor should run blood tests to obtain hormone levels. These determine the biological activity of your ovaries.
3. If you are still ovulating and your doctor gets a slightly abnormal scan, you should be re-examined in four to six weeks.
4. If the scan is abnormal, further studies, including possible laparoscopy and/or laparotomy may be performed.

If you are not ovulating, and your ovary is grossly enlarged, a laparoscopy and/or laparotomy should be performed immediately.

Sylvia came into my office for a postmenopausal cervical smear. As a matter of routine, I performed an ultrasound screening and discovered that one ovary was larger than what I would expect to see in a postmenopausal woman. The enlargement was noticeable in relation to her other ovary, which was the normal size. A potential problem in the pelvis was detected.

Sylvia's cervical smear showed that cancer existed, but was inconclusive as to location. In surgery, I discovered that the suspicious ovary was cancerous. I had to perform a radical hysterectomy and oöphorectomy. Her follow-up treatment included chemotherapy. Sylvia's condition was serious; her prognosis guarded. But the cancer had been discovered early.

Corroborating evidence

All changes in medical practice are slow to effectuate. Yet ultrasound may be a preliminary step to finding a screening method for ovarian cancer. Other scientists are now investigating the use of this tool.

One group of researchers found that they could accurately assess the ovaries of 99.4 per cent of the 1,077 women they studied. They concluded that ultrasound 'provides new hope for the early detection of ovarian cancer. We found it to be quick, the average time taken for examination being only five to ten minutes. Being non-invasive, it was well tolerated by our subjects and provided results immediately'.[1]

New frontiers

Although not yet widely available, a new tool has recently been developed to help doctors visualize internal organs. Nuclear magnetic resonance scanning, like ultrasound, looks into your body without the danger of radiation exposure. This new form of medical technology may allow your gynaecologist to see growths on the ovary with much more clarity than ultrasound by detecting the magnetic field of the internal tissue. In the future, nuclear magnetic resonance may surpass the use of ultrasound, and could provide the long-sought answer for ovarian cancer detection.

In addition to the visualization of enlarged ovaries, molecular biologists are now providing even more promising tests to find and eradicate ovarian cancer. One team has been investigating the immunobiology of ovarian cancer. They found that 80 per cent of patients suffering from a particular kind of ovarian cancer (epithelial ovarian cancer) had elevated blood levels of CA-125.[2] This substance is also found in women with endometriosis.

The exact function of CA-125 or why it occurs with these diseases is still under investigation. But this research bodes well, because it indicates that in the future we may develop a blood test to screen for this silent killer.

What happens if you have cancer?

See a gynaecological oncologist—a specialist in cancer of the female system. Treatment for ovarian cancer includes surgery, radiation and/or chemotherapy.

Surgery. Because ovarian cancer is so dangerous, once it is detected, one or both ovaries, the fallopian tubes, and the uterus are often removed. In cases where only one ovary is lost to the disease, you can still bear children provided that the cancer has been arrested.

Certain germ cell tumours (which frequently strike women in their teens) are more amenable to conservative treatment than others. For example, a Stage 1A *dysgerminoma*, a malignant germ cell of low virulence, can be treated by removing the affected ovary and tube. Up to 75 per cent of patients have been treated successfully with this less radical approach, and they have preserved their ability to have children. If the cancer returns, radiation therapy is successful in 90 per cent of cases.[3]

In rare cases, a pregnant woman may develop ovarian cancer. If the tumour has not spread beyond one ovary, that organ can be removed and the pregnancy can be allowed to continue to term.

Radiation. Radiation is a form of X-ray in which rays are directed to the cancer cells in order to destroy them while doing as little damage as possible to the surrounding healthy cells. The rays may originate from an X-ray machine or from a capsule of radioactive material that has been implanted at the cancer site.

This form of treatment has temporary side effects, including skin irritations, nausea, tiredness, and vomiting. Rest and good nutrition help to minimize these unpleasant reactions.

Chemotherapy. Chemotherapy is the use of drugs to kill the cancer cells while doing less harm to normal cells. One or more drugs can be used with or without radiation. Of course, every case is different, so your oncologist will have to determine what is right for you.

Common side effects of chemotherapy include: nausea, vomiting, hair loss, anaemia, reduced blood-clotting ability, lowered resistance to infection, and sores in the mouth. When the chemotherapy is suspended, the side effects cease. If you undergo radiation and chemotherapy, you can help minimize the general effects by using vitamin supplements.

What causes ovarian cancer?

Ovarian cancer is a disease of our society and our era. It occurs in 10 to 12 per 100,000 women in the United States. In non-industrial countries like Paraguay, for example, it is found in only five out of every million women. We also know that it was essentially unheard of in the nineteenth century.[4] Why should this be so? There are many possible factors involved.

Our Lengthening Life Span. Women are the only female creatures who live long enough to experience menopause—all other mammals retain the reproduction function throughout their lives. This is probably not due to a defect in our species but, rather, to our lengthening life expectancy. Other female mammals simply die before they have exhausted their supply of eggs. In fact, we human females have just recently begun to enjoy our post-menopausal years and use them productively.

In early history, women succumbed to the complications of childbirth long before their twenty-fifth birthdays. By the year AD 1, life expectancy for females reached 33 years of age. During Queen Victoria's reign, in the late 1800s, the average woman lived until the age of 48, toward the end of the childbearing years.

Today, because of great advances in modern science, our longevity has been extended into the late seventies. This is wonderful news, of course, but it can accout for why we are seeing a rise in the incidence of ovarian cancer.

Malfunctioning Ovaries. Although it has not yet been fully proven by research, I believe that any process which keeps the ovaries from functioning normally may lead to ovarian cancer. This theory is based on clinical experience and research findings.

Hysterectomy may shut down the blood supply to the ovaries, causing them to be scarred and inactive. Other conditions, such as endometriosis, severe pelvic inflammatory disease, tubal ligation at an early age, a large fibroid, and the mumps may also achieve the same result. Researchers have theorized that any condition that encapsulates the ovaries, causing them to cease functioning normally, may trigger the development of malignancy.[5]

Irregular menstrual cycles and no periods (*amenorrhoea*) also are a risk factor in the development of ovarian cancer. Ironically, birth control pills (oral contraceptives), often feared as the harbinger of death and disease, may have some positive effect in the prevention of ovarian cancer by regularizing the monthly cycle.

The opposite is also true. Women who have never been pregnant and whose ovaries have not been given a 'rest' during the nine months of gestation are at increased risk. The repeated stimulation of incessant ovulation has been well documented as a risk factor as well as a long period of menstruation (ie, early onset of menses and late menopause).[6]

Pregnancy itself, especially before the age of 25, appears to protect you. Pregnancy might create some changes in the pituitary gland, which permanently alter the secretion of certain hormones that stimulate the ovaries.[7] Perhaps the increasing incidence of ovarian cancer in Western countries is related to the decreasing number of children born to successive generations and sociological factors that delay pregnancy, coupled with other factors such as fat intake, diet, and exposure to toxins.

When follicle development in the ovary goes awry, substantially higher levels of oestrogen can be produced. Sometimes many follicles will start to develop, but none will go to maturity and ovulation. In that case, the ovary becomes enlarged, with many follicles or cysts in various stages of development. One form of this is *polycystic ovary disease*, which does carry an increased risk for ovarian cancer.

Racial and Genetic Factors. The mortality rates for all types of ovarian cancer vary widely from country to country. The Japanese, for example, have a low rate, whereas Swedish women have a relatively high rate. In the United States, the rates for white women are higher than for nonwhites. As black women achieve a higher socioeconomic status, however, they bear

fewer children, and consume a diet higher in fat like their Caucasian counterparts, and thus may run a greater risk.[8]

The woman at highest risk for ovarian cancer:

- Has had no children
- Is a Caucasian of northern European descent
- Is living in an industrialized country

The risk is increased if her sister, mother, maternal aunt, or grandmother have had cancer of the breast or ovary, or if she, herself, has had breast cancer. Studies have even shown an increased risk when close relatives have cancer of the colon, lung, and prostate.[9]

There have been documented cases where four and five family members, spanning three generations, fall victim to ovarian cancer. Familial cancers arise at a younger age and affect both ovaries more often than non-familial cancers.[10]

If there is ovarian cancer in your family, should you have your ovaries removed as a precaution? This is a complex issue. Although our awareness of familial ovarian cancer has been increasing, scientists are still uncertain as to whether it is caused by one gene, several genes, or the interaction of the genetic potential with external factors, such as the use of body talc. It has even been suggested that your susceptibility may depend on genetically controlled factors, such as enzymes that regulate the metabolism of chemical compounds in the environment.

If the disease is caused by a single, dominant gene, the 50 per cent risk of developing this cancer may, indeed, warrant a prophylactic oöphorectomy. If, on the other hand, it is dependent on the combination of several genetic and environmental factors, the 2 to 5 per cent risk for developing this cancer would make oöphorectomy less appealing.

Besides, some women whose ovaries were removed because of hereditary factors developed other abdominal cancers.[11] Only time and scientific investigation will reveal more about the hereditary factors in ovarian cancer. Research is currently being conducted into the existence of chromosomal irregularities specific to ovarian cancer and into hereditary factors for identical twins and their daughters. This is exciting news, because such studies may also lead to a more positive way to screen for this disease.[12] *See a geneticist if you have a family history of ovarian cancer.*

Toxins in the Environment. Are you in the habit of dusting your genital area or sanitary napkin with talcum powder? Studies have shown that women who engage in this seemingly innocent, hygienic practice are increasing their risk for ovarian cancer. Talc is chemically related to asbestos, a well-established environmental cause of cancer, and can increase your risk for the disease.[13] Given how dangerous ovarian cancer can be, there is no reason to continue this practice. I even avoid the routine use of baby powder on my daughter.

Scientific investigations have made a positive association between herbicide exposure and certain types of ovarian cancer.[14] As we continue to contaminate our environment, our reproductive organs will suffer.

Diet. I've already discussed how excess body weight can hinder the detection of ovarian cancer by masking the enlargement of postmenopausal ovaries. A woman's diet, itself, has been correlated with the incidence of the disease.

Women with ovarian cancer eat significantly greater amounts of animal fat and significantly less vegetable fat than the women without cancer.[15] Why should this be so? We are not certain. But perhaps, the greater a woman's weight, the more fat in her body. The more fat, the higher the oestrogen levels. The higher the oestrogen, the greater the irregularities in the menses. And irregular cycles are a risk factor.

An earlier study, although not corroborating these findings on dietary fat, did find that pre-menopausal women reporting diets low in fibre and vitamin A from fruit and vegetable sources showed an increased risk for ovarian cancer. Further analysis demonstrated that vitamin A had some protective effect in the 30- to 49-year age group.[16]

Alcoholism has also been shown to be associated with ovarian cancer. Although there is no association between moderate drinking and ovarian disease, women under the age of 55 who consumed more than twenty drinks per week were at higher risk than women who didn't drink at all.[17] Hypertension, diabetes, and underactive thyroid—conditions that may coincide with obesity—have also been correlated to both polycystic ovary disease and ovarian cancer.[18]

Are you at risk for ovarian cancer? A review

Let's review the potential risk factors for ovarian cancer. Do you:

1. Have a family history of ovarian, uterine, or breast cancer?
2. Have no history of pregnancy?
3. Use body talc products?
4. Find yourself frequently exposed to herbicides and environmental toxins, including those in the workplace?
5. Experience irregular or no menstrual cycles, ovarian malfunctions, ovarian tumours, ovarian cysts, polycystic

ovarian disease, Turner's syndrome (a genetic disorder)?

6. Consume a diet high in fat, low in vitamin A?

7. Have hypertension or diabetes?

Ways to prevent ovarian cancer

Of course, there is little you can do to change your heredity or your medical history. But there are some definite and *easy* steps you can take to help discourage ovarian cancer.

Nutrition. Proper diet is essential to helping prevent ovarian cancer. A low-fat diet helps to eliminate the abdominal fat pad that makes detection so difficult.

A fatty diet has also been correlated with other forms of gynaecological cancer, including endometrial and breast cancer. It would be wise to adopt safe eating habits, which would include:

- Eating less animal fats, eggs, and fried foods
- Eating more fruits and vegetables, especially those rich in vitamin A and vitamin E
- Reducing alcohol intake
- Maintaining a healthy body weight

I suggest supplementing your diet with vitamins E and A.

Birth Control Pills. The risk of ovarian cancer is reduced among women who use combination oral contraceptives. The protective effect of the pills persists as long as ten years after you stop using it. In fact, the 500 deaths annually associated with oral contraceptives (which could theoretically be reduced to 70 if contraceptive users over 35 stopped smoking) are offset by the estimated 850 ovarian cancer deaths that are *prevented* by the pill's use.[19]

Irregular menstrual cycles can be regulated with birth control pills, both for women who skip periods and for those who produce too much oestrogen. Like pregnancy, birth control pills suppress ovulation and the release of gonadotropins, which also tend to decrease the risks.

Family History. If ovarian cancer occurs in your family, there is no need to throw up your hands in despair. Cancer education and genetic counselling initiated by the age of 20 or earlier, and careful surveillance (with bimanual examination and ultrasound twice a year) begun at age 30 are good preventative measures. The option of prophylactic oöphorectomy should only be considered if you have an unequivocally high risk of developing the disease. You should have completed childbearing, received genetic and hormonal counselling, and been informed of the irreversible nature of the surgery.

Toxins. Avoid products containing talc, especially in the genital area. This is good advice for your baby, as well. Keep herbicides such as weedkillers out of your environment.

Regular Screening. Regular screening with ultrasound may be a good idea for women over 50. Ovarian cancer is a frightening disease. Remember, by the time your doctor can feel your ovary to be larger than normal, it may be too late. Although all the evidence isn't in yet, it is possible that ultrasound can help. More investigation is needed into refining screening procedures because this is such a rapidly growing cancer.

Why are so many ovaries being removed?

The National Cancer Institute predicts that

in 1986, 5,100 men will develop testicular cancer an 19,000 women will develop ovarian cancer in the United States. Although these two kinds of cancer are entirely different diseases, with varying methods of detection and levels of seriousness, they are somewhat analogous because of the organs' function. The testes produce hormones and sperm that coincides with the ovaries' production of hormones and eggs.

Because there are roughly four times as many cases of ovarian cancer as compared to testicular cancer, you would expect there to be four times as many oöphorectomies as there are testicle removals performed in 1984. That, however, is not the case. According to the National Centers for Health Statistics, there were 498,000 oöphorectomies performed in 1984, on cancerous as well as non-cancerous ovaries[20] versus only 54,000 testicle removals.

Why should this disparity exist? At the age of 40, why don't we see men lining up to get their testicles amputated as a precautionary measure in the same proportion that we see women consenting to such a surgery? And why does this suggestion seem ludicrous to us?

Although it's true that testicular cancer is less dangerous than ovarian because it is more easily detected and treated early on, I believe that a cultural bias exists with regard to female organs. We endow the male's hormone function with more importance than the female's. A man's virility, his strength, and his ability to reproduce are all linked to his testes. We believe that castration disables him psychologically and impairs his ability to function in society.

Wouldn't the castration of women produce the same catastrophic results? I believe so. Yet we don't generally think of oöphorectomy as having analogous effects. We have been taught that after 35 or 40, our ovaries are dispensable—certainly they are less important than the testes, otherwise we wouldn't agree to have them removed so readily. We have come to believe that we can function without our hormones. How can this be true?

Ovaries have a more complex function than merely the manufacture of eggs. The hormones produced by our ovaries enable us to function physically as well as psychologically. The removal of ovaries creates a magnitude of problems that we are just beginning to evaluate, including heart disease, osteoporosis, arthritis, depression, mood disorders, and neurological diseases. Besides, many women are opting to bear children later in life.

Because oöphorectomy and the loss of the ovaries' hormone contribution has such a profound influence on many body functions, and because there are no meaningful data in the scientific literature to support the value of routine oöphorectomy,[21] I stand fast in my belief that removal of the ovaries should be performed *only* when those organs are cancerous and where there is no other option.

CHAPTER 16

Other menstrual and pelvic problems

'All gynaecological operations should be targeted to the problem. Hysterectomy cures only bleeding. Yet few doctors deal with, for example, chronic pelvic inflammatory disease (PID) other than by total hysterectomy. All that needs to be done is to remove the tubes and any surrounding inflammatory tissue—the source of the infection—and the uterus itself can be left alone.'

Professor Stuart Campbell, Head of Department of Obstetrics and Gynaecology, King's College Hospital.

In 1983, the latest year for which figures are available, 109,500 hysterectomies were performed in the United States for dysfunctional uterine bleeding. Premenstrual tension accounted for 13,000 additional hysterectomies. These figures boggle the mind! The vast majority of these surgeries could have been avoided.[1] In the UK dysfunctional menstrual bleeding and 'other' causes including enigmatic pelvic pain accounts for over 46 per cent of operations.

Cutting off your nose . . .

You've heard the expression, 'It's like cutting off your nose to spite your face'. Well, hysterectomy for menstrual problems is more like 'cutting out your uterus to spite your body'. It will stop your menses, but it can make other things worse.

I'm painfully aware that women suffer from heavy or irregular bleeding, debilitating cramps, post-tubal ligation problems, and premenstrual syndrome. But hysterectomy shouldn't be the answer. Today, there is so much we can do to alleviate suffering, including medications, diet, and exercise. Why rush into hysterectomy, given how damaging it can be, when there are so many alternatives?

I think the conservative approach, and by that I mean conserving the organs, is best for your total health. Of course, this may take some sleuthing on your doctor's part, which requires more time and energy. It's easy to cut first and ask questions later. But I believe hysterectomy should be the very end of the line—after all other courses of treatment have been exhausted.

How to find out what's wrong when you're bleeding abnormally

Any irregularities in bleeding patterns should be investigated fully because there is always a danger of cancer. The threat is real, especially in high-risk women who are obese, have a history of missed periods when they were younger, or who are menopausal—that is, they've stopped having their periods but have now begun to bleed. In these cases a D & C is indicated.

Shirley came in to see me in a state of alarm. She was 48 years old and still pre-menopausal. Over the last year, she noticed that her periods were getting heavier and heavier. Sometimes there was clotting. During the two months preceding her visit, she found it necessary to sequester herself because the flow was so extensive that she feared soaking through her tampon and sanitary napkins. She was worried.

I could readily understand Shirley's anxiety. Not only was she inconvenienced, but she recognized that such unusual bleeding could be a sign of uterine cancer. However, abnormal spotting, heavy bleeding at unusual times, for prolonged periods, or with large blood clots, are often caused by hormonal imbalances and stress that occur at or near the menopause.

Just to stay on the safe side with Shirley, who had gained quite a bit of weight recently, I recommended that she have a D & C. We needed to rule out endometrial cancer (In Chapter 10, I discuss this procedure in detail.) I would like to reiterate that a thorough D & C is essential.

I am happy to say that Shirley's pathology report came back negative—her uterus was cancer-free. The unusual bleeding must have been triggered by a different mechanism. We investigated further and discovered an excess of oestrogen, probably due to Shirley's weight problem. I put Shirley on a strict, low-fat diet and within several months her flow returned to normal.

Growths in the uterus

The hysteroscope is another means helpful in diagnosing bleeding problems. With this device I can scan the interior of the uterus for big adhesions, polyps, cancer, fibroids, and other abnormalities of the lining of the uterus.

Your doctor can't just look in and say with any kind of certainty, 'Oh, that's cancer and that's not.' We still need a tissue diagnosis. Tissue can be biopsied through the hysteroscope or a D & C can be performed.

The bleeding from fibroids may be so severe that it can trigger anaemia. Fibroids certainly aren't cancer, however, and they don't require an instant hysterectomy (see Chapter 9).

Other risk factors for unusual bleeding

Any changes in your daily pattern can cause abnormal bleeding. Stress, poor diet, changes in exercise regime can alter your equilibrium and your hormone balance. Anything that affects the pituitary gland, for example, stresses your body and throws your hormones into flux. if an ovarian cyst develops and doesn't rupture, takes weeks to rupture, or ruptures out of sync, the hormones get released inappropriately or not at all. This mistiming can cause bleeding that does not coincide with your usual cycle.

Spotting because of hormone irregularities

Spotting between cycles can come from a variety of sources. Hormonal irregularities during ovulation or from ovarian cysts may cause it to occur. Breakthrough bleeding from birth control pills is common. This usually causes alarm but is of little consequence.

Spotting because of the cervix

Your cervix can be the source of much

spotting and bleeding. Polyps growing there may bleed intermittently. Chronic vaginal and cervical infections erode and inflame the cervix, creating spotting. These infections can be sexually transmitted or could come from contamination of the vagina by rectal bacteria. I've seen many damaged cervices.

Margo had a cervix so inflamed from chronic vaginal infections that if I so much as touched it with a cervical smear stick, it bled. I can just imagine what happened to it during intercourse. I treated her with antibiotics to clear up the infection and the spotting stopped.

Spotting from the uterus

Polyps coming down the uterus and infections within the uterus can both cause spotting. These can be diagnosed and treated easily using an operative hysteroscope. While your surgeon looks inside the uterus, (s)he can insert a laser fibre or instrument capable of removing the polyp or small fibroid from its lining.

The symptoms of endometrial hyperplasia (the proliferation of the uterine lining) and endometrial cancer (see Chapter 10) include spotting; so do the symptoms of cervical cancer (see Chapter 12).

Spotting from 'foreign bodies' and infection

Helen wasn't paying attention and forgot to remove her tampon after her period was over. By the time she remembered, this foreign body had caused a severe infection. When the infection got into the uterus, Helen began to spot and bleed abnormally. She also experienced pain. She had *endometritis*, which is an infection of the uterine lining or endometrium.

Any foreign body inside the uterus can cause spotting. Intrauterine devices (IUD), although not as popular as they were in the 1970s, are still used. The IUD, even without infection, can cause abnormal bleeding by continually rubbing on the uterine lining.

Bleeding can come from lesions on the vagina, and ulceration from a tampon left in too long. Cancer of the vagina and venereal warts in the vagina are also culprits.

Roberta came in with a remarkable number of venereal warts. The warts started breaking off and becoming infected, and as a result, she bled. Herpes in the vagina and on the cervix, chlamydia—in fact, all of the sexually transmitted diseases—can cause abnormal bleeding and spotting.

No periods

Insufficient food consumption may cause menstrual irregularities. Jill was a 25-year-old aerobics enthusiast who had a five-year history of no periods. Working out every day, she weighed in at 101 pounds on a 5'6" frame. She was a vegetarian to boot. Was Jill prematurely menopausal? Doubtful. She was protein and fat deficient, and therefore oestrogen deficient. As a result, Jill's hormones were not cycling. She was amenorrhoeic, just like the runners and the ballerinas whom I often see with this problem.

You may feel relieved to be free of your periods and may not view amenorrhoea as a matter of concern, but this is a mistake. Intensive exercise and insufficient calorie intake shut down the hormones and inhibit menstruation. Your body needs withdrawal bleeding—it's part of your natural cycle. Amenorrhoea can predispose you to infertility and the lack of oestrogen can exacerbate osteoporosis, especially if you're athletic.

In order to get Jill menstruating again I explained why her life-style needed alteration. We discussed adding more fat and protein to her diet and an easing of her rigorous exercise regimen. Oestrogen with progesterone supplements can also be used to help balance the deficiency. I've successfully treated several women with vitamins and amino acid supplements.

Food supplements to help reduce abnormal uterine bleeding

It is possible that some minor life-style changes, including altering your diet, may help to reduce abnormal uterine bleeding. A word of caution, however: these dietary interventions should in no way replace a visit to your gynaecologist. It is most important that you ascertain the reason for the bleeding, because there is a risk of cancer here. Make sure to have the function of your thyroid checked. Thyroid abnormalities often create menstrual problems.

Dysmenorroea—severe pain with periods

This is a common affliction. It's a qualitative call as to how much pain a woman suffers during her menstrual cycle. Terri takes to bed once a month, doubled up in agony. I, on the other hand, am fortunate not to experience any pain when I bleed. But I do know what menstrual cramps feel like! I had uterine contractions during the birth of my daughter. I can easily imagine women experiencing that kind of severe pain every month and can understand why they would want to be free of the torture. I can understand it, but I can't condone hysterectomy as the first-choice solution.

Drugs have been used for years to battle the symptoms of dysmenorroea. We've all seen the ads for pain-relieving drugs like Ibuprofen directed at girls approaching and experiencing puberty. Aspirin, analgesics like Tylenol (acetaminophen), codeine and, in the United States, habit-forming analgesics like Demerol (meperide hydrochloride) as well as the benzodiazepine derivatives like Valium have all been prescribed in varying dosages. Most of these are narcotic (habit-forming) or narcotic-like in action; that is, they numb and dull the system.

We now know that *prostaglandins* act on the uterus to create contractions. They are produced by the uterus and are also found, in high concentrations, in sperm. It is possible that women who experience severe cramps have an excess of these chemicals produced by the uterus.

Your non-habit-forming pain control programme for any chronic pelvic pain

Chronic pain of the female organs can be more intense than the acute pain of surgery. It is a gnawing, deep, almost nauseating sensation. There is hope, however, for alleviating this pain. The following are some safe suggestions which, of course, avoid hysterectomy.

Menstrual Pain. It is possible to curtail your menstrual cramps with non-narcotic, antiprostaglandin drugs that inhibit the action of the prostaglandins. Antiprostaglandins should be started before the first twinges of pain, however. Once the cramps have gone on for hours, it takes a long time for the drug to become effective.

Habit-forming opiates like morphine and its derivatives have been prescribed to control pain. Our bodies, however, secrete their own opiates. The amino acids, D-phenylalanine, D-leucine, and L-tryptophan, products of the digestion of proteins, are effective in fighting chronic pelvic pain.

How do the amino acids work? It's rather a complicated story. *Enkephalin* is a protein within your central nervous system that decreases pain. Any substance that maintains or increases enkephalin production would help to reduce pain. *Enkephalinase*, on the other hand, is an enzyme that breaks down enkephalin, rendering it ineffective.

D-phenylalanine inhibits the action of enkephalinase, maintaining the enkephalin level, and so reduces the response and degree of pain. It also acts as an anti-inflammatory.[2] Clinically, I have used D-phenylalanine for five years in conjunction with calcium and magnesium and other vitamins to assist in pain control.

The pain threshold is an important factor in pain control. Many substances that control pain sensation alter the threshold mechanism of pain. Each of us has her own threshold. If, for example, my threshold is 5, then whenever I experience a sensation greater than 5, I will feel pain. But if my body is manufacturing its own endorphins and opiates, these will raise my threshold to, say, 8. Then a stimulus of 6 would not be perceived as painful by my body. The amino acid, L-tryptophan, a precursor of the neurotransmitter serotonin, increases the pain threshold.[3]

For centuries, herbs were used to control menstrual pain, and old herb books show how we can smooth out the lining of the uterus and decrease pain using natural agents. I have found that a herbal tea brings some relief in alleviating cramps. The tea may be effective and I see no reason not to try it.

I believe that women who experience debilitating cramps can be helped by vitamin and mineral supplements, herbs, and dietary changes. It is my hunch that the amino acid, D-phenylalanine, vitamin B_6, magnesium, zinc, calcium, and raspberry tea may all be helpful. This regimen is effective in relieving pain from endometriosis and other pelvic problems.

Exercise has been shown to greatly decrease cramping. It is thought that it may, in some way, inhibit the action of prostaglandins or increase the action of the endorphins, the body's natural painkillers.

Obese women tend to produce too much oestrogen which, in turn, creates heavy periods with large blood clots and extensive shedding of the endometrial lining. The obvious solution is to lose weight in order to lessen the flow of oestrogen. Many women may require progesterone therapy as well.

There's always the chance of error

Hanna had severe endometriosis of the bowel. Every month, like clockwork, she suffered intense abdominal pain with her period. She complained to her gynaecologist and he removed her uterus, ovaries, and fallopian tubes.

Hanna's monthly pains continued, even without her reproductive organs, because Hanna's doctor prescribed oestrogen replacement therapy after her surgery to alleviate the hot flushes and depression. But the endometriosis in her intestines remained, so every month, spurred on by the oestrogen, the endometrial implants swelled and bled as if her reproductive organs were still intact. The real issue was never addressed. And now, not only did Hanna have the discomfort, but she also had to contend with the problems inherent in a surgical menopause.

The truth is, there are no guarantees in

this game. Medical science is just not advanced enough to have all the answers. We simply can't make the claims that by taking out the uterus, we will save a woman from severe cramps. It's not always that simple. We need to know the cause of her pain before we undertake surgery as serious as a hysterectomy.

Hanna's case is tragic but it's not unusual. Other problems like intestinal cramps, Crohn's disease, and functional bowel disease can also mimic the symptoms of dysmenorrhoea and endometriosis. Removing the uterus cannot guarantee freedom from pain.

Post-tubal ligation syndrome

We have grown accustomed to accepting tubal sterilization as an easy, consequence-free form of contraception. Having one's 'tubes tied' seems the thing to do. Even the terminology 'Band-Aid sterilization' serves to diminish the import and the possible serious consequences of the procedure. In fact, in the United States, approximately 650,000 women of reproductive age undergo tubal sterilization each year.[4]

I find it difficult to take tubal ligation lightly. In fact, my patients have to fight me for this form of birth control and fight hard. I perform it infrequently because I've seen so many women with post-tubal problems. Maryanne was bleeding and in pain for six years after her tubal. Many post-tubal patients who come to my office seeking relief complain bitterly of more severe cramps, heavier, longer periods, dysfunctional uterine bleeding, pain with intercourse, and pelvic pain or pressure.

My clinical observations have been borne out by scientific investigations. Many studies confirm the existence of post-tubal ligation syndrome and show that existing menstrual problems can be aggravated by tubal sterilization.[5] Three theories explain why these problems occur:

1. Tubal ligation destroys the blood supply to the ovaries.
2. Certain types of tubal sterilization procedures are more likely to result in endometriosis.
3. An increase in the blood pressure within the ovarian artery can create an oestrogen-progesterone imbalance.

Many studies confirm finding varicosities (abnormal swelling or enlargements) in ovarian veins, hormonal imbalances, and fistulas of the fallopian tubes, which are associated with endometriosis in women who have been sterilized.[6]

The most frequent type of sterilization in the 1970s involved burning the tubes during laparoscopy. Not only does this run the risk of burning the bowels but it creates massive tissue damage and adhesions. If a patient of mine chooses to have her tubes tied, I prefer clipping the tubes closed, because this method presents fewer post-operative problems. More research is needed to improve sterilization and decrease its symptoms.

I believe that the fallopian tubes need to be open and working. In a tubal ligation, we burn or clip them closed. If retrograde or backup bleeding occurs during menstruation (see Chapter 8), the tubes blow up and become swollen and inflamed. The ovaries need to be nourished by oxygen and blood. In many cases, fertility cannot be re-established even after the ligation is reversed because of damage to the ovaries.[7]

Probably one of the most serious consequences of post-tubal ligation syndrome is that it may lead to hysterectomy.[8] There is a terrible irony in this. Imagine going in to have your tubes tied, thinking that this will finally take care of all your contraception needs, only to discover months later that your cramps are worse, the bleeding more intense. And from your complaints comes the recommendation for hysterectomy. Studies have shown that post-tubal problems worsen with time. One investigation in Scotland found that the annual hysterectomy rate for sterilized women was 9.3 per cent as opposed to 2.5 per cent in their control population.[9]

Until some long-range follow-up investigations are completed, we can only guess at how many women seek an end to their post-tubal ligation symptoms through hysterectomy. A woman who already has chosen a surgical method of contraception may be likely to choose a surgical solution to her menstrual complaints or to symptoms from endometriosis. I don't believe women are given true options. They are simply told that hysterectomy is the only answer.

Women need to know

Although many governments now require informed consent for sterilization, I believe we are not doing an adequate job in educating women about the potential problems following tubal ligation, including the possibility of hysterectomy.

And we are definitely remiss in screening potential tubal ligation patients. I've seen women in my practice with fibroids and endometriosis whose tubes were tied. If you are already suffering from dysmenorrhoea, heavy bleeding, or irregular cycles, you are not a prime candidate for having your tubes tied. You run the risk of compounding your pain and problems with the procedure. You may dramatically increase your chances for a hysterectomy in the near future.

Premenstrual syndrome: a non-syndrome

From the time that Suzanna was a college student in the 1960s, she recognized that she had cyclic but profound changes in mood. Some days she was happy, excited about life, energetic, sexual, optimistic. Other days, she was depressed, exhausted, weepy, aggressive, irritable, dulled. Until she learned the cause and patterns of her mood swings, they played havoc with her life and relationships.

Suzanna was suffering from a hormonal imbalance. For centuries, women were thought of as hysterical, crazy, or worse when they went through the 'down' phase of their cycles. Fortunately, medical understanding has come of age; these problems are now being taken seriously. Dr Katherina Dalton, of the Premenstrual Syndrome Institute in the University College Hospital, London, has worked long and hard to educate women and the medical community about Premenstrual Syndrome (PMS).

The labelling of this hormonal disorder has allowed us to understand something very basic: chemical fluctuations during the month associated with the menstrual cycle can create imbalances in the brain which, in turn, result in physiological and behavioural changes. These changes ought not to be viewed as disease or mental illness, but rather as part of the ebb and flow of your normal cycle.

Changes may include:

- Oedema (water retention)
- Breast swelling and pain
- Abdominal distension or bloating
- Fatigue and lethargy
- Increased sleep needs
- Mood disorders, including spontaneous crying spells, anxiety, depression
- Constipation

- Acne or other skin eruptions

The question remains, however, as to whether or not an actual *syndrome* exists. According to Dr Dalton, PMS can occur no earlier than two weeks before the menstrual period and is caused by a deficiency in progesterone. A progesterone cottage industry has sprung up around her advocacy of progesterone therapy. I, however, have seen women who suffer from PMS symptoms for up to three weeks (only feeling balanced during menstruation) and others who have symptoms throughout the month. In addition, progesterone therapy works wonders for some women yet not at all for others.

What can this mean? I believe that women have copious varieties of hormonal imbalance disorders. Because scientific investigation has not identified all hormones produced by the female body, we cannot fully diagnose or treat these imbalances as yet. However, research continues on:

- Hormonal release and receptor sites
- Pituitary action
- Excess oestrogen and inadequate progesterone
- Vitamin B_6 deficiency
- Altered glucose tolerance

How to cope when symptoms get out of hand

It's best to record, identify, and group your symptoms month by month. When you discover your own profile, you and your doctor can create an individualized programme to suit your needs. Many women deal with their hormone imbalances by simply recognizing and accepting them, thus integrating the ebb and flow into their lives. This helps to diminish the feeling of 'craziness'.

Some women have had complete resolution with progesterone, whereas others improve with dietary changes and exercise. Amino acids and herbal treatments work for some. You should not feel bound to a particular product (like progesterone) or treatment plan, but rather remain open to new possibilities, realizing that there is no single answer because there is no single disease.

The following are dietary suggestions that may help:

- Avoid caffeine (in coffee, tea, soft drinks, and chocolate) and alcohol. They make matters worse.
- Eat small, frequent meals during the day. Don't go for long periods of time without food. The feeling of starvation contributes to the syndrome.
- Increase protein and fibre in your diet. Bran cereals help relieve constipation.
- Supplement your diet with daily doses of vitamin B_6 and vitamin E.
- Consume more foods high in potassium and magnesium like bananas and oranges.
- Cut down on sodium (salt) in your diet. This contributes to water retention and bloating.

The folly of hysterectomy for PMS

One patient sent this letter to the doctor who performed her hysterectomy, eight months after the operation. It was in her medical file.

Approximately every 28 days for the past 5 months or so, I have been experiencing severe lower back pain. Lack of appetite due to an irregular bowel movement . . . Pain and tenderness in the area of the missing ovaries, alternating from right to left from month to month. I have also been experiencing a change in my emotional or chemical makeup during these periods. These periods seem to last 5 to 7 days. This is all very similar to the monthly menstrual discomfort I was having prior to my hysterectomy. I find it difficult to sleep or relax during this time ...

Scientific studies have shown that neither the presence of the uterus nor menstruation itself are necessary for the manifestation of PMS, which can continue even after the uterus is gone.[10] These investigations now support the view that PMS has a hormonal basis.

Clinically, I have found that PMS gets worse in some patients after hysterectomy. And, for a few, it *begins* after hysterectomy in women who have never had to deal with it while menstruating.

Painful intercourse (dyspareunia)

Sex is not supposed to hurt. On the contrary, pleasure should be your experience. Many women do experience painful intercourse, sometimes as a result of hysterectomy (when the ovaries fall onto the top of the vaginal vault), but often as a result of physiological problems or disease processes.

The following conditions can create pain during entry:

- Infection (especially herpes)
- Monilial vulvitis
- Bartholinitis (infection of the Bartholin gland)
- Atrophic vaginitis (when the vaginal tissue atrophies because of lack of oestrogen)

- Allergy to douches, feminine deodorant sprays, etc.
- A rigid hymen
- Poorly healed episiotomy scar
- Gaping opening or torn muscles from delivery
- Foreign body
- Vaginismus (involuntary contraction of the vaginal muscles)

Pain on deep penetration can be caused by abnormalities in the pelvic cavity. These include:

- Ovarian cysts
- Pelvic inflammatory disease (PID)
- Endometriosis
- Prolapse of female organs
- Adhesions
- Lacerations of the broad ligaments
- Cancer
- Prolapsed ovaries
- Bladder adhering to the vagina after hysterectomy

Although pain during sex can be caused by emotional problems, you can see that there is a whole rash of possible anatomical and physiological causes. All possible organic problems should be ruled out before your problem is labelled psychosomatic. That means a careful history and physical examination should be taken. In the case of cancer, this may be a lifesaving act, but by no means should dyspareunia be a cause for hysterectomy (unless, of course, it is a question of cancer).

If you do experience pain with sex, you may wish to seek out psychological care. This problem can create a good deal of confusion and disruption in your relationships and psychological support can be helpful. Most physiological problems can be cured with less drastic measures, including medication, education, and FRS.

Update: miracle babies

In today's supercharged technological climate, the birth of babies to previously infertile women is becoming commonplace. Yet there is still a large group of women whose concerns have not been addressed: it is one thing to be told that you will have difficulty conceiving due to blocked fallopian tubes and quite another to be informed that you will never have children or be able to add to your family because you must undergo an immediate hysterectomy.

Robin Becker-Menker faced such a possibility. From the start of her menstrual periods as a teenager Robin had suffered from painful, heavy bleeding. Her doctor would occasionally pat her on the shoulder, prescribe another pain medication, and tell her there was nothing to do but learn to live with it.

By age twenty-nine, she had tried everything from holistic diets to exercise programmes to ease her pain. A laparoscopy finally confirmed a sizeable fibroid in the lower left wall of her uterus. At that point, Robin was advised that there was 'nothing to do about it except a hysterectomy', because the fibroid was in such a place that surgery to remove it would be 'very bloody' and doomed to failure. She was told that the fibroid had to be watched because as it increased in size it could cause kidney and bladder problems—and was also likely to cause miscarriages, *if* she were ever able to conceive.

By the autumn of 1985, Robin was engaged to a man who wanted children as desperately as she did. She was distressed to learn that the fibroid was still growing. She

was being told, 'We have to take the uterus out now'.

Joanne Ladjimi, a thirty-seven-year-old orthopaedic nurse in Long Beach, California, saw her gynaecologist after experiencing four years of heavy bleeding and pain between her periods. After ordering an ultrasound and other tests, he called Joanne on the phone and told her that she would never be able to have children; the fibroid was attached to the upper part of her uterus, filling it and blocking the fallopian tubes. 'I kept asking him if it couldn't just be removed. He just flatly said "No." He was very cold and uncaring about it—as if it wasn't important that I have babies. He wouldn't give me any hope and brushed my feelings aside. I had just got married and became hysterical.'

Thuy Nugent, a thirty-eight-year-old engineer in Torrence, California, had been scheduled for a hysterectomy because of her large uterus, the size of a five-month pregnancy. She had been to numerous doctors, all of them stating she had only *one* option. 'It was June, and I was planning to be married in December. I thought of cancelling the wedding. It didn't seem fair to have my fiancé marry a woman who had a hysterectomy.'

After FRS, all three women went on to conceive and carry their pregnancies to term without any complications: Thuy Nugent now has a healthy baby boy—a miracle baby according to those who told her that her uterus needed to be removed; Joanne Ladjimi has now given birth to her second child and is very happy; Robin Becker-Menker states simply '... there are not adequate words to thank for the gift of childbearing. Dr Hufnagel is a miracle worker. I owe her my babies.'

PART IV

Where do we go from here?

CHAPTER 17

Empowering yourself

'Women either don't know or are too frightened to ask very often. Should hysterectomy be carried out for pelvic pain of unknown origin? There may be a valid reason for carrying out hysterectomy even though there is no pathology: it's a clinical decision. Doctors in the UK are very reluctant to follow clinical protocols, and, even with the institution of the White Paper, it is unlikely that they will allow any interference with their clinical decision-making. One of the reasons why clinical protocols are common in the US is that insurance companies demand some sort of standardized approach before they will pay up. Indeed, the control of clinical practice by insurance companies is one of the most important and interesting areas of American medicine.'

UK Head of Obstetrics and Gynaecology

The stories

I have been motivated to do this work and write this book by the physical and emotional pain that I sense around me daily and by the desperation of women who see themselves trapped in a system without hope of escape. In my seven years of private practice as a gynaecological surgeon, I have heard stories—incredible, painful, heart-wrenching stories.

I have shared only a few of these tales with you. I am sure that you have other sad accounts to add to this collection—whether they're your own or those of your grandmother, mother, sister, aunt, cousin, or friend. Eventually, we are all touched by the abuse of unnecessary hysterectomy and other gynaecological surgery that simply removes normal tissues, decreasing fertility and normal functioning.

You must know by now that I feel haunted by the troubled women who come to see me. But no amount of compassion for their plight, no amount of medical or surgical skill can restore organs that have been amputated. Much as I would like to, I can't make up for the emotional pain of the past. At best, I can only offer remedies to counteract some of the losses. And, I can try to prevent future problems for our daughters.

But there is a future—and it is bright. The vast numbers of women facing hysterectomy in the next year, the next decade, the next century can be helped. The practice of medicine, as we know it, can be altered. Alternatives are available, if we only open our eyes to see them. And where alternatives are still lacking, we can create them. We have the skills and technology to do this and even more.

Seize your own power

Much of this book has to do with empowering you—to make informed choices; to participate actively in your own health care; to treat your body and female organs with the respect that they so richly deserve. When you take control of your personal health, you come to terms with your inner strength. You make decisions that are free of fear and follow your intuitive beliefs.

Taking responsibility for your own health may even help your doctors to become better healers. By your active involvement, you can encourage your gynaecologist to progress, to be part of the movement for change.

But you should be warned that the transition from powerless victim to empowered actor in your own situation is not an easy one. There are many factors that may influence how you see yourself in the world. Today, there are few role models to emulate. When no one has taken a prior stand, it's frightening to be the first to say, 'I will agree to hysterectomy if it saves my life. Otherwise, my organs are precious to me—too precious to lose.' Realize that you, too, are *precious*. Our society has not reinforced this position.

Growing up female

You may inadvertently encourage victimization by not educating yourself, by remaining silent, by refusing responsibility for your own medical care. In the doctor's office, you may have been made to act like a frightened, dependent little girl rather than a woman who has the ability to question and demand alternatives.

You may have been conditioned to find fault with yourself: you are too fat, too thin, too ugly, too stupid. If you venture from 'feminine' standards, you are labelled aggressive, hostile, mannish, eccentric, and worse. Single-mindedness, ambition, and independence are discouraged—even though these attributes are perfectly acceptable in men! If you step out of line, you're abnormal.

You may have been socialized to do as you are told. When ordered to get rid of your uterus, you may comply without question, especially if the person giving the orders is older, father-like, and cloaked in the white coat of authority. How can you question this man? You have learned early to respect and revere him. And you want his approval.

You may have been taught that your reproductive organs are of little use 'after childbearing age'.

How do you overcome this training? Only through life experience can you learn that power/authority for its own sake does not deserve your reverence. Hard work, love, and caring earn your respect, but this takes effort on your part and the personal decision to go beyond society's norms. Education is vital.

Indeed, sometimes the threat of hysterectomy can trigger a positive response if you view it as an opportunity to improve the quality of your life. No longer a helpless, hopeless victim of your body and of the tradition-bound medical community, you can take charge, and demand what you feel is right for you. Even the decision to undergo a hysterectomy—when made in full awareness of the potential risks and alternatives and not out of fear—can be a life-affirming experience.

The destructive effects of labelling

One of the first steps to change is stripping away the preconceptions and labels that society and your doctor may impose upon you. Once labelled, you are lost as a human being. Your uniqueness—with all of your concomitant idiosyncrasies, problems, quirks, and needs—is compromised. You are seen merely as a 'nun', a 'case of fibroids', a 'sexpot', 'a lesbian', 'a widow'.

These concepts can be purely an individual matter, based on each doctor's own personal experience and training and not on reality. Perhaps the doctor has had an unsuccessful marriage or is having trouble with a teenage daughter. Perhaps his wife feels threatened or jealous of the time he spends with his patients and expresses bitterness or hatred toward them. Your doctor's personal life can colour how he sees, treats, and labels you.

What can doctors do?

Despite my anger and frustration, it is not my purpose to set you against your doctor or the entire medical profession. Indeed, I only seek amelioration. Your doctor can do much to empower you by humanizing his or her attitudes toward you and the practice of medicine.

How, specifically, can changes be accomplished?

1. Your gynaecologist should never ask you to sign a consent form for exploratory surgery with a 'possible' hysterectomy. In so doing, (s)he deprives you of the opportunity to help take responsibility for the decision-making. The 'possibility' needs to be spelled out completely and in detail. You should be informed of all the potential risks and complications well in advance.

2. In the operating room, your surgeon should always consult the pathologist to discuss the surgical findings. This allows your doctor to have expert guidance during the course of the operation. Any removed tissue should be submitted to the pathologist for immediate review.

3. During the post-operative visit, your gynaecologist can review with you the operative pathology reports.

4. Your doctor needs to make you aware that (s)he is only human and vulnerable to unforeseen circumstances before, during, and after surgery. If you are informed of possible confusions and limitations before surgery, you can better understand any complications that may occur.

There ought to be a law

Only recently have laws been created to protect women who, throughout the world, still struggle for equal status. In the United Kingdom, for example, the statute to prevent sexual discrimination in employment was passed in 1975. Family law has changed only recently. In 1977, Korean women were granted rights of inheritance. Austria permitted divorce after mutual separation in 1978. Married women in Trinidad could not hold property until 1976.

Laws and statutes are needed to protect women from coercion and subjugation. Laws to protect women must address human rights issues, health considerations, and justice and equality. In UK law the concept of 'informed consent' is unknown. Patients must give their signed consent to an operation and this must be obtained 'with due care and formality'. As with all consents of this nature, the primary purpose is to provide evidence that the patient gave consent to the procedure(s) specified should there be any later cause to question what has proceeded. In order to give his/her consent, all patients must be given sufficient explanation of the 'nature and purpose' of the operation or treatment involved to enable them to give that consent—and it is the duty of the doctor to furnish this. Written consent is also needed for the administration of general or other anaesthetic for the purpose of the operation, and, in Australia for the administration of a blood transfusion. Examples of various consent forms in use are given in Appendix 3.

US informed consent laws

In the US, informed consent laws are responsible for actual change in medical practices. By mandate, patients are required to be educated. But the informed consent laws have a secondary benefit—they educate and protect the medical community, as well.

Today, many states have laws requiring informed consent for sterilization. Doctors are now required to inform their patients of alternatives to radical mastectomy in the event of breast cancer. Abusive practices in sterilization and mastectomy have diminished with these important laws. But the gains were hard fought and long overdue.

Hysterectomy is even more firmly entrenched in institutionalized medicine than mastectomy or sterilization. It's part of the feminine legacy, like the pain of childbirth. Changing how we view hysterectomy is a difficult task, but it is a necessary one. And the first step is creating informed consent laws on hysterectomy throughout the United States and beyond.

What you need to be told

Informed consent means that you fully understand:

- What is a hysterectomy?
- How is it performed?
- What are the risks and possible complications to the operation?
- What is oöphorectomy?
- What are its side effects and complications?
- Data on the relative risks and rates of all female cancers.
- What are the medical indications for hysterectomy?
- What are the medical and surgical treatment alternatives for benign diseases?
- What anaesthetic will be used?

These must be communicated to you by your doctor in a language that you understand.

What I'm doing—and what you can do

I have become active politically. I have been working with California State Senator Diane E. Watson, chairperson of the Senate Health and Human Services Committee, in my home state of California, in order to legislate for informed consent. Together, we wrote an informed consent for hysterectomy bill. Senator Watson introduced the bill to the California State legislature. After a gruelling fight, it passed and was signed into law by California Governor George Deukmejian in September 1987. You will find a copy of the bill in the Appendix.

I've also been active on a county level. I testified before the Los Angeles County Human Relations Commission hearings on 'Equity Issues in Health'. As a result of my input, the Los Angeles County Board of Supervisors adopted a resolution to 'make certain women are properly counselled on surgical procedures such as hysterectomies to insure that they are aware of the procedure as well as other alternatives available to them'.

You can make a difference, too.

Empower Yourself with Knowledge. Using the information in this book as a guide, question your gynaecologist about your problems and the alternative solutions. And teach your sons and daughters. Even if they don't grow up to become doctors, they need to learn, as children, about the intrinsic beauty and complexity of the female system.

Simply Refuse to Sign for a Hysterectomy If You Don't Want One. You don't have to be coerced into signing at surgery or your consent can be conditional on whether or not a malignancy is found. You are creating a contract with your surgeon who needs to respect your wishes.

Organize! There is strength in numbers and when voices are raised in unison, they can be heard. I hope that my efforts in California will benefit the women of this state. But wherever you live, I can't think of a better way of constructively venting rage at a system that has done you harm than to advocate publicly for change. And when you do, not only will you feel less resentful, but you will also know that you may have improved the lives of generations of women to come, including your own daughters and granddaughters.

What the medical profession can do

Change is not up to women alone. I believe that we must force a re-examination of society's medical beliefs and practices. Doctors must come to terms with the revolution in women's health care and with their own belief systems.

When I listen to myself instructing my patients about their upcoming surgical experience, I am aware of all of the negative issues I must cover. Yet my patients invariably thank me for taking the time to give them this vital information so that they can make their own choices and participate in their own care.

Many of the pamphlets and commercial patient education materials distributed to women are misleading. I never rely on these. They are written from a *public relations* point of view: they sell surgery, gloss over complications and risks, and paint a rosy, simplistic picture. In an effort to avoid scaring you, they make surgery sound easy and risk free. Yet you are more sophisticated. You want to know. The creation of an informed consent law for hysterectomy can only improve the way in which doctors practice and reduce the problems that arise from inadequate patient education.

From powerless to powerful

I find it curious that a 48-year-old woman can have a face-lift so freely. However, if she wishes to save her reproductive organs, she is ridiculed for being irrational and unstable. Such an attitude devalues not only the organs themselves, but perhaps more important, the truly awe-inspiring complexity of the entire female reproductive system. Remember, this system is not dedicated simply to the propagation of our species. It is tied to nearly every aspect of a woman's health, including her blood chemistry, brain chemistry, neurological system, endocrine system, skeletal system, immune system, body fat, sexuality, and psychological functioning.

I have spent years researching and thinking about how we have come to conclude that the female reproductive system is completely expendable without consequence. I've shared with you some of the historical perspective in Chapter 4. But I suspect the answer may be yet more complex and rooted in some eternal struggle between men and women.

I could cite spiritual issues. For even though I am a scientist, dedicated to careful investigation and scientific method, I cannot deny the fact that women, because of their biology, are in some way connected to the continuum of life. The birth process and menstrual cycle create the link between past and future. This is a link that men may never *fully* understand, because they can't experience the phenomena.

Yet as a scientist, I also see that much of our behaviour is biologically determined. Our moods fluctuate with the cycling of our hormones. Oestrogen and progesterone in some way help to promote our maternal feelings. These emotions are not culturally conditioned. A mother in the jungles of Borneo or the deserts of Ethiopia will react with the same distress if her child is endangered as a mother on the streets of New York. These biological determinants help to create culture and society.

Somehow we have been taught to ignore our biology and diminish its significance to the point where it has become a negative attribute. We allow ourselves to be called the 'weaker' sex. We are seen as being afflicted by our female fluctuations. In the United States 600,000 of us allow our reproductive organs to be removed each year for benign problems. This attitude denies the natural beauty and power of our biological uniqueness, which I believe makes us stronger—not 'weaker'.

It may take a full generation before we, as a society, change our thinking about the female organs and restore to them the importance they deserve. But change we will. We must start with ourselves and our sons and daughters. We must start now.

Update: the laws

In January 1988, Governor Deukmejian (California) signed SB835 into law. The American College of Obstetrics and Gynecology (ACOG) responded to the law by creating a form to be used. It is a start. Doctors may now realize an issue exists. Women have reproductive civil rights—the right to keep their organs, regardless of age or race.

Following publication of the first edition of this book, several articles covering issues concerning Reproductive Health Rights were submitted to *The New York Times*, which published not only the statistical data on hysterectomies but also a letter I had written to the editor. This topic helped to make the nation aware of the desperate need for laws to educate women and doctors on options available and the need for the informed consent for hysterectomy bills.

Members of the legislature in other states called the Institute for Reproductive Health (IRH), requesting research materials that had been put together to establish California's informed consent for hysterectomy bill. We sent out large boxes of papers and books; the Institute became a clearing house of data for the US Senate and groups concerned with health. As of this revision, New York, Pennsylvania, and Oregon have begun work toward state laws to guard against unnecessary hysterectomies. Working toward adoption of these laws has been an enormously uplifting experience. It will take years of work to achieve a national and international awareness of these issues before laws are created establishing these concepts. It will be a long and hard battle. The cost in dollars and time will be enormous. Sometimes fighting for what is God-given seems so futile. Groups that you'd expect to naturally support this crusade—even women who've undergone FRS themselves—get lost in the smoke-screen created by the medical establishment in the hopes of making the issues go away, and the controversy takes over. Those fearing change feed the controversy and distort the entire picture to confuse themselves and others. My desire is relatively simple; to offer women options, nothing more.

CHAPTER 18

What's the next step?

'As a result of the government White Paper perhaps at last we'll start to examine not only what such operations cost but what happens to the patient as a result of them; what might have happened if we'd used a different approach; what might have happened if we'd prevented hysterectomy in the first place . . .'
UK Health Economist

Doctor see, doctor do . . .

My husband likes to tell the story of Dr Joseph Lister. Lister was the first to use antiseptics in the treatment of wounds and during surgery. Indeed, he was the first to scrub his hands with soap and water before operating in Glasgow, about 120 years ago.

Although his work ultimately revolutionized the practice of modern medicine, Lister's ideas were not readily or quickly accepted. In fact, he was considered a heretic and was ridiculed and ostracized for his 'outlandish' ideas. When he visited the United States in 1876, about a decade after his first pronouncements, he was received with indifference. At that time, American surgeons were still consulting the weather report to set the day of their operations. They believed that a wind from the northeast carried certain germs. And they continued to operate in frock coats, not sterile gowns.

Only slowly did Lister's ideas gain accept-ance. One at a time, surgeons began to clip their fingernails and scrub their hands and arms with soap and water before operating. Linen sponges and instruments were boiled. By 1895, all instruments and dressings were sterilized and surgeons operated in rubber gloves.

The difficulty in making a change

For every breakthrough, for every change in convention, there has to be one person who says, 'No. The old way doesn't work. There must be a better approach to this problem.' Indeed, there must be a 'first' person in any field, if change is to occur—otherwise we'd still be letting blood, beating drums, uttering incantations, and watching the weather report.

In medicine, you can always tell the innovator by the arrows sticking out of his back. But arrows can only be hurled because the innovator is in the vanguard—out in front, ahead of the ranks. Only later, after much dust has settled, does the establishment embrace the new idea, as if it was theirs all along.

Scientists in the forefront of their fields, such as Lister, Galileo, and Pasteur, were all condemned for their revolutionary ideas initially. Many people ridiculed them and tried to impede their progress because they questioned and sought to alter the status quo.

In the field of female health, although I have not been the first to state *no more unnecessary hysterectomies*, I am the first to make the point so adamantly and vocally. I have drawn together years of research to support my contention and created surgical techniques to follow up my words with deeds. Thus I've synthesized new options by thought and action, both clinically and politically.

The coming revolution

Just because I am among the first, however, doesn't mean that others won't eventually advocate the preservation of the female organs for benign problems. It is my sincere hope that, informed by this book, you will approach your own doctor and discuss the issues I have raised. Communicate your own needs and wants. Ask for the innovative techniques I have developed and continue to create.

This is the beginning of the revolution in health care, which I mentioned in the first chapter of this book. The medical profession will not change from within. It is up to you, as a consumer, to help create the change with your own questions and even demands. You have empowered yourself with knowledge. Now, you must act.

The struggle for me has been long and hard fought. As you can imagine, my thoughts and beliefs have been attacked by local doctors. This has profoundly affected my life. I have witnessed intrigue, politics, and the misuse of power the likes of which makes soap operas pale in comparison. In fact, I'm planning a book on the difficul-

ties I've encountered in trying to improve women's medicine.

Still, I don't lose hope. I've had support, sometimes from unexpected places. Dr Peter Taleghany, a well-respected gynaecological oncologist trained at Sloan Kettering, was in a position officially to review my work, and proclaimed it technically the best that he had ever seen. Dr Taleghany has come to be one of my staunchest supporters and has joined with me in providing Female Reconstructive Surgery here in Los Angeles.

And I am certain that others will soon follow suit. This is an idea whose time has come. I will continue writing, giving educational seminars, and sharing surgical techniques with other doctors in order to make this technology and these options available to more women throughout the nation.

Finally, I will continue to do surgery. It is my life and my love—a creative art form, like sculpting or painting. I am actually able to change the body and heal it.

The future

The future is ours to have and to shape. I foresee that it may take many years of teaching, but one day change will occur in society. More organs will be saved and, in many cases, this will be beneficial. Women will have the options that they so sorely lack today. I will continue to work toward legislation and to write books to educate women.

Einstein was right. As the heart leads, so technology must follow. Science is merely a tool; it is nothing without a deeper spiritual commitment. It is nothing if it is not used in the service of love and the greater good. *No More Hysterectomies* is our first step in the quest to heal.

APPENDIX 1

Where to go for more information

IMPORTANT WARNING: The self-help approach discussed in this book is not a replacement for consulting with your doctor, nor is it intended to replace normal medical therapy. If you have a medical problem, you should definitely be under the care of your doctor. In addition, before undertaking any self-medication of any kind, you should also consult your doctor.

Regardless of whether your medical problem is mild and occasional or more persistent, you can try a nutritional approach. To obtain further information about nutritional supplements and your reproductive organs, write to:

Institute for Reproductive Health
8721 Beverly Boulevard
Los Angeles, CA 90048
(213) 854 7714

Integrated Health
1661 Lincoln Boulevard
Suite 300
Santa Monica, CA 90404
(213) 452 5197

United Kingdom:

College of Health
18 Victoria Park Square
Bethnal Green
London E2 9PF
01-980 4848

Health Directory (£1) lists health advice telephone service including hysterectomy/women's sexual response. Useful publications include *Guide to Second Opinions*

Endometriosis Society
Ailsa Irving
65 Holmdene Avenue
Herne Hill
London SE24 9LD
01-737 4764

Family Planning Association
27-35 Mortimer Street
London W1N 7RJ
01-636 7866
Will refer women suffering from menopause/post-hysterectomy symptoms to suitable centre

Health Rights
Unit 110
Bon March Building
444 Brixton Road
London SW9 8EJ
01-720 9811
extension 377 or 442
Voluntary organization dealing with patients' rights

Hysterectomy and Endometriosis Support Group (Liverpool)
Carol Naden
28 Manvers Road
Childwall, Liverpool L16 3NP
051-722 5838 after 6pm

Hysterectomy Support Group (London)
Ann Webb
11 Henryson Road
Brockley
London SE4 1HL
01-690 5987
Publishes thrice-yearly newsletter £5; £2.50 unwaged

Hysterectomy Support Group (Wirral)
Judy Vaughan
Rivendell
Warren Way
Lower Heswall
Wirral
Merseyside
051-342 3167

Institute of Psycho-sexual Medicine
11 Chandos Square
Cavendish Square
London W1M 9DD
01-580 0631
01-580 1043 (Thursday only)
Referral list of doctors specializing in psycho-sexual medicine

London Marriage Guidance Council
76A New Cavendish Street
London W1M 7LB
01-580 1087
Offers post-hysterectomy counselling to all couples (not just the married)
Referral service for out-of-London branches of Relate (also in local Directories)

PID Support Group
Jessica Pickard
61 Jenner Road
Stoke Newington
London N16

Women's Health & Reproductive Rights Information Centre
52 Featherstone Street
London EC1Y 8RT
01-251 6580 Helpline & information leaflets
01-251 6332 Register of local contacts

Women's Health Concern (WHC)
Ground floor
17 Earl's Terrace
London W8 6LP
01-602 6669

Women's National Cancer Control Campaign (WNCCC)
1 South Audley Street
London W1Y 5DQ
01-499 7532

Women's Therapy Centre
6 Manor Gardens
London N7 6LA
01-263 6200

Australia:

Key Centre for Women's Health in Society
University of Melbourne Department of Community Medicine
209 Grattan Street
Carlton, Victoria
Australia 3053
613-344 4333
FAX 613-347 4127

How to do your own research

Your local public library as a resource

Learn how to use your local public library to its maximum, looking for lay books and articles and information on women's health issues. You will find, however, that popular magazines may not always present both sides of an issue. The information may be limited by a one-sided approach.

University and medical school libraries

If you can gain access to a university library in your area, you will find that these large institutions with graduate libraries hold a vast number of medical journals and litera- ture. Ask for help from the research librarian in learning how to find information.

You may be given instruction on using the computer retrieval system. This system helps you search for books and articles on a particular subject. Once you become fam- iliar with it, you can ask specific questions on health care subjects and obtain article *abstracts*—brief summaries or descriptions of the journal articles written. This is a great resource used by research doctors, looking up information and data to help in their own work.

You may also call a medical library (usually housed at a teaching hospital-based medical school) and ask for their computer search department. Describe the subject you are researching and the librarian will do the computer search for you. After several days, you will receive a printout of articles and abstracts in your search. You will be charged a flat fee for the connection to the national computer network and a separate on-line fee for the number of minutes of computer time your search requires.

Once you have located journal articles and books on the subject you are research- ing, you can usually find these in the medical or university library. Normally these journals (that are bound in large book-like volumes) can't be checked out, but you can read them there and, with permission, copy some articles on the numerous copying machines available.

Modems: your at-home computer retrieval system

If you are familiar with computers and their use and own a home computer, a home- based computer retrieval system will provide access to medical journals as well as lay publications from your own home. Again, you are charged on a cost per hour basis for use of the system. Various computer systems can be subscribed to for obtaining medical journal data, including: Medline, CINAHL

(Cumulated Index to Nursing and Allied Health) and Blaise.

Update: caution: the FRS 'experts'

Renowned composer Marvin Hamlish called me, asking if I could save a uterus that everyone advised be removed by hysterectomy. I sent him *No More Hysterectomies* and some literature on Female Reconstructive Surgery (FRS) but heard nothing further from him.

One night I got an emergency beep from Marvin himself. Shirley, who was in his employ, had been told by everyone that she needed a hysterectomy. She had been referred to the Chairman of the Department of OB/GYN at a leading New York university medical centre. When she went to see him, she took my book with her. Without even having read it, he told her that he performed the same surgery. He was claiming to be an expert in FRS. Impressed by his position within the medical community both locally and nationally, she agreed to schedule surgery.

On the night before her surgery, she was informed by this doctor that he had ordered several pre-operative blood transfusions because she was anaemic from her bleeding fibroid tumours. Then the nurse came in with a hysterectomy consent for her to sign. The doctor explained he was not sure he could save her uterus and that hysterectomy was probably inevitable. Shirley was now in her hospital bed, terrified and hysterical. She called Marvin Hamlish. Disturbed by the attitudes of these professional medical 'experts', and concerned for Shirley's welfare, he did the only logical thing. He got into a cab, went to the hospital, and packed Shirley up. Shirley came to Los Angeles, where I

performed the FRS for her, successfully removing the multiple tumours and reconstructing her uterus. A few days after that, she flew back to her husband and family in New York.

What was most disturbing about this incident was that another doctor claimed to perform FRS. Local gynaecologists claim to be experts on FRS without ever observing what I actually do, or how I approach this technique. None of them has responded to my open invitation to observe, and most of them totally disregard the fact that it had taken me many years of combining surgical procedures and refining them to develop this term.

Many women recited the same scenario. When their gynaecologists told them they needed a hysterectomy, the women found my book and read it. Feeling more empowered, informed, and educated about their bodies, they were able to ask proper questions and demand answers. These same gynaecologists now stated *they* could perform FRS to conserve their organs, thereby giving them alternatives to their diagnosed hysterectomy, which had previously been denied them. Many of the women had gone on to have inferior surgery, while others ended up with hysterectomies.

A female gynaecologist recently came to Los Angeles to observe the operation. She was the first and only gynaecologist who has been curious enough to want to know exactly *which* procedures are done, and *how* they are performed. The gynaecologist's comment during the operation was, 'You make the impossible look so easy.'

Someday, more gynaecologists will work together as one to exchange varying alternatives and procedures in the conservation of women's reproductive system. My doors remain open.

APPENDIX 3

Health rights

In the UK, the US concept of 'informed consent'—where comprehensive information, about for example any drug used, the trials it has undergone and any possible side effects—is not known in English law. In the UK patients' consent to treatment is nevertheless a prerequisite because treatment or investigations carried out without the consent of the person concerned can amount to an assault and may result in an action for damages. The important part is not getting someone's signature but in making sure they understand the procedure they are about to undergo. In order to decide whether to give his/her consent the patient must be given sufficient explanation of what is entailed—'as much information as a reasonable person would require in order to make a decision' according to the courts—and consent must be obtained with due care and formality and not as in some reported cases a short time before the operation is to take place when the patient has already been given pre-medication.

In the UK, the Department of Health and the various medical defence societies have agreed the working of a multi-purpose 'general consent form' (reproduced below). The primary purpose of the consent form is 'to provide evidence that the patient gave consent to the procedure in question'.

The general consent form should specify the precise procedure you are to undergo. There is a further important proviso and this is that a surgeon can proceed to any treatment considered necessary when this arises from the procedure to which the patient has initially given consent. This further treatment must be seen as necessary to 'preserve the patient's life or health'. In the case of hysterectomy, for example, a woman should only sign a written consent when she is quite clear about what further procedures might or might not be necessary. If she is to have a bilateral salpingo-oöphorectomy, for example, where both her fallopian tubes and ovaries are to be removed, this should be made clear in writing.

It is the responsibility of your doctor not only to explain the procedure to you before gaining your consent but to record in your case notes details of the discussion as well as *details of your own wishes in the matter.* Case notes in fact since they are admissable in court are as, if not more, important in many ways than the consent form alone. In the case of oöphorectomy, for example, there is still debate whether this is advisable or strictly necessary. Obviously if there is cancer or cancer is suspected the operation falls into the latter category. A doctor during your consultation may say that he will remove your ovaries since 'you're over 55 and they're no use to you' (so-called prophylactic reasons) but you may like to question this. In any case if the surgeon intends to do this it must be explained to you and if the oöphorectomy is other than 'strictly necessary' surgeons must get you to sign in advance otherwise you can go to law. In all cases the surgeon should tell you of his *full* intention and if he does not you as the patient should ask.

UK doctors also take note of the extent to which a patient wishes to be informed: ie *the more you ask the more the doctor will tell you.*

A UK general consent form

I, ... of ....
(name and address of person giving consent)

*hereby consent to undergo
OR
*hereby consent to .... undergoing
(name of patient)

the operation/treatment of ....

the nature and purpose of which have been explained to me

by Dr/Mr ....

I also consent to such further or alternative operative measures or treatment as may be found necessary during the course of the operation or treatment and to the administration of general or other anaesthetics for any of these purposes.

No assurance has been given to me that the operation/treatment will be performed or administered by any particular practitioner.

Date .... Signature ....
Patient/parent/guardian*

I confirm that I explained the nature and purpose of this operation/treatment to the person(s) who signed the above form of consent.

Date .... Signature ....
Medical Practitioner

*Delete whichever is inapplicable

An Australian consent form

CONSENT for operative treatment and anaesthesia

Answers I have given to all questions are true to the best of my knowledge and I have not withheld any information.

Following surgery I will be escorted home by a responsible adult, and I have made arrangements for this. I realise that impairment of mental alertness may persist for several hours following anaesthesia, and I will avoid making decisions or taking part in activities which depend upon full concentration or judgement during that period.

*I hereby consent to undergo the operation of .... the effect and nature

of which have been explained to me by Dr................................ and to such further or

alternative operative treatment as may be found necessary, or as a consequence of such

operation.

*I also consent to the administration of local or general anaesthesia for this purpose.

*I also consent to the administration of a blood transfusion if required.

*I understand that, should I require admission to hospital for further care, I will be

responsible for the costs incurred.

Full payment for your stay at .... surgery must be made at the time of your admission.

Dated this.. day of.. 199

(Patient signature) .... (Witness signature) ....

Consent form used at the Center for Female Reconstructive Surgery

INTRODUCTION

A WORD ON INFORMED CONSENT

Informed Consent is a means to educate yourself on risks, options, complications and alternatives to surgery

As we learn more about surgery, Informed Consent will change to include new data.

If there is anything that you feel should be added to the consent form that would be to the benefit of other women, please submit it so that it may be included.

Remember that Informed Consent is not only the collection of these typed papers; it is obtaining multiple professional opinions, the reading of existing medical literature, it is the review of the options you have available, it is discussion with family, it is discussion with women who have had different experiences. Most of all, please realize that you alone are the responsible party for all of your care.

Information on hysterectomy is included because it represents a grouping of possible complications that may or may not occur with that operation. However, though hysterectomy represents an extreme of the spectrum, some degree of complication(s) may occur with any gynecological procedure. These may be to a lesser degree in the actual number of complications or may represent a partial development of a complication.

The following forms are to assist you in understanding the possible risks, complications and options in gynecological surgery, including hysterectomy. Please read all of the material several times before signing.

It is mandatory that you have completed the following tasks prior to your requesting a surgical procedure:

[ ] Have sought out several medical opinions
[ ] Viewed multiple surgeries
[ ] Reviewed all issues surrounding surgery with multiple experts including a psychotherapist
[ ] Met with the nurse to discuss surgery
[ ] Discussed with clergy (Rabbi, priest, etc.)

[ ] Have read on your own and researched your particular medical problem extensively
[ ] Reviewed interview tapes of other women's experiences
[ ] Reviewed Informed Consent video
[ ] Spoke with others with varying opinions

Sign................................ Date................................

Patient Concepts and Desires

My primary desire is the conservation of my female reproductive organs. I am requesting this after thoroughly researching all aspects of all of the current treatment available. I have had multiple physical exams and opinions concerning my condition. I am making this choice while I am in a psychologically sound stable state, without fear or anxiety, without any coercion, and fully understand all aspects of surgery including risks, options, alternatives and complications (both short and long term). I have asked questions and reviewed all issues prior to making a decision to conserve my organs. I am aware that hysterectomy is available to me. I do not, however, desire a hysterectomy at this time and understand all of the ramifications of this as my personal choice and decision. I understand that this decision is solely my responsibility and no one else's.

Patient Comments: ....

....

....

....

....

....

....

Signed: .... Date ....

INFORMED CONSENT OF GYNECOLOGICAL SURGICAL PROCEDURES INCLUDING FEMALE RECONSTRUCTIVE SURGERY

A MESSAGE TO PATIENTS ABOUT SURGICAL RISKS

Surgery is generally safe, helpful and often lifesaving. However, medical or surgical procedures of any type involve the taking of risks, ranging from minor to serious (including the risk of death). It is important to be aware of the following possible risks before receiving the treatment you and your physician are planning. The following may be the reactions of your body to medical/surgical operations or procedures.

1) INFECTION: Invasion of tissue by bacteria or other germs occurs to some degree whenever a cut, incision or puncture is made. In most instances, through the natural defense mechanisms of the body, healing of the affected area occurs without difficulty. In some instances antibiotic medicines are prescribed and at times additional surgical measures may be necessary to combat infection.

2) HEMORRHAGE: The cutting of blood vessels causes bleeding and this occurs in every surgical incision. This bleeding is usually controlled without difficulty. At times, blood transfusions are required to replace blood loss. If blood transfusions are given, there are additional risks of liver inflammation, hepatitis, and the possibility of receiving Acquired Immune Deficiency Syndrome (AIDS). There is no absolutely reliable way to predict these unwanted reactions, some of which may be quite serious and even lead to death.

3) DRUG REACTIONS: Unexpected allergies, lack of proper response to medications or illness caused by the prescribed drugs are possibilities, it is important for you to inform your physician and your anesthesiologist or certified registered nurse anesthetist of any problem you or your family have had with reactions to drugs and which medications you have taken in the past six months, including over-the-counter drugs, especially aspirin.

4) ANESTHESIA REACTIONS: There may be unusual or unexpected responses to the gases, drugs or methods used to anesthetize you which can lead to difficulties with lung, heart or nerve function. Eating or drinking before anesthesia increases the risk of vomiting which may cause significant complications. Inform your anesthesiologist or certified registered nurse anesthetist of problems you and your family have had with anesthesia.

5) BLOOD VESSEL INFLAMMATION AND CLOTTING: It is impossible to predict the occurrence of blood vessel inflammation and clotting problems. If blood clots form, they can move from where they formed to other areas of the body and cause injury.

6) INJURY TO OTHER ORGANS: Because of the closeness of other organs to the area being operated on, there may be injury to other organs. The stress of surgery or the procedure may also harm other organ systems of the body.

7) OTHER RISKS: It is not possible to list all the possible risks and complications, and their variations, that may arise in any surgical operation or medical procedure. Each situation depends upon the purpose and nature of the operation or procedures. Your physician is willing to discuss further with you various details about other risks.

Sign .... Date ....

PreOp Major
for all Gynecological Procedures

Informed Consent for Treatment, Surgical Care and Diagnostic Procedures

I hereby authorize and direct .... with associates or assistants of his/her choice, to perform the following marked treatment(s) and/or procedure(s) on myself [patient name] ....

My diagnosis, or suspected diagnosis is:

....

I am aware that no pathology or different pathology may be found at time of surgery.

....

The operation to be performed is:

[ ] Laparotomy (incision or opening of the body)
[ ] Myomectomy (removal of fibroid tumor(s))
[ ] Hysterectomy (removal of uterus if cancer is found or if uterus is not salvageable)
[ ] Oöphorectomy (removal of ovary(ies) if definite cancer is found or if not salvageable)
[ ] Salpingectomy (removal of fallopian tube(s) if definite cancer is found or if not salvageable)
[ ] Removal of adhesions
[ ] Suspension(s) (uterine, ovarian, bladder, etc)
[ ] Biopsies
[ ] Appendectomy (inversion, etc.)
[ ] Video
[ ] Cystectomy (removal of ovarian cysts)
[ ] Laser
[ ] D & C
[ ] Removal of definitive cancerous tissue(s)

Some common complications of surgery are:

[ ] Mortality (death)
[ ] Bleeding
[ ] Drug reaction(s)
[ ] Multiple surgeries required after initial operation
[ ] Infection
[ ] Anesthetic complication(s)

[ ] Need for blood transfusion(s)
[ ] Failure to heal as anticipated
[ ] Morbidity (severe or chronic illness; includes such things as stroke, pneumonia, pulmonary emboli, blood clots, phlebitis, etc.)
[ ] Failure to have anticipated outcome

Sign .... Date ....

Other possible complications of surgery are:

[ ] Uncontrollable leakage of urine
[ ] Sterility/Infertility (inability to conceive)
[ ] Injury to bowel, ileus or intestinal obstruction
[ ] Hormone deficiency
[ ] Femoral nerve damage
[ ] Adhesion formation
[ ] Loss of normal ovarian hormonal function
[ ] Injury to bladder
[ ] Injury to tube between the kidney and bladder

[ ] Loss of kidney
[ ] Possible loss of sexual desire, orgasm or other sexual response
[ ] Increased risk of osteoporosis
[ ] Possible increased risk of heart disease
[ ] Current symptoms/problems may not be alleviated by surgery
[ ] Hysterectomy may be necessary in the future for the same, recurring, or newly developed problems

ALTERNATIVES TO TREATMENT

Although you and your doctor have decided upon this procedure, do not hesitate to discuss the reasons for the choice and the alternatives available for treatment of your condition. In addition, be sure to ask your doctor any other questions you may have about your treatment.

I understand that there are alternatives to this treatment such as:

[ ] Hysterectomy
[ ] Alternative medical treatment
[ ] Treatment with chemicals, drugs or medications, experimental protocol for treatment
[ ] Alternative surgical treatment

[ ] No treatment
[ ] Continued observation
[ ] Conservative surgery
[ ] Use of devices to avoid surgery
[ ] Other(s)...
....

This is an elective procedure. The possible consequences if this treatment is not followed are:

[ ] Continued pain and discomfort
[ ] Possible infertility
[ ] May be no problems
[ ] Resolution of problems without treatment
[ ] No further progression of problems
[ ] Other..
....

[ ] Continued bleeding
[ ] Tumor growth
[ ] Failure to diagnose other unsuspected pathology
[ ] May require more extensive treatment in the future

Sign .... Date ....

SURGICAL CONSENT INFORMATION

IMPORTANT INFORMATION POINTS
CONCERNING GYNECOLOGICAL SURGERY
INCLUDING HYSTERECTOMY

NOTE: These problems could exist in some lesser form for all gynecological procedures.

[ ] Sexual response may be negatively affected by hysterectomy. Some women may only experience uterine orgasm, and have complete loss of orgasm upon the removal of the uterus. Sexual response may either diminish, or may not be affected at all.

[ ] Despite careful surgical techniques to preserve the ovaries, they may fail to function immediately after hysterectomy; their functional capabilities may diminish, or the life span of the ovaries may be shortened. Any surgical procedure on or near the ovary may diminish its function through adhesion formation and other postoperative processes.

[ ] Residual Ovary Syndrome
After hysterectomy, the ovary(ies) may become enlarged and painful, requiring further medical and/or surgical treatment, including their removal.

[ ] After hysterectomy, hormones may be prescribed by your physician to treat clinical symptoms of menopause (hot flashes, lack of libido, mood swings, insomnia, etc.). Hormones may also be prescribed as a preventative measure against heart disease and osteoporosis.

[ ] Hormone Replacement Therapy can not be guaranteed as being problem free. Some women experience allergies or unpleasant responses to these medications. Some hormones that are deficient may not have medications available currently.

[ ] There are possible psychological changes that may occur as a result of hormonal changes associated with hysterectomy, noting various reports of the uterus as an endocrine organ, as well as changes that may occur with diminished ovarian function. Concepts such as maternal instinct and femininity may be associated with hormones produced by the female reproductive organs.

[ ] Possible development of fistula. These are abnormal openings that occur between two adjacent organs (i.e. vagina, bladder, uterus, rectum, etc.). Example: A fistula between the vagina and rectum would allow feces to enter into the vagina. This can occur during hysterectomy, Female Reconstructive Surgery and other gynecological procedures. (i.e. perineal repairs, vaginal repairs, bladder repairs, etc.)

Sign.................................. Date...................................

[ ] I understand that I may elect for general or regional anesthesia. I will be consented by the anesthesiologists concerning the choice of anesthesia, risks and possible complications. It is my responsibility to discuss this with the anesthesiologist.

[ ] A suspected diagnosis may not be confirmed at surgery. This is not the physician's responsibility. This is a common occurrence in all areas of medical practice and no blame exists when this occurs.

[ ] The uterus' role in your overall general health has not been fully documented. The uterus does make hormones, co-factors and receptors. The full role of these agents has not been fully established.

[ ] A patient's refusal to take hormones or other medications prescribed by the physician may result in irreparable damage and is not the physician's responsibility.

[ ] At surgery, if expected pathology is not found, the surgeon may stop the operation without the removal of any tissues.

[ ] After a hysterectomy, I will still need pap smears and have routine checkups with my gynecologist regardless of my age. There are other female genital cancers that could occur and problems that require routine care.

[ ] Possible financial costs involved with post hysterectomy and other gynecological procedure care including hormone replacement, future medical care and other forms of therapy may be required for lifetime.

[ ] Prolapse of the vagina and bladder may reoccur after hysterectomy which was performed to correct these problems initially. Prolapse of the uterus and other organs may occur after any surgical procedure to correct or improve prolapse. Medications and devices such as a pessary may treat prolapse problems without surgical intervention. Surgically, there are numerous surgical procedures that exist for these problems. I have investigated on my own these various approaches and have elected for the one(s) my physician will perform.

[ ] After hysterectomy, the vagina may be narrowed or shortened. This may negatively affect sex and other functions.

[ ] Endometriosis may not be cured by hysterectomy.

[ ] Chronic pelvic pain may not be cured by hysterectomy.

[ ] Pre-Menstrual Syndrome may not be cured by hysterectomy.

[ ] Fistula formation may occur post hysterectomy as a complication.

Sign.................................... Date....................................

[ ] Possible development of menopause may occur after hysterectomy, either immediately after surgery or acceleration of menopause with its associated problems and symptoms may occur:

decreased libido   insomnia   osteoporosis
personality changes   numbness   migraine headaches
loss of self esteem   hot flashes   dry skin
depression   loss of vaginal lubrication

[ ] Adhesions may develop after any major surgery. These can cause pain, result in digestive problems, bowel obstruction, and/or alter anatomy to create chronic pain. This may require hospitalization and/or further surgery.

[ ] After hysterectomy the abdomen may protrude and push outward with chronic bloating.

[ ] Hysterectomy may be associated with an increased incidence of certain neuropathies (i.e. carpal tunnel syndrome)

[ ] Increase in rheumatoid arthritis and other various joint problems.

[ ] Foreign materials are not routinely placed in my body without my consent. I am aware that accidents may occur in emergency life threatening situations in which an object may inadvertently be left by accident; this may require a second operation to remove said object.

[ ] Concept of Definitive Cancer: During surgery the pathologist may, on frozen section, state whether a particular biopsy is benign or malignant. Several days later, when the permanent sections are finalized, the original diagnosis is susceptible to change. Two situations can occur:

1) Tissues that were examined and thought to be benign can later be identified as cancerous, requiring further surgery to remove additional tissues.

2) Tissues removed because they were believed to be malignant are later found to be benign.

Sign .... Date ....

PreOp—Laparoscopy/Pelviscopy
following
Female Reconstructive Surgery

Following Female Reconstructive Surgery, it is suggested that you have a Second-Look Laparoscopy/Pelviscopy.

During this procedure one can evaluate how your body has healed. Adhesions often will form inside the body following surgery. If the adhesions are not extensive they can be removed during laparoscopy. Irrigation solutions can be used at this time. Adhesions may reform despite attempts at removal.

This surgery may answer several questions concerning your post operative recovery. It can help in the evaluation of adhesions, ovarian function, recurrence of fibroid tumors, endometriosis, etc.; evaluation for possible in vitro fertilization, fallopian tube function and whether or not there is a need for additional surgery for fertility or other reasons.

Second-Look Laparoscopy is especially important to women who wish to try to conceive.

Using laparoscopy to evaluate surgical outcome and the ability to use pelviscopy to perform surgical procedures is offered and encouraged for all patients. It is however the patient's responsibility to request and schedule these procedures.

Failure to undergo laparoscopy could result in multiple problems, including:
1) Problems that could result in obstetrical catastrophe which could have been identified during laparoscopy (i.e. ruptured uterus)
2) Failure to identify blocked fallopian tube (resulting in ectopic pregnancy)
3) Failure to lysis (remove) adhesions by pelviscopy that may later require a major surgery
4) Failure to identify need for alternative procedures i.e. in vitro fertilization, additional surgery

A separate and complete informed consent for minor surgery, laparoscopy and pelviscopy is required prior to the procedure.

Sign .... Date ....

FERTILITY SURGERY
AND/OR
PROCEDURES TO CORRECT INFERTILITY

Various procedures and techniques to advance surgical techniques in the area of correcting infertility are ongoing constantly. Surgeons may be doing different things in different parts of the country and the world. Some techniques are abandoned over time as others are adopted as routine procedures.

It is a patient's responsibility to get multiple opinions and make her own personal decision on the choice of procedure(s) and physician(s).

Numbers and statistics on fertility success can be gathered, however, each patient will heal and respond to surgical intervention differently. It is important that all women who seek such a surgery to conceive be informed that there is no guarantee that conception will occur.

Problems that can routinely occur during surgical procedures to correct infertility are:

1)   Complete failure of surgery. Example: Surgery is done on blocked fallopian tubes to open them. They may remain closed or may even have increased damage from attempts to open them.

2)   Severe adhesions may form post surgically.

3)   Repeated surgeries may be required.

4)   Other technology is needed, such as in the case of in vitro fertilization.

5)   Past or present disease states may prevent fertility (i.e. endometriosis, chronic inflammatory response). These may be chronic or recurring.

Sign .... Date ....

The following are some of the negative aspects of surgical intervention to correct infertility and they include:

[] Cost

[] Stress on body from surgical and medical treatment(s)

[] Risks of complications from surgery

[] High failure rates

[] Psychological stress including increased problems that may occur with multiple procedures

[] Increased need for additional surgeries

[] Need for Second-Look Laparoscopy/Pelviscopy

[] Surgery may actually diminish existing fertility potential

[] Lost time spent in surgical attempts when adoption may have been initiated earlier

Basically, a woman who is motivated to undergo surgery for fertility is doing so motivated by hope. Guarantees of a positive outcome cannot be given to anyone.

A successful conception is a remarkable and blessed event. However, it is important to remember that neither the physician nor the technology used can guarantee a pregnancy.

Be informed that women who do conceive after conservative or reconstructive surgery often have high risk pregnancies and must be aware of the possible complications and risks such as: possible miscarriage(s), ectopic pregnancy, stillborns, problem pregnancies and deliveries. Many women, because of previous surgery, may require delivery by caesarean section.

The final outcome of a live healthy baby is a truly blessed event. Medicine and surgery may only assist, for having a healthy baby is blessed beyond technology.

Sign .... Date ....

CONSENT TO GYNECOLOGICAL PROCEDURES

1) HYSTERECTOMY IRREVERSIBLE. I am satisfied with my understanding that the hysterectomy operation is permanent and its effects can not be reversed.
   a) I will no longer have monthly periods
   b) I will no longer be able to have children

2) POSSIBLE BENEFITS. I am satisfied with my understanding of the reason(s) for the operation.
   I understand my diagnosis is ....
   and that the following benefits may be anticipated from the performance of the gynecological surgery: ....

3) GENERAL RISKS AND COMPLICATIONS. I am satisfied with my understanding of the more common risks and complications which are described in this form and include the infection, bleeding, pain, anesthesia risks and death. I am also aware of the possible short and long term complications that may be directly related to gynecological surgery.

4) LENGTH OF HOSPITALIZATION. My doctor has informed me that my approximate length of hospital stay is .... days, assuming no unforeseen complications. Complications often result in further hospitalization, medical treatment, transfusion, and further surgery.

5) LENGTH OF RECOVERY. My doctor has informed me that my approximate length of recovery is .... days, assuming no unforeseen complications.

6) ALTERNATIVE METHODS OF TREATMENT. I am satisfied with my understanding of alternative procedures or treatments and their possible benefits and risks including:
   ....

7) ANESTHESIA. I understand that I will probably receive a .... anesthetic. I understand the anesthesiologist or certified registered nurse anesthetist will select and administer my anesthetic. I understand I should discuss with them the risks and benefits associated with the anesthesia they select.

8) NO TREATMENT. I am satisfied with my understanding of the possible consequences, outcomes or risks if no treatment is rendered.

9) SECOND OPINION. I have been offered the opportunity to seek a second opinion concerning the need for my gynecological surgery.

Sign .... Date ....

10) ADDITIONAL OR DIFFERENT PROCEDURES DURING CARE AND TREATMENT. I understand that unforeseen conditions may arise and that it may be necessary to perform operations and procedures different from, or in addition to, the gynecological surgery described. I authorize and consent to the performance of such additional or different operations and procedures as are considered necessary and advisable.

11) FEES. My doctor has informed me that his or her fee for the gynecological surgery is approximately $ ...., assuming no unforeseen complications. I understand that in addition to my doctor's fee, there will be other charges, such as hospital or facility costs, anesthesiologist's fees, laboratory and possibly other physicians' fees. I understand that not all of these charges may be paid by my insurance company and that I am responsible for paying any part of these charges not paid by my insurance company.

12) FREE TO WITHHOLD OR WITHDRAW CONSENT. I understand that I am free to withhold or withdraw my consent at any time before the gynecological surgery without affecting the right to future care or treatment and without loss or withdrawal of any state or federally funded program benefits to which I might be otherwise entitled.

13) NO GUARANTEES. I understand there are risks involved in any procedure or treatment, and it is not possible to guarantee, warrant or in any way to give an assurance of a successful result.

14) SPECIFIC RISKS, COMPLICATIONS AND DISCOMFORTS. I am satisfied with my understanding of the specific risks, possible risks, and discomforts of the gynecological surgical procedure including: ....
....

15) OTHER QUESTIONS. I am satisfied with my understanding of the nature of the procedure and all of my questions about the procedure have been answered.

I have read and been given a copy of this form.

DATE: .... TIME: .... AM/PM PHYSICIAN ....

SIGNATURE: .... WITNESS: ....
       (PATIENT)

Informed consent law in California

The people of the State of California do enact as follows:

1. SECTION 1. Chapter 6.5 (commencing with Section 1690) is added to Division 2 of the Health and Safety Code, to read:

1690. (a) Prior to the performance of a

hysterectomy, physicians and surgeons shall obtain verbal and written informed consent. The informed consent procedure shall ensure that at least all of the following information is given to the patient verbally and in writing:

1) Advice that the individual is free to withhold or withdraw consent to the procedure at any time before the hysterectomy or treatment and without affecting the right to future care or treatment and without the loss or withdrawal of any state or federally funded program benefits to which the individual might be otherwise entitled.

2) A description of the type or types of surgery and other procedures involved in the proposed hysterectomy, and a description of any known available and appropriate alternatives to the hysterectomy itself.

3) Advice that the hysterectomy procedure is considered to be irreversible, and that infertility will result; except as provided in subdivision (b).

4) A description of the discomforts and risks that may accompany or follow the performing of the procedure, including an explanation of the type and possible effects of any anesthetic to be used;

5) A description of the benefits or advantages that may be expected as a result of the hysterectomy;

6) Approximate length of hospital stay;

7) Approximate length of time for recovery;

8) Financial cost to the patient of the physician and surgeon's fee.

(b) A woman shall sign a written statement prior to the performance of the hysterectomy procedure, indicating she has read and understood the written information provided pursuant to subdivision (a), and that this information has been discussed with her by her physician and surgeon, or his or her designee. The statement shall indicate that the patient has been advised by her physician or designee that the hysterectomy will render her permanently sterile and incapable of having children shall accompany the claim, unless the patient has previously been sterile, or is postmenopausal.

(c) The informed consent procedure shall not pertain when the hysterectomy is performed in a life-threatening emergency situation in which the physician determines prior written informed consent is not possible. In this case, a statement, handwritten and signed by the physician, certifying the nature of the emergency, must accompany the claim.

(d) The State Department of Health Services may develop regulations establishing verbal and written informed consent procedures that shall be obtained prior to performance of a hysterectomy, that indicate the medically accepted justifications for performance of a hysterectomy, pursuant to this chapter.

1691. The failure of a physician and surgeon to inform a patient by means of written consent, in layman's language and in a language understood by the patient of the alternative efficacious methods of treatment which may be medically viable, when a hysterectomy is to be performed, constitutes unprofessional conduct within the meaning of Chapter 5 (commencing with Section 2000) of Division 2 of the Business and Professions code.

Bibliography and other resources

Many hundreds of hours went into research-ing and writing *No More Hysterectomies* so that you would be presented with the most up-to-date picture of female health care to date. In order to facilitate your reading of this book, however, many of the footnote refer-ences have been removed from the text. They can be found here, in the order in which the subject appears. You may find them helpful, especially if you wish to carry on any further research into hysterectomies and female disorders.

Chapter 1. The revolution in women's health care

For information on the history of gynaecology:

Speert, H., *Obstetrics and Gynecology in America: A History*, Chicago, Ill., The American College of Obstetricians and Gynecologists, 1980.
Kerr, J.M.M., Johnstone, R.W., Phillips, M.H. (Eds) *Historical Review of British Obstetrics and Gynaecology 1800-1950*, Livingstone, 1954.

For information on the continued function of the ovaries after menopause and some of the aftereffects of hysterectomy:

Asch, R.H., Greenblatt, R.B., 'Steroido-genesis in the Postmenopausal Ovary', *Clin. in Obstet. and Gynae.*, April 1977, Vol. 4, No. 1, p. 85.

Judd, H.L., Judd, G.E., Lucas, W.E. et al., 'Endocrine Function of the Postmeno-pausal Ovary: Concentration of Andro-gens and Estrogens in Ovarian and Peripheral Vein Blood', *J. Endocr. Metab.*, 1974, Vol. 39, p. 1020.

Chapter 2. What is a hysterectomy?

For information on persistence of problems following hysterectomy:

Kapadia, S.B., Russak, R.R., O'Donnell, W.F. et al., 'Postmenopausal Uretal Endometri-osis with Atypical Adenomatous Hyper-plasia Following Hysterectomy, Bilateral Oophorectomy, and Long-term Estrogen Therapy', *Obstet. Gynecol.*, 1984, Vol. 64, No. 3 Suppl., pp. 60s-63s.

For information on obstetric catastrophies necessitating hysterectomy:

Phelan, Jeffrey, 'Placenta Accretia', in *Management of Common Problems in Obstetrics and Gynecology*, Mishell, D.R., Jr., and Brenner, P.F., eds., 1984, Medical Economics Books, Oradell, N.J., p. 117.

For US national statistics on the rates and types of hysterectomies:

National Center for Health Statistics, Pokras, R., Hufnagel, V.G., 'Hysterectomy in the United States: 1965–1984', *Vital and Health Statistics*, 1987, Series 13, No. 92. DHHS Pub. No. (PHS) 87-1753. Public Health Service, Washington, DC, US Government Printing Office.

For information on vaginal vault prolapse following hysterectomy:

Symmonds, R.E., Williams, T.J. et al., 'Post-hysterectomy Enterocele and Vaginal Vault Prolapse', *Am. J. Obstet. and Gynecol.*, August 15, 1981, Vol. 140, No. 8, pp. 852-859.

Grundsell, H., Larrson, G., 'Operative Management of Vaginal Vault Prolapse Following Hysterectomy', *Br. J. Obstet, Gynaecol.*, 1984, vol. 91, No. 8, pp. 808-811.

For more information on the effects of hysterectomy on ovarian function:

Janson, P.O., Jansson, I., 'The Acute Effect of Hysterectomy on Ovarian Blood Flow', *Am. J. Obstet. Gynecol.*, Feb. 1977, Vol. 127, No. 4, pp. 349-352.

Cutler, W.B., Garcia, C-R., 'The psycho-neuroendocrinology of the Ovulation Cycle of Women', *Psychoneuroendo-crinology*, 1980, Vol. 5, p. 89.

Jones, Howard, W., Jones, Georgeanna Seegar, eds., *Novak's Textbook of Gynecology*, Tenth Edition. Baltimore, Williams and Wilkins, 1981, p. 28.

Souza, A.Z., Fonseca, A.M., Izzo, V.M. et al., 'Ovarian Histology and Function after Total Abdominal Hysterectomy', *Obstet. Gynecol.*, Dec. 1986, Vol. 68, No. 6, p. 847.

Gray, R., St. Louis, E., Grosman, H. et al., 'Postoperative Residual Ovary Syndrome: An Uncommon Cause of Pelvic Mass', *J. Can. Assoc. Radiol.*, Mar. 1983, Vol. 34, No. 1, pp. 56-58.

Kletzky, O.A., Davajan, V., 'Differential Diagnosis of Secondary Amenorrhea', *Management of Common Problems in Obstetrics and Gynecology*, Mishell, D.R., Jr., and Brenner, P.F., eds, 1984, Medical Economics Books, Oradell, N.J., p. 354.

Chapter 3. Why I believe you should know about the alternatives to hysterectomy

You may find more information on the complications following hysterectomy in the articles listed below.

Operative and post-operative complications:

Blood transfusions and haemorrhage:

Palmer, H.R., Kane, J.G., Churchill, W.H. et al., 'Cost and Quality in the Use of Blood Bank Services for Normal Deliveries, Cesarean Sections, and Hysterectomies', *JAMA*, July 11, 1986, Vol. 256, No. 2, p. 220.

Urinary tract disruptions:

Demos, T.C., Churchill, R., Flisak, M.E. et al., 'The Radiologic Diagnosis of Complications Following Gynecologic Surgery: Radiography, Computed Tomography, Sonography, and Scintigraphy', *CRC Crit. Rev. Diagn. Imaging*, 1984, Vol. 22, No. 1, pp. 43-94.

Hibbard, L.T., 'Surgical Injury to the Ureter', in *Management of Common Problems in Obstetrics and Gynecology*, Mishell, D.R, Jr., and Brenner, P.F., eds, 1984, Medical Economics Books, Oradell, N.J., pp. 263-235.

General complications, febrile morbidity, and infections:

Dicker, R.C., Greenspan, J.R., Strauss, L.T., et al. 'Complications of Abdominal and Vaginal Hysterectomies Among Women of Reproductive Age in The United States', *Am. J. Obstet. Gynecol.*, 1982, Vol. 144, p. 841.

Ledger, W.J., Child, M.A., 'The Hospital Care of Patients Undergoing Hysterectomy: An Analysis of 12,026 Patients from the Professional Activity Study', *Am. J. Obstet. Gynecol.*, 1973, Vol. 117, p. 423.

Roy, S., 'Prevention of Post Operative Gynecologic Infection', in *Management of Common Problems in Obstetrics and Gynecology*, Mishell, D.R., Jr., and Brenner, P.F., eds. 1984, Medical Economics Books, Oradell, N.J., p. 208.

Willson, J.R., Black, J.R., 'Ovarian Abscess', *Am. J. Obstet. Gynecol.*, Vol. 90, No. 34, 1964.

Ledger, W.J., Campbell, C., Willson, J.R., 'Postoperative Adnexal Infections', *Obstet. Gynecol.*, Jan. 1968, Vol. 31, No. 1, pp. 83-89.

Livengood, C.H., III, Addison, W.A., 'Adnexal Abscess as a Delayed Complication of Vaginal Hysterectomy', *Am. J. Obstet. Gynecol.*, July 1, 1982, Vol. 143, No. 5, pp. 596-567.

Vaginal vault disruption:

Kellogg, S.F., 'Cause and Repair of Vaginal Evisceration Following Total Abdominal Hysterectomy', *Int. Corresp. Soc. of Obstet. and Gyn.*, Aug. 1986, Vol. 27, No. 8, pp. 6-8.

Hacker, N.F., Charles, E.H., Savage, E.W., 'Postcoital Posthysterectomy Vaginal Vault Disruption with Haemorrhagic Shock', *Aust. NZ J. Obstet. Gynaecol.*, Aug. 1980, Vol. 20, No. 3, pp. 182-184.

Neurological damage:

Kvist-Poulsen, H., Borel, J., 'Iatrogenic Femoral Neuropathy Subsequent to Abdominal Hysterectomy: Incidence and Prevention', *Obstetrics and Gynecology*, Oct. 1982, Vol. 60, No. 4, pp. 516-520.

Waldemar, G., Werdelin, L., Boysen, G., 'Neurologic Symptoms and Hysterectomy: A Retrospective Survey of the Prevalence of Hysterectomy in Neurologic Patients', *Obstet. Gynecol.*, 1987, Vol. 70, No. 4, pp. 559-563.

Prolapse of fallopian tubes:

Thomson, J.D., 'Fallopian Tube Prolapse After Abdominal Hysterectomy', *Aust. NZ J. Obstet. Gynaecol.*, Aug. 1980, Vol. 20, No. 3, pp. 187-188.

Long-term losses:

Adhesions:

Ratcliff, J.B., Kapernick, P., Brooks, G.G., 'Small Bowel Obstruction and Previous Gynecologic Surgery', *South. Med. J*, Nov. 1983, Vol. 11, pp. 1349-1350, p. 1360.

Osteoporosis:

Riggs, B.L., Wahner, H.W., Dunn, W.L. et al., 'Differential Changes in Bone Mineral Density of the Appendicular and Axial Skeleton with Aging', *J. Clin. Invest.*, 1981, Vol. 67, pp. 328-335.

Schiff, I., Ryan, K., 'Benefits of Estrogen Replacement', *Obstet. and Gynecol. Survey Supplement*, 1980, Vol. 35, No. 6, pp. 402-403.

Hot flushes:

Judd, H.L., Cleary, R.E., Creasman, W.T., 'Estrogen Replacement Therapy', *Obstet. Gynecol.*, Sept. 1981, Vol. 58, No. 3, p. 268.

Emotional and sexual losses:

Depression:

Greenblatt, R.B., Nezhat, C., Roesel, R.A. et al., 'Update on the Male and Female Climacteric', *J. Am. Geriat. Soc.*, Nov. 1979, Vol. 27, pp. 481-484.

Depression and tryptophan:

Alyward, M., 'Plasma Tryptophan Levels and Mental Depression in Postmenopausal Subjects. Effect of Oral Piperazineoestrone Sulphate', *Med.Sci.*, 1973, Vol. 1, p. 30.

Sexual losses:

Dennerstein, L., Burrows, G.D., Hyman, G., 'Sexual Response Following Hysterectomy and Oophorectomy', *Obstet. Gynecol.*, 1977, Vol. 49, p. 92.

Chapter 4. The conspiracy against the uterus

For information on ancient beliefs concerning the uterus:

Precope, John, *Medicine, Magic, and Mythology*. London, William Heinemann Medical Books, 1954, p. 14.

Thorwald, Jurgen, *Science and Secrets of Early Medicine*, Trans. by Richard and Clara Winston. New York, Harcourt Brace Jovanovich, 1962.

Speert, Harold, MD, *Iconographia Gyniatrica: A Pictorial History of Gynecology and Obstetrics*, Philadelphia, F.A. Davis Company, 1973, p. 8.

Ricci, James, V., *The Development of Gynaecological Surgery and Instruments*, Philadelphia, The Blakiston Company, 1949, p. 7.

Chapter 5. The hysterectomy industry

for information on the difficulties of obs-gynae practice:

'Economic, Legislative, and Demographic Trends: Implications for Obstetrics and Gynecology in 1987', *Economic Impact: Health Care Delivery, Financing, and Reimbursement*, Jan. 1987, The American College of Obstetricians and Gynecologists, Washington, DC, p. 4.

Hysterectomies in the US vs. England and Europe:

Burchell, R.C., Harris, B., Marik, J.J., 'Hysterectomy: For Whom, When, How?', *Patient Care*, June 15, 1980, p. 29.

Easterday, C.L., Grimes, D.L., Riggs, J.A., 'Hysterectomy in the United States', *Obstet. Gynecol.*, Aug. 1983, Vol. 62, No. 2, p. 203.

Chapter 7. Why is the uterus important

For information on miscarriage and abnormal chromosome complements:

Sachs, E.S., Jahoda, M.G., Van Hemel, J.O. et al., 'Chromosome Studies of 500 Couples with Two or More Abortions', *Obstet. Gynecol.*, March 1985, Vol. 65, No. 3, pp. 375-378.

For information on prostaglandins and arthritis:

Kunkel, S.L., Ogawa, H., Conran, P. B.A. et al., 'Suppression of Acute and Chronic Inflammation by Orally Administered Prostaglandins', *Arthritis Rheum.*, Sept. 1981, Vol. 24, No. 9, pp. 1151-1158.

On the conflicting research regarding hysterectomy and sexuality:

Bernhard, L., 'Methodology Issues in Studies of Sexuality and Hysterectomy', *J. of Sex Research*, Feb. 1986, Vol. 22, No. 1, pp. 108-128.

Chapter 8. Clarifying the mysteries of endometriosis and adenomyosis

You will find additional information on endometriosis and adenomyosis in the following medical articles.

On endometriosis after hysterectomy:

Kapadia, S.B., Russak, R.R., O'Donnell, W.F. et al., 'Postmenopausal Uretal Endometriosis with Atypical Adenomatous Hyperplasia Following Hysterectomy, Bilateral Oophorectomy, and Long-term Estrogen Therapy', *Obstet. Gynecol.*, 1984, Vol. 64, No. 3, Suppl., pp. 60s-63s.

On the advantages of laser surgery for endometriosis:

Chong, A.P., Baggish, M.S., 'Management of Pelvic Endometriosis by Means of Intraabdominal Carbon Dioxide Laser', *Fertil. Steril.*, Jan. 1984, Vol. 41, No. 1, pp. 70-74.

Pittaway, D.E., Daniell, J.F., Maxson, W.S., 'Ovarian Surgery in an Infertility Patient as an Indication for a Short-Interval Second-Look Laparoscopy: A Preliminary Study', *Fertil. Steril.*, Nov. 1985, Vol. 44, No. 5, pp. 611-614.

On the effectiveness of danazol to treat endometriosis:

Greenblatt, R.B., Tzingounis, V., 'Danazol Treatment of Endometriosis: Long-Term Follow-Up', *Fertil. Steril.*, Nov. 1979, Vol. 32, No. 5, pp. 518-520.

Meldrum, D.R., Pardridge, W.M., Karow, W.G., 'The Hormonal Effects of Danazol and Medical Oophorectomy in Endometriosis', *Obstet. Gynecol.*, Oct. 1983, Vol. 62, No. 4, pp. 480-485.

Doberl, A., Bergqvist, A., Jeppsson, S. et al., 'Regression of Endometriosis Following Shorter Treatment with Lower Dose of Danazol', *Acta Obstet. Gynecol. Scand.*, Suppl, 1984, Vol. 123, pp. 51-58.

Wood, G.P., 'Clinical Assessment of Danazol for Endometriosis', *Contemporary Ob/Gyn*, March 1976, Vol. 7, p. 28.

On the use of Depo-Provera to treat endometriosis:

The Subcommittee on Reproductive Endocrinology for the American College of Obstetricians and Gynecologists, 'Depot Medroxyprogesterone Acetate Used as a Contraceptive', paper, October 31, 1981.

Rosenfield, A., Maine, D., Rochat, R. et al., 'The Food and Drug Administration and Medroxyprogesterone Acetate', *JAMA*, June 3, 1983, Vol. 249, No. 21, pp. 2922-2928.

On the risks for developing endometriosis:

'Management of Endometriosis', *ACOG Technical Bull.*, March 1985, No. 85, p. 1.

Sanfilippo, J.S., Wakim, N.G., Schikler, K.N., 'Endometriosis in Associaiton with Uterine Anomaly', *Am. J. Obstet. Gynecol.*, Jan. 1986, Vol. 154, No. 1, pp. 39-43.

Tang, L.C., Ngan, H.Y., Tang, M.H., 'Rudimentary Uterine Horn with Adenomyosis and Pelvic Endometriosis in 23-Year-Old Girl', *J. Adolesc. Health Care*, July 1986, Vol. 7, No. 4, pp. 265-267.

Lamb, K., Hoffman, R.G., Nichols, T.R., 'Family Trait Analysis: A Case Control Study of 43 Women with Endometriosis and their Best Friends', *Am. J. Obstet. Gynecol.*, March 1986, Vol. 154, No. 3, pp. 596-601.

On menstrual cycle as a factor in endometriosis:

Dramer, D.W., Schiff, I., Berger, M.J. *JAMA*, Aug. 1986, Vol. 255, No. 14.

On prostaglandins and endometriosis:

Nelson, G.H., 'Prostaglandins and Reproduction', in *Current Problems in Obstetrics and Gynecology*, Vol. IV, No. 4, October 1980, Yearbook Medical Publishers, Chicago, p. 19, 26.

Drake, T.S., O'Brien, W.F., Ramwell, P.W. et al., 'Peritoneal Fluid Thromboxane B$_2$ and 6-keot-prostaglandin F$_{1n}$ in Endometriosis', *Am. J. Obstet. Gynecol.*, 1981, Vol. 140, p. 401.

Difficulties in diagnosing adenomyosis before hysterectomy:

Rao, B.N., Persaud, V., 'Adenomyosis Uteri: Report on a 15-Year (1966–1980) Study at the University Hospital of the West Indies', *W.I. Med. J.*, 1982, Vol. 31, pp. 205-207.

New diagnostic tools for adenomyosis:

Mark, A.S., Hricak, H., Heinrichs, L.W., 'Adenomyosis and Leiomyoma: Differential Diagnosis with MR Imaging', *Radiology*, May 1987, Vol. 163, No. 2, pp. 527-529.

For the risks in developing adenomyosis:

Nikkanen, V., Punnonen, R., 'Clinical Significance of Adenomyosis', *Annales Chirurgiae of Gynaecologiae.* 1980, Vol. 69, pp. 278-280.

Azziz, R., 'Adenomyosis in Pregnancy. A Review', *Journal of Reprod. Med.*, April 1986, Vol. 31, No. 4, pp. 224-227.

Blum, M., 'Adenomyosis: Study in a Jewish Female Population', *Int-Surg.*, Oct-Dec. 1981, Vol. 66, No. 4, pp. 341-343.

Bird, C.C., McElin, T.W., 'Adenomyosis and Other Benign Diffuse Englargements of the Uterus', *Clinical Gynecology*, Vol. 1, Chap. 37, p. 2.

Vora, I.M., Raizada, R.M., Rawal, M.Y., 'Adenomyosis: A Retrospective Study of 105 Cases', *Journal of Postgraduate Medicine*, 1981, Vol. 27, No. 1, pp. 7-11.

Chapter 9. The case against monitoring fibroids

For fibroids growing in other parts of the pelvis:

Sutherland, J.A., Wilson, E.A., Edger, D.E. et al., 'Ultrastructure and Steroid-binding Studies in Leiomyomatosis Peritonealis Disseminata', *Am. J. Obstet. Gynecol.*, April 15, 1980, Vol. 136, No. 8, pp. 992-996.

Common symptoms associated with fibroids:

Omu, A.E., Ihejerika, I.J., Tabowei, G., 'Management of Uterine Fibroids at the University of Benin Teaching Hospital', *Trop. Doct.*, 1984, Vol. 14, No. 2, pp. 82-85.

Van Son, R.N., Sedlis, Ca., 'Massive Hemorrhage in Fibroid with Cystic Degeneration', *NY State J. Med.*, 1965, vol. 65, No. 23, pp. 2938-2940.

The effect of fibroids on pregnancy:

Jewelewicz, R., Husami, N., Wallach, E.E., 'When Uterine Factors Cause Infertility', *Contemp. Ob/Gyn*, 1980, Vol. 16, p. 95.

Behrman, S.J., Kistner, R.W., *Progress in Infertility*, Second Edition, Boston, Little, Brown, 1975, p. 91.

Chapter 10. Endometrial hyperplasia and endometrial cancer

You may find the following articles helpful in understanding endometrial hyperplasia, endometrial cancer, and hormone replacement therapy.

On the difficulties in diagnosing endometrial hyperplasia:

Fu, Y-S., in 'Symposium: Detecting Endometrial Cancer and Precursor Lesions',

Contemporary Ob/Gyn, Sept. 1983, pp. 239-247.

Ferenczy, A.M., in 'Symposium: Detecting Endometrial Cancer and Precursor Lesions', *Contemporary Ob/Gyn*, Sept. 1983, p. 233.

Gusberg, S.B., 'Current Concepts in the Control of Carcinoma of the Endometrium', CA, July/Aug. 1986, Vol. 36, No. 4, p. 245.

On excess oestrogen endometrial hyperplasia/cancer:

Flowers, C.E., Wilborn, W., Hyde, B.M., 'Mechanisms of Uterine Bleeding in Postmenopausal Patients Receiving Estrogen Alone or with Progestin', *Obstet. Gynecol.*, Feb. 1983, Vol. 61, No. 2, pp. 135-143.

Coulam, C.B., 'Why Ca Risk Is Higher in Anovulatory Women', *Contemporary Ob/Gyn*, May 1984, p. 87.

Smith, D.C., Prentice, R., Thompson, D.J. et al., 'Association of Exogenous Estrogen and Endometrial Carcinoma', *N. Eng. J. Med.*, 1975, Vol. 293, p. 1164.

Ziel. H.K., Finkle, W., 'Increased Risk of Endometrial Carcinoma Among Users of Conjugated Estrogens', *N. Eng. J. Med.*, 1975, vol. 293, p. 1167.

Robboy, S.J., Miller, A.W., Kurman, R.J., 'The Pathologic Features and Behavior of Endometrial Carcinoma Associated with Exogenous Estrogen Administration', *Path. Res. Pract.*, 1982, Vol. 174, pp. 250-252.

On hormone replacement therapy:

Goldfein, A., 'Estrogen Replacement Therapy in Postmenopausal Women', *Rational Drug Therapy*, Jan. 1977, Vol. 11, No. 1, p.2.

Nachtigall, L.E., Nachtigall, R.H., Nachtigall, R.D. et al., 'Estrogen Replacement Therapy I: A 10-Year Prospective Study in the Relationship to Osteoporosis', *Obstet. Gynecol.*, 1979, vol. 53, No. 3, pp. 277-281.

Chapter 11. Prolapse

For more information on the history of the causes and treatment of uterine prolapse:

Speert, Harold, MD, *Iconographia Gyniatrica: A Pictorial History of Gynecology and Obstetrics*. Philadelphia, F.A. Davis Company, 1973, p. 463.

Hayes, Albert, *Physiology of Woman and Her Diseases*. Boston, Peabody Medical Institute, 1869, p. 316.

Stage, S., *Female Complaints*. New York, W.W. Norton and Co., 1979, p. 77.

On secondary and vaginal prolapse following hysterectomy:

Acharin. R.F., 'Pulsion Enterocele: Review of Functional Anatomy of the Pelvic Floor', *Obstet. Gynecol.*, Feb. 1980, Vol. 55, No. 2, pp. 135-140.

Symmonds, R.E., Williams, T.J. et al., 'Posthysterectomy Enterocele and Vaginal Vault Prolapse', *Am. J. Obstet. Gynecol.*, Aug. 15, 1981, Vol. 140, No. 8, p. 855.

Chapter 12. Cervical cancer

For cervical cancer statistics and death rates:

Silverberg, E., Lubera, J., 'Cancer Statistics, 1987', *CA-A Cancer Journal for Clinicians*, 1987, Vol. 37, pp. 2-19.

Mortality, Vol. 2 in *Vital Statistics of the United States, 1976*. National Center for Health Statistics, 1976, part A.

On the importance of a yearly cervical smear:

Jones, W., Saigo, P., 'The "Atypical"

Papanicolaou Smear', *CA-A Cancer Journal for Clinicians*, July/Aug. 1986, Vol. 36, No. 4, p. 239.

On understanding your cervical smear:

Nelson, J.H., Hervy, A.E., Richart, R.M., 'Dysplasia, Carcinoma in Situ, and Early Invasive Cervical Carcinoma', *CA*, Nov. 1984, Vol. 34, No. 6, pp. 306-318.

On how often you should have a cervical smear:

Bearman, D.M., MacMillan, J.P., Creasman, W.T., 'Papanicolaou Smear History of Patients Developing Cervical Cancer: An Assessment of Screening Protocols', *Obstet. Gynecol.*, Feb. 1987, Vol. 69, No.2, pp. 151-155.

On the importance of cervical smears for older women:

Celentano, D.D., Shapiro, S., Weisman, C.S., 'Cancer Prevention Screening Behavior Among Elderly Women', *Prev. Med.*, 1982, Vol. 11, pp. 454-463.
Riesenberg, D.E., 'Editorial: The Papanicolaou Test in Elderly Women', *JAMA*, July 18, 1986, Vol. 256, No. 3, p. 393.
Mandelblatt, J., Gopaul, I., Wistreich, M., 'Papanicolaou Smear Testing in Elderly Women', Letter, *JAMA*, Nov. 28, 1986, Vol. 256, No. 20, pp. 2818-2819.

On colposcopy for diagnosis:

Townsend, D.E., Richart, R.M., 'Can Colposcopy Replace Conization?', *CA-A Cancer Journal for Clinicians*, 1982, Vol. 32, No. 2, pp. 85-91.
Nelson, J.H., Hervy, A.E., Richart, R.M., 'Dysplasia, Carcinoma in Situ, and Early Invasive Cervical Carcinoma', *CA*, Nov. 1984, Vol. 34, No. 6, p. 308.

On laser surgery and biopsy for dysplasia:

Stanhope, R.C., Phibbs, G.D., Stuart, G.C. et al., 'Carbon Dioxide Laser Surgery', *Obstet. Gynecol.*, May 1983, Vol. 61, No. 5, pp. 624-627.
Drescher, C.W., Peters, W.A., III, Roberts, J.A., 'Contribution of Endocervical Curettage in Evaluating Abnormal Cervical Cytology', *Obstet. Gynecol.*, Sept. 1983, Vol. 62, No. 3, pp. 343-347.
Larsson, G., Alm, P., Grundsell, H., 'Laser Conization Versus Cold Knife Conization', *Surg. Gynecol. Obstet.*, Jan. 1982, Vol. 154, No. 1, pp. 59-61.
Bekassy, Z., Alm, P., Grundsell, H. et al., 'Laser Miniconization in Mild and Moderate Dysplasia of the Uterine Cervix', *Gynecol. Oncol.*, 1983, Vol. 15, p. 357.

On conization with laser for CIS:

Bekassy, Z., Alm, P., Grundsell, H. et al., 'Laser Miniconization in Mild and Moderate Dysplasia of the Uterine Cervix', *Gynecol. Oncol.*, 1983, Vol. 15, p. 357.
Wright, V.C., Davies, E., Riopelle, M.A., 'Laser Cylindrical Excision to Replace Conization', *Am. J. Obstet. Gynecol.*, Nov. 1984, Vol. 150, No. 6, pp. 704-709.

On follow-up for dysplasia and CIS:

Tsukamoto, N., 'Treatment of Cervical Intraepithelial Neoplasia With the Carbon Dioxide Laser', *Gynecol. Oncol.*, July 1985, Vol. 21, No. 3, pp. 331-336.

On treatments for venereal warts:

Stanhope, R.C., Phibbs, G.D., Stuart, G.C. et al., 'Carbon Dioxide Laser Surgery', *Obstet. Gynecol.*, May 1983, Vol. 61, No. 5, pp. 624-627.
Sillman, F.H., Boyce, J.G., Macasaet, M.A., '5-Fluorouracil/Chemosurgery for Intraepithelial Neoplasia of the Lower Genital Tract', *Obstet. Gynecol.*, Sept. 1981, Vol. 58, No. 3, pp. 356-360.

Crum, C.P., Levine, R.U., 'Cervical Condyloma and CIN: How Are They Related?' *Contemp. Ob/Gyn.*, Sept. 1983, pp. 116-137.

On poor hygiene and cervical cancer:

American Cancer Society, 'Report on the Cancer-Related Check-up: Cancer of the Cervix', *CA*, 1980, Vol. 30, pp. 215-223.

On cervical cancer and smoking:

Sassoon, I.M., Haley, N.J., Hoffman, D. et al., 'Cigarette Smoking and Neoplasia of the Uterine Cervix: Smoke Constituents in Cervical Mucus', *N. Eng. J. Med.*, 1985, Vol. 312, pp. 315-316.

Holly, E.A., Petrakis, N.L., Friend, N.F. et al., 'Mutagenic Cervical Mucus in Women Smokers', abstracted, *Am. J. Epidemiol.*, 1985, Vol. 122, p. 518.

Chapter 13. Understanding your ovaries

On ovarian anatomy:

Goldfein, A., 'Estrogen Replacement Therapy in Postmenopausal Women', *Rational Drug Therapy*, Jan. 1977, Vol. 11, No. 1, p. 1.

Healy, D.L., Hodgen, G.D., 'The Endocrinology of Human Endometrium', *Obstetrical and Gynecological Survey*, 1983, Vol. 38, No. 8, S510.

Chapter 14. The ovarian cyst: is it time for surgery?

On diagnosing ovarian cysts:

Hutcherson, P.W., in *International Correspondence Society of Ob/Gyn.*, May 1984, p. 77.

On oral contraceptives to suppress follicular cysts:

'Should OCs Be Prescribed to Prevent Adnexal mass?' *Contraceptive Technology Update*, Sept. 1982, Vol. 3, No. 9, pp. 116-118.

Chapter 15. Ovarian cancer—detecting the silent killer

For facts and statistics on ovarian cancer:

Barber, Hugh, R.K., 'Ovarian Cancer', *CA-A Cancer Journal for Clinicians*, May/June 1986, Vol. 36, No. 3, p. 150.

On diet and ovarian cancer:

Snowdon, D.A., 'Diet and Ovarian Cancer', *JAMA*, 1985, Vol. 254, pp. 356-357.

On oral contraceptives as a preventive for ovarian cancer:

'OCs May Play a Protective Role', *Adv. in Reprod. Med.*, Sept. 1, 1982, Vol. 1, No. 7, p. 2.

On precautions if you are genetically at risk:

Lynch, H.T., Albano, W.A., Lynch, J.F., 'Surveillance and Management of Patients at High Genetic Risk for Ovarian Carcinoma', *Obstet. Gynecol.*, May 1982, Vol. 59, No. 5, pp. 589-596.

Chapter 16. Other menstrual and pelvic problems

On tubal ligation syndrome and its risks:

Huggins, G.R., Sondheimer, S.J., 'Complications of Female Sterilization, Immediate and Delayed', *Fertility and Sterility*, March 1984, Vol. 41, No. 3, pp. 337-355.

Notes

Chapter 1: The revolution in women's health care

1. Coulter, A., McPherson, K., Vessey M. Do British women undergo too many or too few hysterectomies? *Soc. Sci. Med.*, Vol. 27, No. 9, 1989, 987-994.

2. 'Referral for Psychological Effects of Hysterectomy', *Ob. Gyn. News*, Vol. 19, No. 20, Nov. 15-30, 1984, p. 2.

3. Lee, N.C., Dicker, R.C., Rubin, G.L., 'Confirmation of the Preoperative Diagnoses for Hysterectomy', *Am. J. Obstet. Gynecol.*, Oct. 1, 1983, Vol. 150, pp. 283-287.

4. Hufnagel, V., 'Uses and Application of Intraoperative Ultrasound (abst.)', *Program of the Reproductive Health Care International Symposium*, Hawaii, October 1982, p. S28.

Chapter 2: What is hysterectomy?

1. Bell, J. Sevin, B-U, Averette, H., 'Vaginal Cancer After Hysterectomy for Benign Disease: Value of Cytologic Screening', *Obstet. Gynecol.*, Vol. 64, No. 5, Nov. 1984, pp. 699-702.

Stuart, G.C., Allen, H.H., Anderson, R.J., 'Squamous Cell Carcinoma of the Vagina Following Hysterectomy', *Am. J. Obstet. Gynecol.*, Feb. 1981, Vol. 139, No. 3, pp. 311-315.

2. Grattarola, R., Secreto, G., 'Breast Cancer Years After Hysterectomy and Bilateral Ovariectomy and Increased Androgenic Activity', *Oncology*, 1980, Vol. 37, No. 1, pp. 37-40.

3. Korenbrot, C., Flood, A.B., Higgens, M. et al., 'Case Study #15: Elective Hysterectomy: Costs, Risks, and Benefits', in *The Implications of Cost-Effectiveness Analysis of Medical Technology, Background Paper #2: Case Studies of Medical Technologies*, Congress of the United States, Office of Technological Assessment, October 1981, p. 9.

Amirikia, H., Evans, T., 'Ten-year Review of Hysterectomies: Trends, Indications, and Risks', *Am. J. Obstet. Gynecol.*, June 1979, Vol. 134, No. 4, p. 433.

Livengood, C.H., III, and Addison, W.A., 'Adnexal Abscess as a Delayed Complication of Vaginal Hysterectomy', *Am. J. Obstet. Gynecol.*, July 1, 1982, Vol. 143, No. 5, pp. 596-597.

4. Glavecke, L., 'Korperliche und Veranderungen im Weiblichen Korper nach kunstlichem Verlust der Ovarien einerseits und des Uterus andererseits', *Arch. Gynaekol*, Vol. 35, 1889, p. 1.

Mond, R., 'Kurze Mitteilungen uber die Behandlung der Beschwerden bei naturlichen oder durch Operationen veranlabter Amenorrhoen mit Eierstocksconserven', *Munch Med Wochenschr*, Vol. 14, 1896, p. 314.

Sessums, J.V., Murphy, D.P., 'Hysterectomy and the Artificial Menopause', *Surg. Gynecol. Obstet.*, Vol. 55, 1932, p. 286.

5. Riedel, H., Lehmann-Willenbrock, E., Semm, K., 'Ovarian Failure After Hysterectomy', *The Journal of Reproductive Medicine*, Vol. 31, No. 7, July 1986, pp. 597-600.

Korenbrot, C., Flood, A.B., Higgens, M. et al., p. 13.

Garcia, C-R., Cutler, W., 'Preservation of the Ovary: A Reevaluation', *Fertility and Sterility*, Oct. 1984, Vol. 42, No. 4, p. 511.

Beavis, E.L.G., Brown, J.B., Smith, M.A., 'Ovarian Function after Hysterectomy with Conservation of the Ovaries in Premenopausal Women', *J. Obstet. Gynaecol. Br. Commonw.*, 1969, Vol. 76, p. 969.

6. Riedel, H., Lehmann-Willenbrock, Semm, pp. 597-600.

Greenblatt, R.B., Professor Emeritus of Endocrinology, Medical College of Georgia, Augusta, GA, in a letter to Dr Leon Zussman, Long Island Jewish-Hillside Medical Center, New Hyde Park, NY, April 21, 1978.

7. Riedel, H., Lehmann-Willenbrock, Semm, p. 599.

Chapter 3: Complications

1. McKinlay, S.M., McKinlay, J.B., 'Health Status and Health Care Utilization by Menopausal Women', in Mastroianni, L., and Paulsen, C.A., eds. *Aging, Reproduction, and the Climacteric.* New York: Plenum Publishing Co., 1985.

McKinlay, J.B., McKinlay, S.M., Brambilla, D.J., 'Health Status and Utilization Behavior Associated with Menopause', *Am. J. Epidemiol.*, Jan. 1987, Vol. 125, No. 1, pp. 110-121.

2. Easterday, C.L., Grimes, D.A., Riggs, J.A., 'Hysterectomy in the United States', *Obstet. Gynecol.*, Aug. 1983, Vol. 62, No. 2, p. 203-212.

Korenbrot, C., Flood, A.B., Higgens M. et al., 'Case Study #15: Elective Hysterectomy: Costs, Risks, and Benefits', in *The Implications of Cost-Effectiveness Analysis of Medical Technology, Background Paper #2: Case Studies of Medical Technologies*, Congress of the United States, Office of Technological Assessment, October 1981, p. 9.

3. Roos, N.P., 'Hysterectomies in One Canadian Province: A New Look at Risks and Benefits', *Am. J. Public Health*, Jan. 1984, Vol. 74, No. 1, pp. 39-46.

4. Ehrenreich, Barbara, English, Deirdre. *For Her Own Good: 150 Years of the Experts' Advice to Women*, London: Pluto Press, 1979, p. 110.

5. Korenbrot et al., p. 10.

6. Gambrell, R.D., Massey, F.M., Castaneda, T.A. et al., 'The Use of Progestogen Challenge Test to Reduce the Risk of Endometrial Cancer', *Obstet. Gynecol.*, 1980, Vol. 55, pp 732-738.

7. Vandenbroucke, J.V., *JAMA*, March 14, 1986, quoted in *American Medical News*, March 14, 1986, p. 51.

Holmdahl, R., Jansson, L., Andersson, M., 'Female Sex Hormones Suppress Development of Collagen-Induced Arthritis in Mice', *Arthritis Rheum.*, Dec. 1986, Vol. 29, No. 12, pp. 1501-1509.

8. Cole, P., Berlin, J., 'Elective Hysterectomy', *Am. J. Obstet. Gynecol.*, 1977, Vol. 129, p. 117.

Centerwall, B.S., 'Premenopausal Hysterectomy and Cardiovascular Disease', *Am. J. Obstet. Gynecol.*, Jan. 1981, Vol. 139, No. 1, pp. 58-61.

Easterday, p. 209.

Rosenberg, L., Hennekens, C.H., Rosner, B. et al., 'Early Menopause and the Risk of Myocardial Infarction', *Am. J. Obstet. Gynecol.*, Jan. 1981, Vol. 139, No. 1, p. 47.

Colditz, G.A., Willett, W.C., Stampfer, M.J., 'Menopause and the Risk of Coronary Heart Disease in Women', *N. Eng. J. Med.*, April 1987, Vol. 316, No. 18, pp. 1105-1110.

Sheldon, J.D., 'Prostacyclin from the Uterus and Woman's Cardiovascular Advantage', *Prostaglandins Med.*, 1982, Vol. 8, p. 459.

9. Gordon, R., Kannel, W.B., Hoortland, M.C., McNamara, P.M., 'Menopause and cardiovascular disease'. *Ann. Intern. Med. 89*, 1978, 157-61.

Centerwell, B.S., 'Premenopausal hysterectomy and cardiovascular disease'. *Am. J.*

Obstet. Gynecol., 139, 1981, 58-61.

10. Studd, J.W., Thom, M.H., 'Ovarian Failure and Aging', *Clin. in Endocrin. and Metabol.*, March 1981, Vol. 10, No. 1, p. 102.

Kase, N., Judd, H.L., Mishell, D.R., 'Managing the "Surgical Menopause"', *Highlights from a Round-Table Discussion: The Clinical Management of the Perimenopause*, 1981, Upjohn Co., p. 3.

11. Turpin, T.J., Heath, D.S., 'The Link Between Hysterectomy and Depression', *Can. J. Psychiatry*, 1979, Vol. 24, p. 247.

Dennerstein, L., Burrows, G., Cox, L., Wood, C., *Gynaecology, Sex and Psyche*, Melbourne; Melbourne University Press, 1978, p. 169.

Richards, D.H., 'Depression after Hysterectomy', *Lancet 2*, 1973, Vol. 25, pp. 430-433.

Sloan, D., 'The Emotional and Psychosexual Aspects of Hysterectomy', *Am. J. Obstet. Gynecol.*, July 15, 1978, Vol. 131, No. 4, pp. 598-605.

——, 'Referral for Psychological Effects of Hysterectomy', *Ob. Gyn. News*, Vol. 19, No. 22, Nov. 15-30, 1984, p. 2.

Korenbrot et al., p. 12.

12. Hibbard, L.T., 'Chronic Pelvic Pain', *Management of Common Problems in Obstetrics and Gynecology*, Mishell, D.R., Jr., and Brenner, P.F., eds, 1984, Oradell, N.J.: Medical Economics Books, p. 214.

13. Dennerstein, L., Laby, B., Burrows, G.D. et al., 'Headache and Sex Hormone Therapy', *Headache*, 1978, Vol. 18, p. 146.

Moaz, B., Durst, N., 'Psychology of the Menopause', in *Female and Male Climacteric*, P.A. van Keep, D.M. Serr, and R.B. Greenblatt, eds., Lancaster, England: MTP Press, Ltd., 1979, pp. 9-16.

14. Zussman, Leon, Zussman, S., Sunley, R., Bjornson, E., 'Sexual Response After Hysterectomy-Oophorectomy: Recent Studies and Reconsideration of Psychogenesis', *Am. J. Obstet. Gynecol.*, Vol. 140, August 1981.

15. Ricci, James, V., *The Genealogy of Gynaecology*, Philadelphia: The Blakiston Co., 1950, p. 246.

16. Raboch, J., Boudnik, V., Raboch, J., Jr., ['Sex Life Following Hysterectomy'], *Geburtshilfe und Frauenheikunde*, Jan. 1985, Vol. 45, No. 1, pp. 48-50.

Utian, W., 'The True Clinical Features of Postmenopause and Oophorectomy, and Their Response to Oestrogen Therapy', *S. Afr. Med. J.*, June 3, 1972, Vol. 46, p. 732.

17. Dennerstein, L., Burrows, G.D., Wood, C. et al., 'Hormones and Sexuality: Effect of Estrogen and Progestogen', *Obstet. Gynecol.*, Sept. 1980, Vol. 56, No. 3, p. 321.

18. Greenblatt, R.B., Perez, D.H., 'Problems of Libido in the Elderly', in *The Menopausal Syndrome*, R.B. Greenblatt, V.B. Mahesh, and P.G. McDonough, eds., Medcom, Inc., 1974, p. 95.

Chakravarti, S., Collins, W.P., Newton, J.R. et al., 'Endocrine Changes and Symptomatology after Oöphorectomy in Premenopausal Women', *Brit. J. Obstet. Gynaec.*, 1977, Vol. 84, p. 773.

19. Dennerstein, Burrows, Cox, Wood, p. 169.

20. Jaszczak, S.E., Evans, T.N., 'Intrafascial Abdominal and Vaginal Hysterectomy: A Reappraisal', *Obstet. Gynecol.*, April 1982, Vol. 59, No. 4, p. 441.

Kilkku, P., Gronroos, M., Hirvonen, T. et al., 'Supravaginal Uterine Amputation vs. Hysterectomy. Effects on Libido', *Acta Obstet. Gynecol. Scand.*, 1983, Vol. 62, No. 2, pp. 147-152.

21. Jones, Howard, Jones, Georgeanna Seegar, eds., *Novak's Textbook of Gynecology*, Tenth Edition, Baltimore, Williams and Wilkins, 1981, p. 162.

Chapter 4: The conspiracy against the uterus

1. Grant, J.M., and Hussein, I.Y., 'An audit of abdominal hysterectomy over a decade in a

district hospital'. *Brit. J. Obstet. Gynae.*, Vol. 91, 1984, pp. 73-77.

2. Sloan, D., 'The Emotional and Psychosexual Aspects of Hysterectomy', *Am. J. Obstet. Gynecol.*, July 1978, Vol. 131, No. 6, pp. 598-605.

3. National Center for Health Statistics. Pokras, R., Hufnagel, V.G., 'Hysterectomy in the United States: 1965-1984', *Vital and Health Statistics*, 1987, Series 13, No. 92. DHHS Pub. No. (PHS) 87-1753. Public Health Service, Washington, DC, US Government Printing Office.

4. Spellacy, W.N., Miller, S.J., Winegar, A., 'Pregnancy after 40 Years of Age', *Obstet. Gynecol.*, Oct. 1986, Vol. 68, pp. 452-454.

5. Quoted in Barker-Benfield, G.J., *The Horrors of the Half-Known Life: Male Attitudes Towards Women and Sexuality in Nineteenth-Century America*, New York: Harper & Row, 1976, p. 124-125.

6. Speert, Harold, MD. *Iconographia Gyniatrica: A Pictoral History of Gynecology and Obstetrics*, Philadelphia, F.A. Davis Company, 1973, p. 10.

7. Ibid. p. 9.

8. Greer, Germaine, *The Female Eunuch*, New York: McGraw-Hill Book Company, 1971, p. 40.

9. Ibid. p. 40.

10. Speert, p. 455.

11. Ehrenreich, Barbara, English, Deirdre. *For Her Own Good: 150 Years of the Experts' Advice to Women*, London: Pluto Press, 1979, pp. 93-97.

12. Speert, p. 469.

Hollick, Fredrick, MD. *The Diseases of Women, Their Causes and Cure Familiarly Explained*, New York: T.W. Strong, 1848, quoted in Ehrenreich, Barbara and Deirdre English, p. 108.

Dirix, M.E., MD. *Woman's Complete Guide to Health*, New York: W.A. Townsend and Adams, 1869, pp. 23-24, quoted in Ehrenreich, Barbara and Deirdre English, p. 110.

13. Stage, Sarah, *Female Complaints*, New York: W.W. Norton and Co., 1979, p. 70.

14. Bliss, W.W., *Woman and Her Thirty Years Pilgrimage*, Boston: B.B. Russell, 1870, p. 96, quoted in Ehrenreich, Barbara and Deirdre English, pp. 109, 111-112.

15. Battey, Robert, 'Extirpations of the Functionally Active Ovaries for the Remedy of Otherwise Incurable Diseases', *Transactions of the American Gynecological Society*, Vol. I, 1876, p. 102, in Stage, Sarah, p. 80.

16. Quoted in Barker-Benfield, G.J., *The Horrors of the Half-Known Life: Male Attitudes Towards Women and Sexuality in Nineteenth-Century America*, New York: Harper & Row, 1976, pp. 124-125.

17. Stage, Sarah, p. 81.

Quoted in Ehrenreich, Barbara and Deirdre English, p. 111.

18. Henrotin, Ferdinand, MD., 'Conservative Surgical Treatment of Para and Peri Uterine Septic Disease', *Transactions of the American Gynecological Society*, Vol. XX, 1895, p. 225, in Stage, Sarah, p. 81.

19. Korenbrot, C., Flood, A.B., Higgens, M. et al., *Case Study #15: Elective Hysterectomy: Costs, Risks, and Benefits*, in *The Implications of Cost-Effectiveness Analysis of Medical Technology, Background Paper #2: Case Studies of Medical Technologies*, Congress of the United States, Office of Technological Assessment, October 1981, p. 5.

Wright, R.C., 'Hysterectomy: Past, Present, and Future', *Obstet. Gynecol.*, 1969, Vol. 33, p. 560.

Chapter 5: The hysterectomy industry

1. Nicholl, J.P., Beeby, N.R., Williams, B.T., 'Comparison of the activity of short stay independent hospitals in England and Wales, 1981 and 1986', *Brit. Med. J.*, Vol. 298, 28 Jan., 1989, pp. 239-242.

2. Dennerstein, L., Burrows, G., Cox, L., Wood, C., *Gynaecology, Sex and Psyche*, Melbourne: Melbourne University Press, 1978, p. 166.

3. Barker-Benfield. *The Horrors of the Half-Known Life: Male Attitudes Toward Women and Sexuality in Nineteeth-Century America*, New York: Harper & Row, 1976, p. 125.

4. Domenighetti, G., Luraschi, P., 'Hysterectomy and Sex of the Gynecologist', [letter], *N. Eng. J. Med.*, Dec. 5, 1985, p. 1482.

5. Coulter, A., McPherson, K., and Vessey, M., 'Do British women undergo too many or too few hysterectomies?' *Soc. Sci. Med.*, Vol. 27, No. 9, 1989, pp. 987-994.

6. Coulter, A., and McPherson, K., 'The Hysterectomy Debate', *Quarterly Journal of Social Affairs*, 2, Economic and Social Research Council, 1986.

7. Selwood, T., and Wood. C., 'Incidence of hysterectomy in Australia'. *Med. J. of Aust.*, 2, 1978, pp. 201-204.

8. Dyke, F.J., Murphy, F.A., et al., 'Effect of surveillance on the number of hysterectomies in the province of Saskatchewan'. *New Engl. J. Med.*, 296, 1977, pp. 1326-1328.

9. Domenighetti, G., Luraschschi, P., Casabianca, A., et al., 'Effect of information campaign by the mass media on hysterectomy rates'. *Lancet*, Dec. 24/31, 1989.

10. National Center for Health Statistics, Pokras, R., Hufnagel, V.G., 'Hysterectomy in the United States: 1965-1984', *Vital and Health Statistics*, 1987, Series 13, No. 92. DHHS Pub. No. (PHS) 87-1753. Public Health Service, Washington, DC, US Government Printing Office.

11. 'Referral for Psychological Effects of Hysterectomy', *Ob. Gyn. News*, Vol. 19, No. 20, Nov. 15-30, 1984, p. 2.

12. Zussman, Leon et al., 'Sexual Response after Hysterectomy-Oophorectomy: Recent Studies and Reconsideration of Psychogenesis', *Am. J. Obstet. Gynecol.*, August 1981, Vol. 140, p. 725.

13. Dunn, M., 'Blacks Have Many More Hysterectomies', *The Daily Breeze*, June 25, 1986, p. D2.

14. National Center for Health Statistics, Pokras, R., Hufnagel, V.G., 1987.

15. Korenbrot, C., Flood, A.B., Higgens, M. et al., 'Case Study #15: Elective Hysterectomy: Costs, Risks, and Benefits', in *The Implications of Cost-Effectiveness Analysis of Medical Technology, Background Paper #2: Case Studies of Medical Technologies*. Congress of the US, office of Technological Assessment, October 1981, p. 6.

16. McPherson, K., Strong, P.M., Epstein, A., Jones, L., 'Regional variation in the use of common surgical procedures within and between England and Wales, Canada and the USA', *Soc. Sci. & Med.*, 15A, 1981, pp. 273-288.

17. Amirikia, H., Evans, T.N., 'Ten year review of hysterectomies: trends, indications and risks', *Amer. J. of Obs. & Gyn.*, 134, 1979, pp. 431-437.

Grant, J.M., Hussein, I.Y., 'An audit of abdominal hysterectomy over a decade in a district hospital', *Brit. J. of Obs. & Gyn.*, 91, 1984, pp. 73-77.

18. Opit, L.J., Gadiel, D., 'Hysterectomy in New South Wales: an evaluation of its use and outcome', *Office of Health Care Finance, NSW*, 1982.

19. Coulter, A., McPherson, K., 'The Hysterectomy debate', *Quarterly Journal of Social Affairs*, 2, Economic and Social Research Council, 1986.

20. Ibid.

21. Cava, E.F., 'Hysterectomy in a Community Hospital', *Am. J. Obstet. Gynecol.*, 1975, Vol. 122, p. 434.

22. Lee, N.C., Dicker, R.C., Rubin, G.L., 'Confirmation of the Preoperative Diagnoses for Hysterectomy', *Am. J. Obstet. Gynecol.*, Oct. 1, 1983, Vol. 150, pp. 283-287.

23. 'Hysterectomy Costs Vary Widely in US, New Report Indicates', *Contraceptive Technology Update*, April 1986, p. 43.

24. Coulter, A., McPherson, K., Vessey, M.,

'Do British women undergo too many or too few hysterectomies?' *Soc. Sci. Med.*, Vol. 27, No. 9, 1988, pp. 987-994.

25. Easterday, C.L., Grimes, D.A., Riggs, J.A., 'Hysterectomy in the US', *Obstet. Gynecol.*, Aug. 1983, Vol. 62, No. 2, p. 210.

Korenbrot, et al., pp. 16-17.

26. Easterday, C.L., pp. 210-211.

Chapter 6: What is female reconstructive surgery

1. Magos, A., Baumann, R. and Turnbull, Sir A., 'Transcervical resection of the endometrium (TCRE): elegy of the hysterectomy for menorrhagia.' *Brit. J. of Obs. & Gynae.*, Vol. 96, No. 10, Oct. 1989. Paper presented at the Royal College of Obstetrics and Gynaecology meeting, Apr. 1989.

2. Chong, A.P., Baggish, M.S., 'Management of Pelvic Endometriosis by Means of Intra-abdominal Carbon Dioxide Laser', *Fertil. Steril.*, Jan. 1984, Vol. 41, No. 1, pp. 70-74.

McLaughlin, D.S., 'Metroplasty and Myomectomy with the CO_2 Laser for Maximizing the Preservation of Normal Tissue and Minimizing Blood Loss', *J. Reprod. Med.*, Jan. 1985, Vol. 30, No. 1, pp. 1-9.

Chapter 7: Why is the uterus important?

1. 'Premenopausal hysterectomy and risk of cardiovascular disease', *Lancet*, May 16, 1987 (letter).

2. Burchell, R.C., Harris, B., Marik, J.J., 'Hysterectomy: For Whom, When, How?' *Patient Care*, June 15, 1980, p. 29.

3. Healy, D.L., Hodgen, G.D., 'The Endocrinology of Human Endometrium', *Obstetrical and Gynecological Survey*, 1983, Vol. 38, No. 8, S509-530.

4. Tseng, L., Mazela, J., Mann, W.J. et al., 'Estrogen Synthesis in Normal and Malignant Endometrium', *J. Clin. Endocrinol. Metab.*, 1982, Vol. 55, p. 1029.

5. Petraglia, F., Facchinetti, F., M'Futa, K. et al., 'Endogenous Opioid Peptides in Uterine Fluid', *Fertil. Steril.*, Vol. 46, No. 2, Aug. 1986, pp. 247-250.

Cowan, B.D., North, D.H., Whitworth, N.S., 'Identification of a Uteroglobin-like Antigen in Human Uterine Washings', *Fertil. Steril.*, Vol. 45, No. 6, June 1986, pp. 820-823.

6. Centerwall, Brandon, S., 'Premenopausal Hysterectomy and Cardiovascular Disease', *Am. J. Obstet. Gynecol.*, 1981, Vol. 139, No. 58, pp. 58-61.

Fribourg, S., 'Risk of Cardiovascular Disease After Hysterectomy', [letter] *Am. J. Obstet. Gynecol.*, Jan. 1, 1982, p. 120.

Rosenberg, L., Hennekens, C.H., Rosner, B. et al., 'Early Menopause and the Risk of Myocardial Infarction', *Am. J. Obstet. Gynecol.* Jan. 1981, Vol. 139, No. 1, p. 47.

Centerwall, B.S., 'Reply to Dr Fribourg', [letter], *Am. J. Obstet. Gynecol.*, June 1, 1981, Vol. 140, No. 3, p. 356.

7. Stokes, N.M., *The Castrated Woman*, New York: Franklin Watts, 1986.

8. Munnell, E.W., 'Total Hysterectomy', *Am. J. Obstet. Gynecol.*, 1947, Vol. 54, p. 31.

9. Zussman, L., Zussman, S., Sunley, R., Bjornson, E., 'Sexual Response After Hysterectomy-Oophorectomy: Recent Studies and Reconsideration of Psychogenesis', *Am. J. Obstet. Gynecol.*, Aug. 1981, Vol. 140, p. 725.

10. Zussman et al., p. 725.

Utian, W.H., 'Effect of Hysterectomy, Oophorectomy, and Estrogen Therapy on Libido', *Int. J. Gynaecol. Obstet.*, 1975, Vol. 13, p. 97.

11. Salmon, U.J., Geist, S.H., 'Effects of Androgens upon Libido in Women', *J. Clin. Endocrinol.*, 1943, Vol. 3, p. 235.

Asch, R.H., Greenblatt, R., 'Steroidogenesis in the Post-Menopausal Ovary', *Clin. Obsts. Gynecol.*, 1977, Vol. 4, No. 1, p. 85.

12. Salmon and Geist, p. 235.

Studd, J.W.W., Thom, M.H., 'Ovarian Failure and Aging', *Clin. Endocrinol. Metab.*, 1981, Vol. 10, p. 1.

13. Asch and Greenblatt, p. 85.

14. Kinsey, A., *Sexual Behavior in the Human Female*, Philadelphia: W.B. Saunders, 1953.

15. Zussman et al., p. 729.

16. Masters, W.H., Johnson, V., *Human Sexual Response*, Boston: Little, Brown, & Co., 1966, pp. 116-119, 126, 238.

17. Hite, Shere., *The Hite Report*, New York: Macmillan Publishing Co., 1976, pp. 81, 95-99.

18. ——, 'Referral for Psychological Effects of Hysterectomy', *Ob. Gyn. News*, Nov. 15-30, 1984, Vol. 19, No. 22, p. 2.

Alzate, H., 'Vaginal Eroticism: A Replication Study', *Arch. Sex Behavior*, Dec. 1985, Vol. 14, No. 6, pp. 529-537.

Alzate, H., 'Vaginal Eroticism and Female Orgasm: A Current Appraisal', *J. Sex. Marital Ther.*, Winter 1985, Vol. 11, No. 4, pp. 271-284.

Alzate, H., Lodono, M.L., 'Vaginal Erotic Sensitivity', *J. Sex. Marital Ther.*, Spring 1984, Vol. 10, No. 1, pp. 49-56.

19. Sakai, K., Yamamoto, T., Kamiya, H., 'Female Sexual Response after Hysterectomy', *Nippon Sanka Fujinka Gakkai Zasshi. Acta Obstetrica et Gynaecologica J.*, June 1983, Vol. 35, No. 6, pp. 757-763.

20. Masters, R.H., Johnson, V., p. 118.

21. Zussman et al., p. 729.

Chapter 8: Endometriosis and adenomyosis

1. National Center for Health Statistics, Pokras, R., Hufnagel, V.G., 'Hysterectomy in the United States: 1965-1984', *Vital and Health Statistics*, 1987, Series 13, No. 92, DHHS Pub. No. (PHS) 87-1753. Public Health Service, Washington, DC, US Government Printing Office.

2. Redwine, D.B., 'Age-related Evolution in Color Appearance of Endometriosis', Presented at the Annual Meeting of Districts VIII-IX of The American College of Obstetricians and Gynecologists, Oct. 31, 1984, Scottsdale Az., and the Forty-First Annual Clinical Meeting of the American Fertility Society, Sept. 28, 1985, Chicago, Ill.

3. Reich, H., McGlynn, F., 'Treatment of Ovarian Endometriomas Using Laparoscopic Surgical Techniques', *J. Reprod. Med.*, July 6, 1986, Vol. 31, No. 7, p. 583.

Reich, H., personal communication, Sept. 18, 1987.

4. Blumenkrantz, M.J., Gallagher, N., Bashore, R.A. et al., 'Retrograde Menstruation in Women Undergoing Chronic Peritoneal Dialysis', *Obstet. Gynecol.*, May 1981, Vol. 57, No. 5, pp. 667-670.

Halme, J., Hammond, M.G., Hulka, J.F., 'Retrograde Menstruation in Healthy Women and in Patients with Endometriosis', *Obstet. Gynecol.*, August 1984, Vol. 64, No. 2, pp. 151-154.

5. Koninckx, P.R., Ide, P., Vandenbroucke, W., 'New Aspects of the Pathophysiology of Endometriosis and Association Infertility', *J. Reprod. Med.*, 1980, Vol. 24, p. 257.

diZerega, G.S., Barber, D.L., Hodgen, G.D., 'Endometriosis: Role of Ovarian Steroids in Initiation, Maintenance and Suppression', *Fertil. Steril.*, 1980, Vol. 33, p. 649.

6. Dmowski, W.P., Steele, R.W., Baker, G.F., 'Deficient Cellular Immunity in Endometriosis', *Am. J. Obstet. Gynecol.*, 1981, Vol. 141, p. 377.

Halme, J., Becker, S., Wing, R.D., 'Accentuated Cyclic Activation of Peritoneal Macrophages in Patients with Endometriosis', *Am. J. Obstet.*

Gynecol., 1984, Vol. 148, p. 85.

Mathur, S., Peress, M.R., Williamson, H.O. et al., 'Autoimmunity to Endometrium and Ovary in Endometriosis', *Clin. Exp. Immunol.*, Nov. 1982, Vol. 50, No. 2, pp. 259-266.

Lamb, K., Hoffman, R.G., Nicols, T.R., 'Family Trait Analysis: A Case Control Study of 43 Women with Endometriosis and Their Best Friends', *Am. J. Obstet. Gynecol.*, March 1986, Vol. 154, No. 3, pp. 596-601.

Olive, D.L., Henderson, D.Y., 'Endometriosis and Mullerian Anomalies', *Obstet. Gynecol.*, March 1987, Vol. 69, No. 3, Part 1, pp. 412-414.

Nelson, G.H., 'Prostaglandins and Reproduction', in *Current Problems in Obstetrics and Gynecology*, Vol. IV, No. 4, Oct. 1980, Yearbook Medical Publishers, Chicago, p. 25.

Koninckx, P.R. et al., p. 257.

7. Owolabi, T.O., Striclker, R.C., 'Adenomyosis: A Neglected Diagnosis', *Obstet. Gynecol.*, Oct. 1977, Vol. 50, No. 4, pp. 424-427.

Tsukahara, Y., Sakai, Y., Kotani, T. et al., 'A Case of Ovarian Endometroid Carcinoma and Malignant Transformation of Adenomyosis Uteri', *Nippon Sanka Fujinka Gakkai Zasshi*, Oct. 1981, Vol. 33, No. 10, pp. 1767-1770.

Hernandez, E., Woodruff, J.D., 'Endometrial Adenocarcinoma Arising in Adenomyosis', *Am. J. Obstet. Gynecol.*, Dec. 1, 1980, Vol. 138, pp. 827-832.

Woodruff, J.D., Erozan, Y.S., Genadry, R., 'Adenocarcinoma Arising in Adenomyosis Detected by Atypical Cytology', *Obstet. Gynecol.*, Jan. 1986, Vol. 67, No. 1, pp. 145-148.

Nikkanen, V., Punnonen, R., 'Clinical Significance of Adenomyosis', *Annales Chirurgiae of Gynaecologiae*, 1980, Vol. 69, pp. 278-280.

Greenwood, S.M., 'The Relation of Adenomyosis Uteri to Coexistent Endometrial Carcinoma and Endometrial Hyperplasia', *Obstet. Gynecol.*, July 1976, Vol. 48, No. 1, pp. 68-72.

8. Israel, L.S., Woutersz, T.B., 'Adenomyosis, a Neglected Diagnosis', *Obstet. Gynecol.*, 1959, Vol. 14, pp. 168-173.

Molitor, J.J., 'Adenomyosis—A Clinical and Pathological Appraisal', *Am. J. Obstet. Gynecol.*, 1971, Vol. 110, pp. 257-284.

Bird, C.C., McElin, T.W., Manalo-Estrella, P., 'The Elusive Adenomyosis of the Uterus—Revisited', *Am. J. Obstet. Gynecol.*, March 1972, Vol. 112, No. 5, p. 587.

Kilkku, P., Erkkola, R., Gronroos, M., 'Nonspecificity of Symptoms Related to Adenomyosis. A Prospective Comparative Survey', *Acta Obstet. Gynecol. Scand.*, 1984, vol. 63, No. 3, pp. 229-231.

9. Molitor, J.J., p. 275-284.

Weseley, A.C., 'The Preoperative Diagnosis of Adenomyosis', *Diag. Gyn. Obstet.*, Summer 1982, Vol. 4, No. 2, pp. 105-106.

Blum, M., 'Adenomyosis Study in a Jewish Female Population', *Int.-Surg.*, Oct.-Dec. 1981, Vol. 66, No. 4, pp. 341-343.

Chapter 9: Fibroids

1. National Center for Health Statistics, Pokras, R., Hufnagel, V.G., 'Hysterectomy in the United States: 1965-1984', *Vital and Health Statistics*, 1987, Series 13, No. 92. DHHS Pub. No. (PHS) 87-1753. Public Health Service, Washington, DC, US Government Printing Office.

2. Jones, H.W., Jones, G.S., 'Sarcoma of the Uterus', in *Novak's Textbook of Gynecology*, Tenth Edition, Baltimore; Williams and Wilkins, 1981, p. 452.

3. Macleod, D., Hawkins, J., *Bonney's Gynaecological Surgery*, New York: Hoeber Medical Division, Harper & Row, 1964, pp. 360-361.

4. Buchi, K., Keller, P.J., 'Estrogen Receptors in Normal and Myomatous Human Uteri', *Gynecol. Obstet. Invest.*, 1980, Vol. 11, pp. 59-60.

Wilson, E.A., Yang, F., Rees, E.D., 'Estradiol

and Progesterone Binding in Uterine Leiomyomata and in Normal Uterine Tissues', *Obstet. Gynecol.*, Jan. 1980, Vol. 55, No. 1, pp. 20-23.

Tamaya, T., Fujimoto, J., Okada, H., 'Comparison of Cellular Levels of Steroid Receptors in Uterine Leiomyoma and Myometrium', *Aceta Obstet. Gynecol. Scand.*, 1985, Vol. 64, No. 4, p. 307.

5. Stevenson, C.S., 'Myomectomy for Improvement of Fertility', *Fertil. Steril.*, 1964, Vol. 15, p. 367.

Rosenfeld, D.L., 'Abdominal Myomectomy for Otherwise Unexplained Infertility', *Fertil. Steril.*, Aug. 1986, Vol. 46, No. 2, p. 329.

6. Rosenfeld, p. 328-330.

Garcia, C-R, Tureck, R.W., 'Submucosal Leiomyomas and Infertility', *Fertil. Steril.*, 1984, Vol. 42, p. 16.

Chapter 10: Endometrial hyperplasia and endometrial cancer

1. Kurman R.J., in 'Symposium: Conservative or Aggressive Management of Early Ca?', *Contemporary Ob/Gyn.*, May 1984, pp. 261-265.

McBride, J.M., 'Premenopausal Cystic Hyperplasia and Endometrial Carcinoma', *J. Obstet. Gynaecol. Br. Commw.*, 1959, Vol. 66, p. 288.

2. Kurman, 1984, p. 265.

3. Kurman, R.J., Kaminski, P.F., Norris, H.J., 'The Behavior of Endometrial Hyperplasia: A Long-Term Study of "Untreated" Hyperplasia in 170 Women', *Cancer*, July 15, 1985, Vol. 56, No. 2, p. 403.

Gusberg, S.B., 'Current Concepts in the Control of Carcinoma of the Endometrium', *CA*, July/Aug. 1986, Vol. 36, No. 4, p. 245.

Gusberg, S.B., Kaplan, A.L., 'Precursors of Corpus Cancer. IV. Adenomatous Hyperplasia as Stage 0 Carcinoma of the Endometrium', *Am.*

J. Obstet. Gynecol., 1963, Vol. 87, pp. 662-678.

4. Richart, R., in 'Symposium: Detecting Endometrial Cancer and Precursor Lesions', *Contemporary Ob/Gyn.*, Sept. 1983, pp. 231, 239.

Kurman, R., in 'Symposium: Detecting Endometrial Cancer and Precursor Lesions', *Contemporary Ob/Gyn.*, Sept. 1983, p. 239.

5. Gambrell, R.D., Massey, F.M., Castaneda, T.A. et al., 'The Use of Progestogen Challenge Test to Reduce the Risk of Endometrial Cancer', *Obstet. Gynecol.*, 1980, Vol. 55, pp. 732-738.

6. Schneider, J.H., Bradlow, H.L., Strain, G., 'Effects of Obesity on Estradiol Metabolism: Decreased Formation of Nonuterotropic Metabolites', *Obstetrical and Gynecological Survey*, 1983, Vol. 38, No. 10, p. 616.

Gambrell, R., 'Estrogen Therapy and Endometrial Cancer', *Audio-Digest Obstet. Gyn.*, April 5, 1983, Vol. 30, No. 7, 1983, p.1.

Schneider, J.H. et al., p. 619.

7. La Vecchia, C., DiCarli, A., Fasoli, M. et al., 'Nutrition and Diet in the Etiology of Endometrial Cancer', *Cancer*, March 1986, Vol. 57, No. 6, pp. 1248-1253.

8. Smith, E.M., Sowers, M.F., Burns, T.L., 'Effects of Smoking on the Development of Female Reproductive Cancers', *JNCI*, August 1984, Vol. 73, No. 2, pp. 371-376.

9. Flowers, C.E., Wilborn, W., Hyde, B.M., 'Mechanisms of Uterine Bleeding in Postmenopausal Patients Receiving Estrogen Alone or with Progestin', *Obstet. Gynecol.*, Feb. 1983, Vol. 61, No. 2, pp. 135-143.

Whitehead, M.I., Townsend, P.T., Pryse-Davies, J. et al., 'Effects of Estrogen and Progestins on the Biochemistry and Morphology of the Postmenopausal Endometrium', *N. Eng. J. Med.*, 1981, Vol. 305, p. 1599.

Campbell, S., McQueen, J., Minardi, J. et al., 'The Modifying Effect of Progestogen on the Response of the Postmenopausal Endometrium to Exogenous Estrogens', *Postgrad. Med. J.*, 1978, Vol. 54, p. 59.

Hammond, C., Jelovsek, F.R., Lee, K.L. et al., 'Effects of Long-term Estrogen Replacement Therapy. II. Neoplasia'. *Am. J. Obstet. Gynecol.*, 1979, Vol. 133, p. 537.

Gambrell, R.D., Jr., Maier, R.C., Sanders, B.I., 'Decreased Incidence of Breast Cancer in Postmenopausal Estrogen-Progesterone Users', *Obstet. Gynecol.*, Oct. 1983, Vol. 62, No. 4, p. 440.

Gambrell, R.D. et al., 1980, pp. 732-738.

Gambrell, R.D., 1983, p. 1.

10. Ferenczy, in 'Symposium: Conservative or Aggressive Management of Early Ca?', *Contemporary Ob/Gyn.*, May 1984, p. 266.

11. Kurman, 1984, p. 259.

The Cancer and Steroid Study of the Centers for Disease Control and the National Institute of Child Health and Human Development. 'Combination Oral Contraceptive Use and the Risk of Endometrial Cancer', *JAMA*, Feb. 13, 1987, Vol. 257, No. 6, pp. 796-800.

12. Farhi, D.C., Nosanchuk, J., Silverberg, S.G., 'Endometrial Carcinoma in Women Under 25 Years of Age', *Obstet. Gynecol.*, Dec. 1986, Vol. 68, No. 6, pp. 741-745.

Chapter 11: Prolapse

1. Speert, Harold Iconographia Gyniatrica: A Pictorial History of Gynecology and Obstetrics, Philadelphia, F.A. Davis Company, 1973, p. 463.

2. Kauppila, O., Punnonen, R., Teisala, K., 'Prolapse of the Vagina after Hysterectomy', *Surg. Gynecol. Obstet.*, July 1985, Vol. 161, No. 1, pp. 9-11.

3. Symmonds, R.E., Pratt, J.H., 'Vaginal Prolapse Following Hysterectomy', *Am. J. Obstet. Gynecol.*, 1960, Vol. 79, p. 899.

4. Symmonds, R.E., Williams, T.J. et al., 'Posthysterectomy Enterocele and Vaginal Vault Prolapse', *Am. J. Obstet. Gynecol.*, Aug. 15, 1981, Vol. 140, No. 8, pp. 852-859.

5. Freese, M.P., Levitt, E.E., 'Relationships Among Intravaginal Pressure, Orgasmic Function, Parity Factors, and Urinary Leakage', 'Arch. Sex. Behav., 1984, Vol. 13, No. 3, pp. 261-268.

6. Hayes, Albert. *Physiology of Woman and Her Diseases*, Boston: Peabody Medical Institute, 1869, p. 316, quoted in Stage, Sarah, *Female Complaints*, New York: W.W. Norton and Co., 1979, p. 79.

7. Sinha, B., Quadros, M., 'Chronic Inversion of the Uterus Due to Submucous Fibroid', *J. Indian Med. Assoc.*, 1979, Vol. 73, No. 1, pp. 16-17.

Chapter 12: Cervical cancer

1. Morell, N.D., Taylor, J.R., Snyder, R.N. et al., 'False-Negative Cytology Rates in Patients in Whom Invasive Cervical Cancer Subsequently Development', *Obstet. Gynecol.*, July 1982, Vol. 60, No. 1, pp. 41-45.

2. Bogdanich, W., 'Lax laboratories: The Pap Test Misses Much Cervical Cancer Through Labs' Errors', *The Wall Street Journal*, Nov. 2, 1987, p. 1.

3. Swanson, G.M., Bell, S.H., Young, J.L., 'US Trends in Carcinoma of the Cervix: Incidence, Mortality, and Survival', in Hafez, E.S., Smith, J.P., eds., *Carcinoma of the Cervix: Biology and Diagnosis*. The Hague: Martinus Nijhoff Publishers, 1976, pp. 1-9.

4. Mandelblatt, J., Gopaul, I., Wistreich, M., 'Gynecological Care of Elderly Women: Another Look at Papanicolaou Smear Testing', *JAMA*, July 18, 1986, Vol. 256, No. 3, p. 367.

5. Bell, J., Sevin, B-U., Averette, H., 'Vaginal Cancer After Hysterectomy for Benign Disease: Value of Cytologic Screening', *Obstet. Gynecol.*, Nov. 1984, Vol. 64, No. 5, pp. 699-702.

Townsend, D.E., 'Intraepithelial Neoplasia of the Vagina', in *Gynecologic Oncology: Fundamental Principles and Clinical Practice*, Edinburgh: Churchill Livingstone, 1981, p. 340.

6. Meisels, A., Fortin, R., Roy, M., 'Condylo-

matous Lesions of the Cervix II. Cytologic Colposcopic and Histopathologic Study', *Acta Cytol.*, 1977, Vol. 21, No. 3, pp. 379-390.

7. LiVolsi, V., in 'Evaluation of Condylomatous Changes', *International Correspondence Society of Ob/Gyn.*, 1984, Vol. 25, No. 8, pp. 63-64.

8. Berman, M.L., 'Cervical Intraepithelial Neoplasia (CIN) and Cancer', *Audio-Digest Obstet./Gynecol.*, June 3, 1986, Vol. 33, No. 11, Side B.

Ferenczy, A., 'Using the Laser to Treat Vulvar Condylomata Acuminata and Intraepidermal Neoplasia', *Can. Med. Assoc. J.*, 1983, Vol. 128, p. 135.

9. Grundsell, H., Alm, P., Larsson, G., 'Cure Rates after Laser Conization for Early Cervical Neoplasia', *Ann. Chir. Gynaecol.*, 1983, Vol. 72, No. 4, pp. 218-222.

10. Nelson, J.H., Hervy, A.E., Richart, R.M., 'Dysplasia, Carcinoma In Situ, and Early Invasive Cervical Carcinoma', *CA*, Nov. 1984, Vol. 34, No. 6, p. 319.

11. Sall, S., Creasman, W., Richart, R., 'Premalignant Lesions of the Cervix', *ACOG Update*, 1978, Vol. 4, No. 5, p. 4.

12. Olsen, S.J., Love, R.R., 'A New Direction in Preventative Oncology: Chemoprevention', *Seminars in Oncology Nursing*, Vol. 2, No. 3, Aug. 1986, pp. 211-221.

Butterworth, C.E., Hatch, K.D., Gore, H. et al., 'Improvement in Cervical Dysplasia associated with Folic Acid Therapy in Users of Oral Contraceptives', *Am. J. Clin. Nutr.*, 1982, Vol. 35, pp. 73-82.

Butterworth, C.E., Norris, D., 'Folic Acid and Vitamin C in Cervical Dysplasia' [letter] *Am. J. Clin. Nutr.*, Feb. 1983, Vol. 37, No. 2, pp. 332-333.

13. Nelson et al., p. 320.

14. Kessler, I.I., 'Human Cervical Cancer as a Venereal Disease', *Cancer Res.*, 1976, Vol. 36, pp. 783-791.

Alexander, E.R., 'Possible Etiologies of Cancer of the Cervix other than Herpesvirus', *Cancer Res.*, June 1973, Vol. 33, pp. 1485-1496

15. Campion, M.J., Singer, A., Clarkson, P.K. et al., 'Increased Risk of Cervical Neoplasia in Consorts of Men with Penile Condylomata Acuminata', *Lancet*, April 1985, Vol. 1, No. 8435, pp. 943-946.

16. Meisels, A., Morin, C., 'Human Papillomavirus and Cancer of the Uterine Cervix', *Gynecol. Oncol.*, 1981, Vol. 12, S111.

Nash, J.K., Burke, T.W., Hoskins, W.J., 'Biologic Course of Cervical Human Papilloma Virus Infection', *Obstet. Gynecol.*, Feb. 1987, Vol. 69, No. 2, pp. 160-162.

Schneider, A., Sawada, E., Gissmann, L., Shah, K., 'Human Papillomaviruses in Women with a History of Abnormal Papanicolaou Smears and in their Male Partners', *Obstet. Gynecol.*, April 1987, Vol. 69, No. 4, p. 554.

——, 'Test Detects HPV Strains Tied to Cancer', *Medical World News for Obstetricians, Gynecologists, Urologists*, June 11, 1987, p. 33.

Fujii, T., Crum, C., Winkler, B. et al., 'Human Papillomavirus Infection and Cervical Intraepithelial Neoplasia: Histopathology and DNA Content', *Obstet. Gynecol.*, Jan. 1984, Vol. 63, No. 1, pp. 99-104.

——, 'Genital Human Papillomavirus Infections', *ACOG Technical Bulletin*, No. 105, June 1987.

Kaufman, R., Koss, L.G., Kurman, R.J. et al., 'Statement of Caution in the Interpretation of Papillomavirus-associated Lesions of the Epithelium of Uterine Cervix', *Am. J. Obstet. Gynecol.*, 1983, Vol. 146, p. 125.

Syrjanen, K.J., Heinonen, U.M., Kauraniemi, T., 'Cytologic Evidence of the Association of Condylomatous Lesions with Dysplastic and Neoplastic Changes in the Uterine Cervix', *Acta Cytol.*, 1981, Vol. 25, pp. 17-22.

Meisels, A., Roy, M., Fortier, M. et al., 'Human Papillomavirus Infection of the Cervix', *Acta Cytol.*, 1981, Vol. 25, pp. 7-16.

17. Crum, C.P., Levine, R.U., 'Cervical

Condyloma and CIN: How Are They Related?' *Contemp. Ob/Gyn.*, Sept. 1983, pp. 116-137.

18. Smotkin, D., Berek, J., Fu, Y.S. et al., 'Human Papillomavirus Deoxyribonucleic Acid in Adenocarcinoma and Adenosquamous Carcinoma of the Uterine Cervix', *Obstet. Gynecol.*, Aug. 1986, Vol. 68, No. 2, pp. 241-244.

Nelson et al., p. 313.

Crum, C.P., Levine, R.U., pp. 121-122.

——, 'Evidence Supports Papillomavirus, Cervical Ca Tie', *Ob. Gyn. News*, Oct. 15-31, 1984, Vol. 19, No. 20, p. 52.

——, 'Treatment for Genital Tract Condyloma Focus of Debate', *Ob. Gyn. News*, Oct. 15-31, 1984, Vol. 19, No. 20, p. 53.

19. Sillman, F.H., Boyce, J.G., Macasaet, M.A., '5-Fluorouracil/Chemosurgery for Intraepithelial Neoplasia of the Lower Genital Tract', *Obstet. Gunecol.*, Sept. 1981, Vol. 58, No. 3, pp. 356-360.

Krebs, H-B., 'Prophylactic Topical 5-Fluorouracil Following Treatment of Human Papillomavirus-Associated Lesions of the Vulva and Vagina', *Obstet. Gynecol.*, Dec. 1986, Vol. 68, No. 6, pp. 837-841.

20. Nelson et al., pp. 306-325.

'Sex at Early Age Held Major Cervical Neoplasia Factor', *Ob. Gyn. News*, Nov. 15-30, 1984, Vol. 19, No. 22, p. 2.

Draper, G.J., Cook, G.A., 'Changing Patterns of Cervical Cancer Rates', *Br. Med. J.*, 1983, Vol. 287, pp. 510-512.

MacGregor, J.E., 'Rapid Onset Cancer of the Cervix', *Brit. Med. J.*, 1982, Vol. 284, No. 6314, pp. 441-442.

Grunebaum, A.N., Sedlis, A., Sillman, F. et al., 'Association of Human Papillomavirus Infection with Cervical Intraepithelial Neoplasia', *Obstet. Gynecol.*, Oct. 1983, Vol. 62, No. 4, pp. 448-455.

21. Graham, S., Priore, R., Graham, M. et al., 'Genital Cancer in Wives of Penile Cancer Patients', *Cancer*, Nov. 1979, Vol. 44, pp. 1870-1874.

Smith, P.G., Kinlen, L.J., White, G.C., 'Mortality of Wives of Men Dying with Cancer of the Penis', *Br. J. Cancer*, March 1980, Vol. 41, No. 3, pp. 422-428.

22. Coppleson, M., 'The Origin and Nature of Premalignant Lesions of the Cervix Uteri', *Intern. J. Gynaecol. Obstet.*, 1970, Vol. 8, pp. 539-550.

Coppleson, M., Reid, B., *Preclinical Carcinoma of the Cervix Uteri: Its Nature, Origin and Management*, Oxford, England: Pergamon Press, 1967.

Alexander, E.R., 'Possible Etiologies of Cancer of the Cervix other than Herpesvirus', *Cancer Research*, 1973, Vol. 33, pp. 1485-1496.

23. ——, 'Herpes Simplex Virus Infections', *ACOG Technical Bulletin*, No. 102. March 1987.

24. Ibid.

Nelson et al., p. 313.

25. Alexander, E.R., 1973, p. 1487.

Berggren, O., 'Association of Carcinoma of the Uterine Cervix and Tricomonas Vaginalis Infestations', *Am. J. Obstet. Gynecol.*, 1969, Vol. 105, pp. 116-168.

26. Mandelblatt, J. et al., July 1986, p. 369.

Warnecke, R.B., Graham, S., 'Characteristics of Blacks Obtaining Papanicolaou Smears', *Cancer*, 1976, Vol. 37, pp. 2015-2125.

Diaz-Bazan, N., 'Cervical Carcinoma in El Salvador', in Hafex, E.S., Smith, J.P., eds., *Carcinoma of the Cervix: Biology and Diagnosis*, The Hague: Martinus Nijhoff Publishers, 1976.

DeBritton, R.C., Reeves, W.C. et al., 'Cervical Carcinoma in Panama', in Hafez, E.S., Smith, J.P., eds., *Carcinoma of the Cervix: Biology and Diagnosis*, The Hague: Martinus Nijhoff Publishers, 1976.

Dabanans, A., 'Cervical Cancer and Detection in Chile', in Hafez, E.S., Smith, J.P., eds., *Carcinoma of the Cervix: Biology and Diag-*

nosis, The Hague: Martinus Nijhoff Publishers, 1976.

Christopherson, W.M., Parker, J.E., 'A Study of the Relative Frequency of Carcinoma of the Cervix in the Negro', *Cancer*, 1960, Vol. 13, pp. 711-713.

27. Lynch, H.T., Krush, A.J., 'The Cancer Family Syndrome and Cancer Control', *Surg. Gynecol. and Obstet.*, Feb. 1971, Vol. 132, No. 2, pp. 247-250.

Andrews, F.J., Linehan, J.J., Melcher, D.J., 'Cervical Carcinoma in Both Mothers and Daughters', *Acta Cytol.*, Jan.-Feb. 1981, Vol. 25, No. 1, pp. 3-4.

Way, S., Hetherington, J., Galloway, D.C., 'Simultaneous Cytological Diagnosis of Cervical Cancer in Three Sisters', *Lancet 2*, 1959, p. 890.

Rotkin, I.D., 'Further Studies in Cervical Cancer Inheritance', *Cancer*, Sept. 1966, Vol. 19, No. 9, pp. 1251-1268.

28. Briton, L.A., Schairer, M.S. et al., 'Cigarette Smoking and Invasive Cervical Cancer', *JAMA*, June 20, 1986, Vol. 255, No. 23, p. 3268.

Lyon, J.S., Gardner, J.W., West, D.W., 'Smoking and Carcinoma in Situ of the Uterine Cervix', *Am. J. Public Health*, 1983, Vol. 73, p. 558.

29. Spriggs, A.A., 'Cancer of the Cervix', *Journal of Clinical Pathology*, Nov. 1972, Vol. 25, No. 11, p. 1008.

Chapter 13: Understanding your ovaries

1. Wells, S., Hegar, A., Battey, R., 'Castration in Nervous and Mental Diseases', *JAMA*, 1886, Vol. 7, pp. 547-549 in 'JAMA 100 Years Ago', Elizabeth Knoll, ed., Nov. 21, 1986, Vol. 256, No. 19.

2. National Center for Health Statistics, Pokras, R., Hufnagel, V.G., 'Hysterectomy in the United States: 1965-1984'. *Vital and Health Statistics*, 1987, Series 13, No. 92. DHHS Pub.

No. (PHS) 87-1753. Public Health Service, Washington, DC, US Government Printing Office.

Garcia, C.R., Cutler, W.B., 'Preservation of the Ovary: A Reevaluation', *Fertil. Steril.*, Vol. 42, No. 4, October, 1984, pp. 510-514.

3. Jones, Howard, W., Jones, Georgeanna, Seegar, eds., *Novak's Textbook of Gynecology, Tenth Edition*, Baltimore: Williams and Wilkins, 1981, p. 37.

Vandenbroucke, J.V., *JAMA*, March 14, 1986, quoted in *American Medical News*, March 14, 1986, p. 51.

Centerwall, B.S., 'Premenopausal Hysterectomy and Cardiovascular Disease', *Am. J. Obstet. Gynecol.*, Jan. 1, 1981, Vol. 139, No. 1, pp. 58-61.

4. Asch, R.H., Greenblatt, R.B., 'Steroidogenesis in the Postmenopausal Ovary', *Clin, in Obstets. and Gynaec.*, April 1977, Vol. 4, No. 1, p. 85.

5. Longcope, C., 'Steroid Production in Pre- and Postmenopausal Women', *The Menopausal Syndrome*, eds., Greenblatt, R.B., Mahesh, V.B., McDonough, P.G., NY: Medcom, Inc., 1974, p. 6.

6. Studd, J.W.W., 'The Climacteric Syndrome', in *Female and Male Climacteric*, van Keep, P.A., Serr, D.M., Greenblatt, R.B., eds., Lancaster, England: MPT Press Ltd., 1979, pp. 23-24.

Chapter 14: The ovarian cyst

1. Snowden, R., and Christian, B., eds., 'Patterns and Perceptions of Menstruation', A WHO International Collaborative Study, WHO and Croom Helm, London.

2. Speert, Harold, MD, *Iconographia Gyniatrica: A Pictorial History of Gynecology and Obstetrics*, Philadelphia: F.A. Davis Company, 1973, p. 455.

3. Spanos, W.J., 'Preoperative Hormonal Therapy of Cystic Adnexal Masses', *Am. J.*

Obstet. Gynecol., 1973, Vol. 116, pp. 551-556.

"Should OCs Be Prescribed to Prevent Adnexal Mass?" *Contraceptive Technology Update*, Sept. 1982, Vol. 3, No. 9, p. 117.

4. Ibid.

5. Spanos, W.J., 'Counseling Tips Can Help Manage Patient Fears about OCs, Cancer', *Contraceptive Technology Update*, 1986, Vol. 7, No. 9, pp. 109-112.

6. Schlaerth, J.B., 'Management of Ovarian Germ-Cell Tumors', in *Management of Common Problems in Obstetrics and Gynecology*, Mishell, D.R., Jr., Brenner, P.F., eds., 1984, Oradell, NJ, Medical Economics Books, p. 326.

Chapter 15: Ovarian cancer

1. Campbell, S. et al., 'Real Time Ultrasonography for Determination of Ovarian Morphology and Volume: A Possible Early Test for Ovarian Cancer?' *Lancet*, Feb. 20, 1982, p. 425.

Hall, D.A. et al., 'Sonographic Visualization of the Normal Postmenopausal Ovary', *J. Ultrasound Med.*, January 1986, Vol. 5, No. 11.

Goswamy, R.K. et al., 'Screening for Ovarian Cancer', *Clinics in Obstetrics and Gynaecology*, Vol. 10, No. 3, p. 621.

2. Barbiari, R.L., 'CA-125 in Patients with Endometriosis', *Fertil. Steril.*, June 1986, Vol. 45, No. 6, p. 767.

Bast, R.C., Jr., Klug, T.L., St. John, E. et al., 'A radioimmunoassay Using a Monoclonal Antibody to Monitor the Course of Epithelial Ovarian Cancer', *N. Engl. J. Med.*, 1983, Vol. 309, p. 883.

3. DiSaia, P.J., 'Germ Cell Tumors and Fertility', *The Female Patient*, Aug. 1983, p. 27.

4. Personal communication, May 29, 1987, Donald J. Woodruff, MD, Director, Gynecologic Pathology, Johns Hopkins University, Baltimore, Md.

5. Koch, M., Starreveld, A.A., Hill, G.B., Jenkins, H., 'The Effect of Tubal Ligation on the Incidence of Epithelial Cancer of the Ovary', *Cancer Prevention*, 1984, Vol. 7, pp. 241-245.

Cramer, D.W., Welch, W.R., Cassells, S., Scully, R.E., 'Mumps, Menarche, Menopause, and Ovarian Cancer', *Am. J. Obstet. Gynecol.*, Sept. 1983, Vol. 147, No. 1, pp. 1-6.

Cramer, D.W., Welch, W.R., 'Determinants of Ovarian Cancer Risk. II. Inferences Regarding Pathogenesis', *JNCI*, Oct. 1983, Vol. 71, No. 4, pp. 717-721.

6. Heintz, A.P., Hacker, N.F., Lagasse, L.D., 'Epidemiology and Etiology of Ovarian Cancer: A Review', *Obstet. Gynecol.*, July 1985, Vol. 66, No. 1, pp. 127-135.

La Vecchia, C., Franceschi, S., Gallus, G. et al., 'Incessant Ovulation and Ovarian Cancer: A Critical Approach', *J. Epidemiol.*, June 1983, Vol. 12, No. 2, pp. 161-164.

7. Greene, M., Clark, J.W., Blayney, D.W., 'The Epidemiology of Ovarian Cancer', *Semin. Oncol.*, Sept. 1984, Vol. 11, No. 3, pp. 209-226.

de Waard, F., 'Hormonal Factors in Human Carcinogenesis', *J. Cancer Res. Clin. Oncol.*, 1984, Vol. 108, No. 2, pp. 177-180.

Cramer, D.W., et al., Oct. 1983, p. 711.

8. Barber, Hugh, R.K., 'Ovarian Cancer', *CA-A Cancer Journal for Clinicians*, May/June 1986, Vol. 36, No. 3, p. 151.

9. Lingemen, C.H., 'Environmental Factors in the Etiology of Carcinoma of the Human Ovary: A Review', *Am. J. Ind. Med.*, 1983, Vol. 4, No. 1-2, pp. 365-379.

Cramer, D.W. et al., Oct. 1983, p. 711.

10. Piver, S.M., Barlow, J.J., Sawyer, D.M., *Obstet. Gynecol.*, 1982, Vol. 60, p. 397.

Simpson, J.L., 'Polygenic Factors May Be At Work', *Advances in Reprod. Med.*, Nov. 1982, Vol. 1, No. 11, p. 3.

11. Parmley, T.H., Woodruff, J.D., 'The Ovarian Mesothelioma', *Am. J. Obstet. Gynecol.*, 1974, Vol. 120, p. 234.

12. Trent, J.M., Salmon, S.E., 'Karyotypic Analysis of Human Ovarian Carcinoma Cells Cloned in Short-Term Agar Culture', *Cancer Genet. Cytogenet.*, June 1981, Vol. 3, No. 4, pp. 279-291.

Wake, N., Hreshchyshyn, M.M., Piver, S.M., Matsui, S., Sandberg, A.A., 'Specific Cytogenetic Changes in Ovarian Cancer Involving Chromosomes 6 and 14', *Cancer Res.*, Dec. 1980, Vol. 40, No. 12, 4512-4518.

Lynch, H.T., Schuelke, G.S., Wells, I.C. et al., 'Hereditary Ovarian Carcinoma. Biomarker Studies', *Cancer*, Jan. 15, 1985, Vol. 55, No. 2, pp. 410-415.

13. Cramer, D.W., Welch, W.R., Scully, R.E., Wojciechowski, C.A., 'Ovarian Cancer and Talc: A Case-Control Study', *Cancer*, July 15, 1982, Vol. 50, No. 2, pp. 372-376.

14. Donna, A., Betta, P.G., Robutti, F. et al., 'Ovarian Mesothelial Tumors and Herbicides: A Case-Control Study', *Carcenogenesis*, July 1984, Vol. 5, No. 7, pp. 941-942.

15. Cramer, D.W., Welch, W.R., Hutchison, G.B. et al., 'Dietary Animal Fat in Relation to Ovarian Cancer Risk', *Obstet. Gynecol.*, June 1984, Vol. 63, No. 6, pp. 833-838.

Naylor Dana Institute, *Cancer*, Dec. 1986, Vol. 58, No. 11, pp. 2732-2381.

16. Byers, T., Marshall, J., Graham, S. et al., 'A Case Control Study of Dietary and Nondietary Factors in Ovarian Cancer', *JNCI*, Oct. 1983, Vol. 71, No. 4, pp. 681-686.

17. Gwinn, M.L., Webster, L.A., Lee, N.C., Layde, P.M., Rubin, G.L., 'Alcohol Consumption and Ovarian Cancer Risk', *Am. J. Epidemiol.*, May 1986, Vol. 123, No. 5, pp. 759-766.

18. Hildreth, N.G., Kelsey, J.L., LiVolsi, V.A. et al., 'An Epidemiological Study of Epithelial Carcinoma of the Ovary', *Am. J. Epidemiol.*, 1981, Vol. 114, No. 3, pp. 398-405.

19. Rosenberg, L., Shapiro, S., Slone, D. et al., 'Epithelial Ovarian Cancer and Combination Oral Contraceptives', *JAMA*, 1982, Vol. 247, p. 3210.

'Making Choices: Evaluating the Health Risks and Benefits of Birth Control Methods', the Alan Guttmacher Institute.

20. Rutkow, I.M., 'Obstetric and Gynecologic Operations in the United States, 1979 to 1984', *Obstet. Gynecol.*, June 1986, Vol. 67, No. 6, pp. 755-759.

21. Garcia, C.R., Cutler, W.B., 'Preservation of the Ovary: A Reevaluation', *Fertil. Steril.*, Oct. 1984, Vol. 42, No. 4, pp. 510-514.

Chapter 16: Other menstrual and pelvic problems

1. Unpublished data. National Center for Health Statistics, Pokras, R., Hufnagel, V.G., 'Hysterectomy in the United States: 1965-1984', *Vital and Health Statistics*, 1987, Series 13, No. 92. DHHS Pub. No. (PHS) 87-1753. Public Health Service, Washington DC, US Government Printing Office.

Roos, N.P., 'Hysterectomies in One Canadian Province: A New Look at Risks and Benefits', *Am. J. Public Health*, Jan. 1984, Vol. 74, No. 1, pp. 39-46.

2. Budd, K., 'Use of D-Phenylalanine, an Enkephalinase Inhibitor, in the Treatment of Intractable Pain', *Ad. Pain Res. Ther.*, 1983, Vol. 5, pp. 305-308.

Ehrenpreis, S., 'D-Phenylalanine and other Enkephalinase Inhibitors as Pharmacological Agents: Implications for Some Important Therapeutic Applications', *Int. J. of Acupuncture and Electro-Therapeutics, Res.*, 1982, Vol. 7, pp. 157-172.

3. Shpeen, S.E., Morse, D.R., Furst, M.L., 'The Effect of Tryptophan on Post-Operative Endodontic Pain', *Oral Surgery*, 1984, Vol. 58, No. 4, p. 446.

4. Moses, V.I., Rubin, G.L., Layde, P.M. et al.,

'Tubal Sterilization Among Women of Reproductive Age, United States, 1979-1980', *Centers for Disease Control, Morbidity and Mortality Weekly Report*, Vol. 32, 1983, p. 9SS.

5. DeStefano, F., Perlman, J.A., Peterson, H.B., 'Long-term Risk of Menstrual Disturbances After Tubal Sterilization', *Am. J. Obstet. Gynecol.*, Aug. 1, 1985, Vol. 152, No. 7 pt. 1, pp. 835-841.

——, 'Factors Seen as Possible Links to Post-tubal Ligation Syndrome', *Contra. Tech. Update*, Feb. 1986, Vol. 7, No. 2, pp. 13-15.

6. El Minawi, M.F., Mashor, N., Reda, M.S., 'Pelvic Venous Changes after Tubal Sterilization', *J. Reprod. Med.*, Oct. 1983, Vol. 28, No. 10, pp. 641-648.

Cattanch, J., 'Oestrogen Deficiency after Tubal Ligation', *Lancet*, April 13, 1985, 1(8433) pp. 847-849.

Hargrove, J.T., Abraham, G.E., 'Endocrine Profile of Patients With Post-tubal Ligation Syndrome', *J. Reprod. Med.*, July 1981, Vol. 26, No. 7, pp. 359-362.

Alvarez-Sanchez, F., Segal, S.J., Brache, V. et al., 'Pituitary Ovarian Function after Tubal Ligation', *Fertil. Steril.*, 1981, Vol. 36, pp. 606-609.

Rock, J.A., Parmley, T.H., King, T.M. et al., 'Endometriosis and the Development of Tuboperitoneal Fistulas after Tubal Ligation', *Fertil. Steril.*, Jan. 1981, Vol. 35, No. 1, pp. 16-20.

7. Hargrove, J.T., pp. 359-362.

Radwanska, E. et al., 'Luteal Deficiency Among Women with Normal Menstrual Cycles, Requesting Reversal of Tubal Sterilization', *Obstet. Gynecol.*, 1979, Vol. 54, p. 189.

8. Stock, R.J., 'Sequelae of Tubal Ligation: An Analysis of 75 Consecutive Hysterectomies', *South. Med. J.*, Oct. 1984, Vol. 77, No. 10, pp. 1255-1260.

Kedrick, J.S., Rubin, G.L., Lee, N.C. et al., 'Hysterectomy Performed Within 1 Year After Tubal Sterilization', *Fertil. Steril.*, Nov. 1985, Vol. 44, No. 6, pp. 606-610.

9. DeStefano, Perlman, pp. 835-841.

Templeton, A.A., Cole, S., 'Hysterectomy Following Sterilization', *Br. J. Obstet. Gynaecol.*, Oct. 1982, Vol. 89, No. 10, pp. 845-888.

10. Backstrom, C.T., Boyle, H., Baird, D.T., 'Persistence of Symptoms of Premenstrual Tension in Hysterectomized Women', *Br. J. Obstet. Gynaecol.*, May 1981, Vol. 88, No. 5, pp. 530-536.

Index